THE GENERAL SURGEON

Recollections from Four Continents

Moshe Schein

tfm publishing Limited, Castle Hill Barns, Harley, Nr Shrewsbury, SY5 6LX, UK
Tel: +44 (0)1952 510061; Fax: +44 (0)1952 510192
E-mail: info@tfmpublishing.com; Web site: www.tfmpublishing.com

Editing, Design & Typesetting: Nikki Bramhill BSc (Hons) Dip Law

Paperback ISBN: 978-1-913755-65-2
E-book editions: © 2026
ePub ISBN: 978-1-913755-66-9
Web pdf ISBN: 978-1-913755-67-6

Printed by Gutenberg Press Ltd., Gudja Road, Tarxien, GXQ 2902, Malta
Tel: +356 2398 2201; Fax: +356 2398 2290
E-mail: info@gutenberg.com.mt; Web site: www.gutenberg.com.mt

Contents

Dedication

I dedicate this book to my wife Heidi and sons Omri, Yariv, and Dan, who shared with me the burden of the long journey. And to the memory of my dear parents and sister.

And finally, I am indebted to the many, many thousands of patients who passed through my hands. They, of all races, ages, social echelons, and nationalities were my best teachers, by trusting to me their lives and bodies. Each of them has a life story, be it tragic or fortunate, which could be the subject of a memoir. It may sound a cliché but it is true!

Prologue

The only things that are important in life are the things you remember.

Jean Renoir

I write because it is my nature so to do, and I can write only what I know, and I know nothing but China, having always lived there.

Pearl S. Buck

[In my case, replace "China" with "Surgery".]

This is how he *imagined* his last day at work to be. No patients are scheduled to operate on or consult. He just walks around, bidding farewell to anyone who recognizes him. His office has already been emptied. Desk clear, walls bare — diplomas, paintings, photographs of his father and family, treatment algorithms — all gone. The last thing he must do is to return his ID tag — he will not be able to access the clinic and hospital anymore. The clinic laptop must go as well. As of now, he does not belong here any longer. Essentially, his surgical career is over.

If asked which key words would define who he is, he would say — a general surgeon. Yes, this is how he describes his persona. For he lived, ate, breathed, dreamed, and slept surgery for forty-five years. Thinking about it, his hands explored the inside of living human bodies over the years, from the scalp to the toes. He removed fractured pieces of the cranium, cleaned clogged carotid arteries, resected lumpy thyroids and parathyroids, and chopped out cancerous esophagi and breasts. He fixed holes in the heart, and sutured torn lungs and ruptured diaphragms. He had walked within abdomens, chopping off, or fixing up, livers, pancreases, stomachs, colons, intestines, and gallbladders — everything. He replaced leaking aortic aneurysms and bypassed occluded arteries in the limbs. He incised gravid uteri to deliver newborn babies. He never shied away from the so-called 'minor' procedures, such as hernias, lumps, bumps, skin cancers, varicose veins, etc. He must have saved many lives. He never counted how many. He only remembers the few lives he has lost or directly contributed to their demise. He inflicted lots of pain to heal and alleviate suffering. He constantly read, pondered, discussed, and dreamed — about surgery.

He will never walk again into the emergency room late at night, approach the suffering patient and his family — all anxiously awaiting him — and introduce himself, "I am the general surgeon." He will not examine the abdomen, look at the CT images and declare, "We have to operate on you now!" He never questioned why many thousands of people permitted him to plunge a knife into their inner parts. Why did they trust him? For him, it was obvious: he knows what he is doing. He is a general surgeon.

He is a surgeon no more. He is seventy-five years old and generally in good shape. So what now? A memoir?

I am that surgeon, and this book is my recollection of surgical life.

* * * * *

This narrative, then, could be considered a surgical memoir. I promise you, however, that you will not find here a typical surgical memoir: a story of a remarkable surgical life written by a distinguished retired surgeon — one of those who, after his eventual death, would deserve a glorifying obituary, written by yet another surgical giant, in a newspaper or a professional journal. I look at the surgical memoirs and autobiographies that occupy the bookshelves in my study — whom do we have here? Edward Churchill, Francis Moore, William Heneage Ogilvie, Geoffrey Keynes, Max Thorek, Allen Whipple, Thomas Starzl, George Crile, Jr., Arthur Hertzler, George Sava, and many others — all great famous masters!

This memoir is different, for its writer is definitely not obituary-eligible. While, at some stage, he strove to be an eminent clinician and a notable academician, he never reached the top of his profession. But who would read and buy a memoir of an ordinary surgeon? How should I promote this piece? *The surgical globetrotter*? *Reminiscences of an international surgeon*? *Memoirs of the errant surgeon*? Each would be an accurate and descriptive proposition. Finally, I chose *The General Surgeon*, paying tribute to my brothers in the trenches — the humble, run-of-the-mill general surgeons worldwide.

Although 'surgical' is its claim to fame, this memoir is aimed not only at surgeons or medical practitioners. Whenever possible, I have tried to portray events and persons against the background and perspective of the various places and times.

According to Gore Vidal, "A memoir is how one remembers one's own life, while an autobiography is history, requiring research, dates, facts double-checked." Cynthia Ozick agrees: "The approaches of a memoirist and a journalist can also be said to differ… memory, at bottom, is an act of imaginative re-creation, not of archival legwork." True, but I hope the reader will agree that the selective use of dates and relevant facts could provide some orientation in time and convey a sense of urgency if not credibility, when needed.

Like some memoirists, I found writing about myself and developing my character challenging — it is so much easier to describe others. Perhaps the ability to deeply expose oneself, to dwell on painful secrets, and to self-analyze comes to the memoirist only later in life. Most probably, if it were to be composed at some time just before my death and/or after the death of a few others, it would be more revealing. I will leave it to the reader to analyze my psychopathology. Gabriel Garcia Márquez wrote: "Everyone has three lives: the public, the private, and the secret." That secret life includes pieces that one wants to forget and ones that one remembers fondly but cannot write about for various reasons. Therefore, part of my secret life is not included in the following pages…

Mordecai Richler said: "If you caricature friends in your first novel they will be upset, but if you don't, they will feel betrayed." A common memoirist's dilemma is whether to write about intimate living friends. No one is perfect; each of us could be easily caricatured, but in this memoir, my close friends, even those who are friends no more, will be spared. This is also, to some degree, true concerning my wife and sons: they will have occasional guest appearances, but this manuscript is for them rather than about them.

For obvious reasons, the names of many people, but not all, who come onto the narrative stage are fictionalized. As no one walks throughout life with a tape recorder in his pocket, most of the dialogues presented have been reconstructed — some based on notes taken early after the described events took place. However, all patients' case histories, although blinded to preserve patients' privacy, are based on true cases. All documents presented are based on originals kept by the author.

Many memoirists tend to exclude daily life from their narrative, leaping instead from one exciting anecdote to another outstanding experience or achievement, as if life is an ongoing series of grand events without the shades of gray or ordinary in between. This I have strived to avoid. At the same time, I took to heart the advice of my good friend Abraham Verghese: "A memoir should represent a string of anecdotes — not be bogged down with those parts of our lives which are mundane."

A memoir could be considered a slide show. Black and white slides in one's mind… memories… With some effort, one can add color and context to each slide. However, many slides must be excluded to avoid being a *nudnik*. Undoubtedly, different slides may be more or less of interest to some readers. So please feel free to skip or scroll over the dull chapters until you find something interesting.

Where, at what point, should I start? Should I follow the example of literary giants like Vladimir Nabokov, Marcel Proust, or Leo Tolstoy, who started their memoirs at an age when memories began recording in their childhood brains?

Or should I take the formalistic approach, beginning with my parents or their parents? Should I proceed chronologically or resort to today's gimmicky jumping forward and backward techniques until the reader loses orientation?

I will start at the beginning and proceed chronologically. So let us return to 1950, to the green marshes of the Island of Wolin, at the mouth of the Oder River, where it empties into the Baltic Sea.

* * * * *

One

Poland

I was born in 1950 in Wolin, a small island where the great Oder River opens to the Baltic Sea. Wolin once belonged to Sweden until the seventeenth century, when it was conquered by the Prussians to become a part of the German Pomerania. After the Second World War, Wolin was annexed to Poland. This was where my father served as a chief surgeon of a secret Polish military hospital, treating Greek communist fighters injured during the civil war that raged in Greece during those years. However, my first retrievable memory is of the Polish city of Łódź — another station in my father's surgical career — where he held the university cathedra of military surgery. I see a toddler jumping on an expansive sofa, laughing hysterically, cuddled, and tickled by our two young house servants (yes, house servants in communist Poland!). My parents must have been away, and the three-year-old Marek (my Polish name) had been left in the large hands of the Latvian Magda and the German Ursula. My taste in women — I like them fair and statuesque — indeed began to develop.

Willa Cather, Nebraska's most noted novelist, said: "Most of the basic material a writer works with is acquired before the age of fifteen." But I must leap forward, bypassing the early Nabokov's *Speak, Memory* motives, or this will become like Henry Roth's three-volume story of his first twenty years of life.

In Poland, where I spent my early childhood, I was unaware of being Jewish until the six-year-old Andrzej called me *zyd* ('kike' in Polish). Andrzej's parents were the janitors in our apartment block, a six-story, gray, Stalin-era building in Warsaw inhabited by members of the elite communist intelligentsia. Andrzej's family lived in the basement; his father stocked the furnace with coal and drank vodka, and his mother cleaned the stairs and supervised the entrance. Andrzej and I played in the yard. That was the winter of 1956, just after the anti-Stalinist Polish leader Gomułka was released from jail and regained power, heralding the early 'thaw' in Poland. Only then was my father allowed to travel to Israel to visit his 'lost' family. He returned to frozen Warsaw with stories (and postcards) of golden oranges, green *kibbutzim*, and camels in yellow deserts. He also brought a bunch of overripe bananas, which were as rare as Beluga caviar on the moon in Poland in those days. I shared the delicious, soft, graying fruit with Andrzej; after munching down his portion, he declared solemnly, "My father says that your father went to visit the *zydzi* in Palestine." He then pointed his sticky finger at me: "You are a *zyd*!"

"I am not!" I burst out crying and ran home to my mother. "Andrzej says I'm a *zyd*."

"Is that so? You do not have to play with him all the time."

A year later, in March 1957, workers assembled a giant wooden container (they called it a "lift") in our backyard. They jam-packed it with whatever property we had — a few selected pieces of heavy furniture which were loaded into it, including my father's oak desk, are still with us in Wisconsin. I remember the officers of the State Border Police sitting at our kitchen table; their job was to see that no original Polish art or mushrooms (cherished by the authorities like gold) would leave the country. They spent the day savoring the vodka, kielbasa, black bread, dill pickles, and cigarettes served up by my mother. The oldest of the bunch, a merry-looking, mustachioed officer, put me on his lap, patted my blond hair, and kidded: "Hey son, you don't look like them *zydzi*, they might not accept you there in Palestine. Ha, ha ha."

A week later, my parents, sister, and I boarded the train at Warsaw's central railway station. All I remember from that journey are the bright streetlights in rainy Vienna; the massive straw-covered flask of Chianti, the cheese and salami sandwiches bartered through the compartment's window when the train stopped in an Italian station; the extended stay at a seaside hotel in Genoa, awaiting the ship, eating spaghetti and ice cream; the small white Israeli ship *Jerusalem* whose Captain — elderly, short, and fat — pinched my cheeks and stuffed me with delicious Swiss chocolates. I remember the misty, cool, and windy early morning, seagulls crying, and passengers crowding the decks, expecting the first glimpse of the Promised Land. Suddenly it appeared on the pale horizon: first the Stella Maris Monastery, the lighthouse on Mount Carmel; then the green mountain itself with the golden cupola of the Bahai Temple, lighted by the sun's rays rising from the eastern hinterland. Finally, the gray houses and white roofs of Haifa came into view. The slow arrival from the sea to what would become his hometown created an image that would forever stay in that seven-year-old boy's mind.

I remember saying in Polish (more likely my parents remembered it for me) to one of my 'new uncles' who were greeting us at the harbor, "I don't want all these *zydzi* (kikes). I want to go back to Poland." We often tend to come up with "what if" questions when thinking about the past. At that time, my father was offered a position in New York and Berlin. What if — what would have become of me if we had emigrated to America or Germany rather than to Israel? I do not know. But I know that I am happy to have become an Israeli. I still consider myself a proud Israeli after all those years wandering around the *golah* (diaspora) — even if I am not too proud of what Israel has become.

* * * * *

I returned to Poland as a tourist precisely fifty years later.

May 2007. A heat wave engulfs Poland. The good old East European summer: no air conditioning, the aroma of sour human sweat permeates the air. My mother had spent the first year of the war here in Krakow. I was a small boy when I left Poland, but the Polish language comes back rapidly; the food is so familiar, like my mother's cooking. A night train to Wolin together with our Polish friends Wojciech and Ewa. The scent of late spring in the Polish countryside enters through the open windows. My sleep is interrupted whenever the train stops: the conductor runs through the corridor, announcing the various stations as if read from the lexicon of the Holocaust. This was a country of over three million Jews; today, there are less than twenty thousand — many still uncomfortable disclosing who they are. The rhythmical clicks of a dark train in the night: what this brings into the mind of a Jew traveling through Poland would sound a cliché.

We arrive at the island of Wolin at the mouth of the Oder River. Calm, swampy waters, lakes, ancient forests, green fields, and sleepy old German resort towns are now carrying Polish names. Pre-war German vacationers called Wolin "the lungs of Berlin" — Berlin being some hundred miles to the southwest. During the war, Wolin had submarines and airbases — we encounter remains of the Nazi infrastructure in the forests and on the coast. From the beach village of Dziwnów we look across the water: a few red brick buildings. "This was the 'Greek Hospital,'" explains Mariusz, a local surgeon. "As you see, it is surrounded by water, accessed by ferry only. What took place there was a top military secret; locals did not know and did not want to ask. Today it is still an off-limit military zone. I look across the calm misty water at the place where I was born fifty-seven years ago. According to my mother, it was at midnight, a few minutes before 1 May, but it was registered as 30 April. Another legend she told was that an error could have occurred as she had given birth surrounded by Greek women. (A DNA test — 100% Ashkenazi Jew — refuted that far-fetched theory of me being swapped for a Greek boy.)

We drive to the adjacent township of Kamień Pomorski. "They have your birth certificate at the town hall," advises Mariusz. "You may want to ask for a copy which would be useful should you decide to obtain Polish citizenship." "Thanks, but I have enough citizenships," I reply.

Another night train, southwards to Warsaw. I do not recognize the railway station through which, together with my father, mother, and sister — they are all gone now — we departed Poland fifty years ago. However, the monstrous Palace of Culture — Stalin's gift to the people of Warsaw, which towers nearby — looks very familiar to me. Warsaw appears like a sprawling Central-European version of Tel Aviv. The heat wave continues: hydrated by liters of cold beer, I wander around, looking for whatever was left from its Jewish past (almost nothing, of course) and my own. With a street map, I search our old house in Nowowiejska 10. This is the residential zone of central Warsaw where little businesses, grocery stores, bakeries, restaurants, bars, barber shops, used bookshops, and coffee houses are intermingled with apartment blocks.

I stand in front of the gate to our old house but do not recognize it; only the inner courtyard leading to the back alley evokes memories — I remember playing here with other toddlers. As I take pictures of the building, people passing by look at me quizzically — what is he photographing? I look up at the third floor, where our apartment was. In my mind, I can see my young mother in her flowery summer dress. I see my father in his dark professional suit. I see myself sitting on the carpet, playing with my wooden toys. I stand in silence for a few minutes, paying tribute to my parents and thanking them for taking me out of this city and this country — a vast cemetery of my people. Still, I feel a particular affinity with this place and its people — not only do I understand their language, but their gestures and body language are familiar. After a week in Poland, I feel I could merge into local daily life — only my vocabulary and accent need improvement. The next day we fly back to Wisconsin.

* * * * *

On vacation with father, mother, and sister Sylvia; winter in Zakopane, summer by the Baltic Sea (1952-1954).

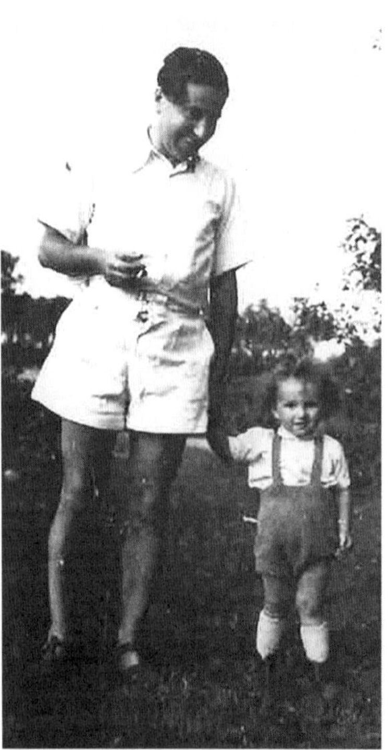

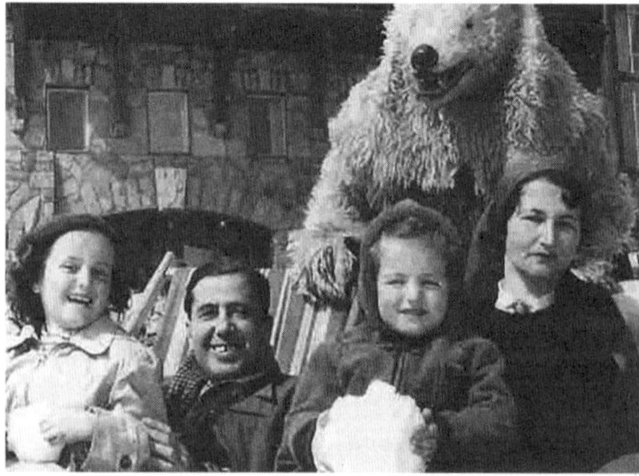

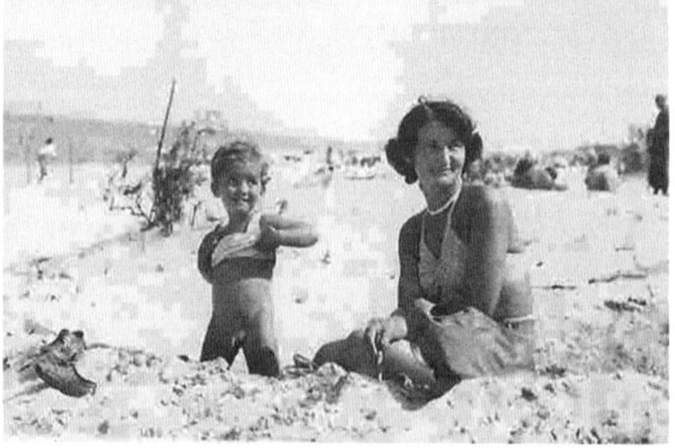

Two

Youth

In 1957, when our ship docked at the port of Haifa, Jewish immigrants, the "surviving burning embers," as defined by the cliché de jour, were received in Israel with warmth and affection. Over half of Israel's population was made of such surviving pieces of driftwood. You could see them everywhere: metal or gold teeth or no teeth in their mouths, concentration camp numbers tattooed on their arms; talking Romanian, Polish, or Yiddish; selling corn on the cob boiled in large pots over open fires on the street corners, schlepping through the neighborhoods with large sacks on their shoulders, screaming: "*Alte sachen kaufen!*" ("Buying old things!"), like they had done before in the *shtetels*, which were no more.

We arrived in Israel as part of the mass exodus of Polish Jewry in 1957. However, we were not exactly 'driftwood' — our circumstances were relatively privileged. My father was related to the 'clan' of Aba Khoushy (1898-1969), then Haifa's most influential mayor; that helped immensely. We were not cramped, like others, into the *maabarot* (temporary dwellings for new immigrants, constructed at the edge of towns to accommodate the arriving masses), but settled in a rented garden cottage on the outskirts of Haifa. A few months later, we moved, ahead of a long waiting list, to a new apartment block at the foot of Mount Carmel. A relatively modest position at an orthopedic outpatient clinic awaited my father from the first month of arrival. However, with his inherent ambition, charisma, and the 'backup,' he started to climb rapidly. We were the first to be connected to a private telephone line in our new suburb, and my father was one of the first owners of a privately imported car in Haifa — this was the end of the austerity era (*tzena*). The vehicle was a British-made Vauxhall Victor, 1958 — a total disaster! Only three years later, my father could afford a large, newly built apartment, in a detached, red-shingled house, on the upper slopes of the Carmel, overlooking the city and port.

However, at those ascetic times, I was not pleased with the relative affluence of my father and the conditions we lived in. The opposite was true: I was timid about what we had compared to those surrounding us. "Your father is stinking rich," my friends in school would accuse me. "No, he's not," I would defend myself. "You have nine rooms in your house," they would mock me. "It is because my father needs space to see his patients," I would retort. "Aba Khoushy, Aba Khoushy gave it all to you," the kids would tease, referring to the almighty mayor. A fistfight would ensue. Times have changed: today's kids are proud of the elevated socioeconomic status of their family, but at that time, in the young, socialistic State of Israel, I was embarrassed by it.

Within two weeks of my arrival, I started the first grade of elementary school. I could not understand a word of Hebrew, nor could I decipher the funny alphabet they drew on the blackboard (I could not solve any alphabet, as in Poland the starting school age was seven). But the kids were nice to me, competing to see who could be kinder to the poor "*oleh chadash*" (newcomer) who had arrived in this warm paradise — the "land of milk and honey" according to the Bible and the popular song taught in kindergarten — from what they conceived to represent the hell of diaspora.

There was only one little problem — my foreskin: in Poland, under the communist regime, traditional circumcision had not been accepted; thus, I arrived in Israel uncircumcised. "You have a funny prick," a boy commented at the school urinal. A few months later, I underwent circumcision under general anesthesia. Subsequently, I demanded that my Polish name, Marek, be changed to a Hebrew one.

"The kids make fun of me," I complained, "they call me *Marak*" (soup in Hebrew). I came up with "Moshe" (Moses) — like the biblical prophet and the famous one-eyed national hero General Moshe Dayan. My parents preferred the name "Meir" but complied.

I had to repeat the first grade, but after a significant intellectual effort during the summer vacation, I passed an examination that landed me in the third grade. It defined my scholastic swan song because, henceforth, I would be an academic catastrophe. My performance had been so appalling that during the final year of elementary school, the director of the school (*Leo Beck*) advised my parents that continuing into high school would be out of the question: "A child with such limited resources should enter a professional school for apprentices, to learn a trade such as carpentry or plumbing." My father, however, tried to accommodate me in another 'good' high school, *Chugim*, where my older sister was already excelling in her studies. I remember the interview with the grave, white-haired headmaster.

"Who is your favorite Hebrew poet?" he asked.

"Hayim Nahman Bialik," I said.

"Which one of his poems do you like best?"

"'My father,' I think…"

"Well, Moshe, take this copybook and write down a brief essay about that poem — anything which comes into your mind. Here, take this pen."

I sat in an empty classroom for an hour, scribbling a few pages. I liked the poem and thought I was writing a masterpiece. I handed the completed 'treatise' to the headmaster. He eyed it rapidly and said sternly, "Excellent, Moshe. Thank you very much. Now go home, and we'll contact your father."

I never discovered what the headmaster had to say to my father verbatim. Still, I was made to understand that my little masterpiece had been considered an utter disaster — the work of someone who is intellectually challenged for his age. I was twelve years old.

My father, who had already established himself in town, managed — I do not know how much effort it involved — to place me in the worst high school in the city. But even there, my performance was atrocious. Many years later, one night in 1992, in Haifa, I was called to operate on a man suffering from intestinal obstruction. I immediately recognized him as Moshiko, a stupid kid from my elementary school. Now, thirty years later, he did not remember me. When I introduced myself, he exclaimed, "You — a surgeon? I thought you were a retard!"

Actually, I excelled in nothing. I was forced to take piano lessons when I was nine or ten years old. I remember the petite, delicate middle-aged lady who used to come each week to our house. She would sit with me by the black German-made *Schimmel* piano we had brought from Poland. "Piano forte," she would command me in a heavy Polish accent. Later, the lessons continued in a conservatorium in a beautiful old Arab house in the downtown section of the German Colony (I never asked myself why that part of town was called "German" and why no Arabs lived in that house). After a few years of piano lessons, the teacher organized a public recital for all her students. I had to play a short piece by Chopin. It was a fiasco. I was flustered and confused. What I played did not sound like Chopin at all. "No more piano for me…" I told my parents.

I did not fare better in sports, although I loved them and tried hard. I adored basketball, and I was shooting hoops for long hours. But I never managed to be in the starting lineup for any school team. I tried my luck with medium distance running, mainly 1500 meters. I represented my school in the interschool athletic competition — it seemed like no other kid was interested. It was a sweltering early summer's day in Haifa's main stadium, and I started much too fast and finished last.

Still today, I dream about failing examinations, being unprepared, being asked questions, and not knowing what to say. I wake up and thank the Lord for not having to go to school anymore. So many times I was called to the blackboard only to be humiliated by the teacher in front of the class. I remember how one of my teachers handed out the results of a test in Hebrew grammar; he put a sardonic smile on his face and said: "And as usual, our Mr. Schein received the lowest score ever recorded in the annals of this school! 17%!" The class erupted in wild laughter. I smiled like a buffoon — I would never show that I was upset. I played the happy imbecile. I was not fond of the days of parent-teacher meetings. My father was the one to attend. I would lock myself in my room, dreading his return. I heard bits and pieces of his report to my mother through the door. "What should we do with the boy?" was a recurrent phrase he used. A line of private tutors was hired to improve my school performance. They were university students in their twenties in need of an extra *shekel*. Rather than letting them help me with math, algebra, or physics, I asked them about their military service or basketball.

However, towards the final year of high school, I took myself into my own hands — as they say in Hebrew — and I started to study seriously for the first time in my life. To everybody's surprise, I managed to matriculate — passing *all* the final examinations. Not with flying colors but with a reasonable average.

What was the clinical etiology of my learning disabilities? An attention deficit disorder? Probably. Perhaps, one day, if I decide to embark on what Günter Grass called "peeling the onion" (of one's life), I will dwell on it.

* * * * *

Our family life? It was a typical new upper-middle-class Ashkenazi Israeli family — what would today be considered as belonging to the 'elite.' My father worked in the hospital, and my mother was a dedicated *hausfrau*. My father would come home at noon, eat a warm lunch, and have a siesta. In the afternoon, he would consult on private patients in his study. My parents frequently entertained at home in Polish style: in summer on the balcony overlooking the sea; in winter inside, the rooms full of cigarette smoke (both my parents smoked like a chimney, and so did their guests), with lots of tasty food (Polish dishes) and booze, Scotch being the favorite. Late at night, through my bedroom walls, I could hear the laughter and rowdy jokes when the men started playing cards (poker). For my parents' generation, it was like being together again in *Mitteleuropa* before or during the war.

My parents were not their children's friends, as many parents today are — as we try to be with our sons. They were warm, loving, and caring but — much more so my father — somewhat aloof. When not busy at work or socializing, he would sit for hours, reading 'heavy' books and smoking. It does not seem to me now that he and I spoke much to each other — if we did, my memory hasn't registered it as significant. He left us before I became mature enough to appreciate and apply his wisdom. But I remember spending long evenings listening to conversations he had with his friends. The general topic was politics — my father was an ardent center-left *Mapai* party member, later becoming the Labor Party. All his life, he was a fierce socialist.

My father was forty years old when I was born. Even as a child, I remember him puffing and panting when walking on the beach or swimming together because of his crippling emphysema. When I was ten years old, he suffered his first heart attack. It was then, when in my child's mind, I began to realize that his life span was limited. Each night in bed, I remember saying, "Please, God, let my father live as long as possible."

The four of us used to lunch and dine together almost daily. Like in Europe, lunch was the main culinary event of the day: always soup, meat or fish, dessert, and wine on Shabbat. In summer, on Saturdays, the family spread out on the beach under the shade of a broad tent; in winter, we often gathered mushrooms on the green slopes of the Carmel Mountain. Saturday was frequently the 'restaurant day' — usually in one of Haifa's, Akko's, or Nazareth's superb Arab eateries.

However, the most fantastic Arab food was served in Samur's house in the Druze-Arab village *Shfaram*, at the foothills of Lower Galilee. After my father had repaired the fractured spine of a young Druze called Samur, we became frequent Saturday guests in his home village. Here we were shepherded from one house to another, each member of the extended Samur family competing as to who will host and feed the great *doktor* from Haifa.

The numerous visits to the village (I was occasionally dispatched to stay a week or so with Samur's family when my parents went vacationing in Europe) left a delightful imprint in my mind. The old stone Arab houses on the slope of the hill basking in the soft, or harsh, sun; sheep, chickens, and little children loitering on the narrow footpaths; old men in baggy, skirt-like white trousers, sitting, smoking on their front porches. That distinctive and alluring smell of an Arab village: a mishmash of dung, vegetation, hay, and wood fire on which, in the little courtyards, the fresh pita bread was baked.

With the little Druze boys, Kamal and Jamal, I would ride on smallish donkeys down to the stony fields where we picked up and ate fresh, green chickpeas. In summer, we would select an enormous watermelon in the field, fracture it with a stone, and gorge ourselves on its cool, sweet, watery innards. Each visit to the village culminated in a prolonged, unforgettable feast in the best Druze-Arab tradition.

Samur and his family occasionally reciprocated with a visit to Haifa: his wife and mother, in traditional Druze attire, would carry baskets loaded with pita bread, homemade olive oil, and various fresh products from the village, and the feast would be repeated on our dining room table. Our neighbors would raise their eyebrows: "What are these village Arabs doing at Professor Schein's house?" But my father cherished such multicultural relationships, and with time he became the unofficial "medical Godfather" of the Druze villages in northern Israel. I believe that the close contact with the Arab village early in my life — the majority of young Israeli Jews never have a chance to interact with Arabs or Druzes socially — helped to develop an attitude of respect (even fondness) for their culture and traditions. Later in my life, I participated in battles and skirmishes with the 'other side' —

they shot at me, and I shot back at them. But I have never felt any hatred or contempt that still prevails on both sides of the chronic conflict.

My parents were secular. We did not observe any Jewish religious laws (my father used to visit the synagogue only once a year — at Yom Kippur, listening to the opening prayer *Kol Nidrei*, not from inside, but through the door or window). And so, on Saturday afternoons, during the soccer season, my father and I regularly attended the games played by the home team *Hapoel Haifa* — my father served as the team's orthopedic surgeon. Whenever one of the players was hurt, my father would be summoned to the field on the stadium's announcement system. It made me very proud, raising my prestige at school, as I could boast to my classmates that my father is the doc of the soccer stars.

At least once a year, my parents vacationed overseas — a luxury in those days. They traveled by boat to Italy and hopped through Europe's usual touristy spots. We, the kids, were left behind: I, at a summer camp or in a kibbutz; my sister — I do not recall where. However, there were strains between my parents. My father was quite a womanizer; this and his poor health and volatile temper must have frazzled my mother. Even as a child, I sensed their sporadic tensions, learning about the details much later. Only when we become adults, we are curious about our parents' inner lives — who they are or were. Then it is too late…

My sister Sylvia, only three years older but much more mature — or so it seemed — was living her life apart, rarely involved in our weekend outings. Unlike me, she did very well in school and had a tremendously active social life, being constantly chased by tall and hirsute young men. Already then, she was extremely moody, susceptible to rages, dramas, and tantrums. I recall glass doors violently slammed, broken, and repeatedly replaced. In retrospect, it heralded a relatively tragic and short life for my poor and bright sister. I believe that my sister and I represented to our parents a constant source of qualms: her behavior, and I due to my 'retardation.' Ample scientific data suggest that children of Holocaust survivors are (like their parents) at an increased risk of post-traumatic stress disorder and its various manifestations. My sister was one such case. Most probably, I am another.

Like most of our generation, we had no grandparents. We had had them, but whatever was left of them remained in the ditches of Eastern Europe before we were born. Similar was the fate of all our uncles and aunts on both sides. Except Aunt Erna — my father's older sister. She, who had immigrated to Palestine well before the war, was the only one to survive. Once a month, on Sabbath morning, I remember, we would drive to Tel Aviv, in my father's Vauxhall Victor — my sister never wanted to join us — to visit Aunt Erna and her third husband, Yechiel Blum. He was a typical Holocaust survivor (his first wife and daughters had perished in the camps): frugal, anxious and self-absorbed. I remember how enthusiastically and loudly he would *shlurf* his chicken soup with *kneidlach*.

We would arrive at their little rent-controlled apartment just off the trendy Dizengoff Street around 10 a.m. After tea and cake, we would walk that street — considered the Fifth Avenue of Tel Aviv — and then go back for lunch of chopped chicken livers, clear chicken soup, and boiled chicken thighs, with boiled potatoes and rosemary. Finally, the ubiquitous compote — fruit cooked in syrup. After lunch, the adults would retire for an hour *schlafstunde* (nap). I would sit on the balcony, which was permanently shuttered against the sun and the wind that blew from the sea, browsing old family albums and war picture albums. Later, coffee and cakes would be served, and then we would drive back on the old Tel Aviv-Haifa road.

Years later, when Uncle Yechiel died, I was in the army. When Aunt Erna died, I was in South Africa. I do not even know where they were buried. Lonely unattended graves. Families. Their histories. Everything is lost. There is no space to tell everything.

* * * * *

According to Ivan Bunin, the human memory not only helps us make some sense of our lives by sifting the significant events in our past from the insignificant, but also poeticizes the past, which acquires a certain legendary quality — the so-called "poetry of life."

So, the tiny Polish boy rapidly shed off his Central 'European-ness,' his 'otherness,' and did whatever he could to fit in. No more long trousers — only khaki ultra-shorts; navy blue or khaki short-sleeved shirts, always hanging loose over the belt; open Biblical sandals, never with socks. He tried to imitate the *kibbutzniks* with whom he used to spend his summer vacations and who he adored. There was nothing more exciting for him than to wake up at dawn before the cruel August sun started baking the Jezreel Valley; to ride on the tractor with his much-admired *kibbutznik* cousins Yossi or Bari (later killed in the reserve army service, 1967), down to the orange groves where, barefooted, ankles deep in mud, they would rearrange the heavy, rusty pipes of the irrigation system. In the late morning, they would ride up, back to the kibbutz, to the communal dining room, where each sun-scorched and famished farmer was elaborately working on his breakfast salad: onions, cucumbers, tomatoes, and radishes chopped into small pieces and some fresh parsley thrown in. Two peeled, hard-boiled eggs were fractured over the salad, which was splashed with a generous helping of olive oil and sour cream, salt, pepper, and hot paprika; a few thick slices of fresh dark bread were smeared with a generous layer of butter. One swallowed a few glasses of fresh milk, the fat still foaming on the surface. Then back to the fields.

In the late afternoon, when the sweltering valley cooled down, he would relax at the kibbutz's swimming pool, watching with evolving interest the deeply bronzed bodies of the yellow-haired northern European beauties, who used, in those days, to volunteer in the kibbutz. Those nymphets, probably, brought back in his subconscious the much earlier images of the fair and statuesque Magda and Ursula, throwing him around on the couch in Łódź. But the boy was timid and awkward regarding the opposite sex. He engaged in a few platonic love affairs — in most instances, the subjects of his 'love' were not aware of it — but it was not until he became a soldier that he had a taste of a woman's body.

When he was sixteen years old, the boy was dispatched by his parents to a summer school in the quaint and rustic Isle of Man, in the middle of the Irish Sea. The purpose was to improve his English language skills and add a worldly layer to his provincial habits. The school was combined with a summer camp for Jewish teenagers from London — packed with heavily made-up promiscuous English girls. He remembers an episode at dinner: a thin and wild-looking girl named Terry suddenly placed her small hand under the table, starting to knead his crotch. He did not realize what she was doing and why. He continued eating. Terry lifted her hand and uttered with disgust: "What a queer!" Later he consulted the dictionary to find out what "queer" stood for. This is how naïve he was. Naïve, shy, and socially awkward.

He was a loner. During those days, Israeli kids belonged to two camps: one of the youth movements like the Scouts, or the so-called "salon movement." Activities in the youth movements included outdoor proficiencies and political discussions based on specific political affiliations. Those belonging to the "salon movement" would meet on Friday nights in one of their parents' living rooms, wear blue jeans, clear the parents' bars, and dance slow dances to the tunes of Elvis Presley or Cliff Richard. He joined the Scouts organization at thirteen (in Israel, it was for girls and boys alike). Soon, however, he became annoyed by the political correctness of the discussions — the way the seventeen-year-old leaders tried to brainwash the kids. He resigned after a year. As he was never invited to any of the "salon" parties, he spent Friday nights alone. He did not possess even a pair of blue jeans, only khakis. A loner.

Gradually he became an ardent patriot. As early as elementary school, the (alleged) last words of national hero Yosef Trumpeldor, who had been fatally injured during a skirmish with Arabs in the Galilee in 1920, were repeatedly drummed into his young brain. The hero, a Russian Jew who had already lost an arm during the Russo-Japanese War, apparently died saying, "Never mind, it is good to die for our country." Influenced by the enthusiasm of the 'young country,' stimulated by tales of heroism emerging from the wars and border skirmishes fought all around at that time, the teenager developed only one ambition — to be a hero when his time arrives. To prime himself, each night, he ran miles around the neighborhood on the slopes of the Carmel and climbed up and down the *wadis* that disfigure the mountain on their way into the sea. When he was eighteen, he was recruited to the Israel Defense Forces.

* * * * *

Top left: with mother (1959). Top right: with father, sister, and mother at the bar mitzvah reception (1963). Bottom left: at the kibbutz (1965). Bottom right: with father and mother at the bar mitzvah reception (1963).

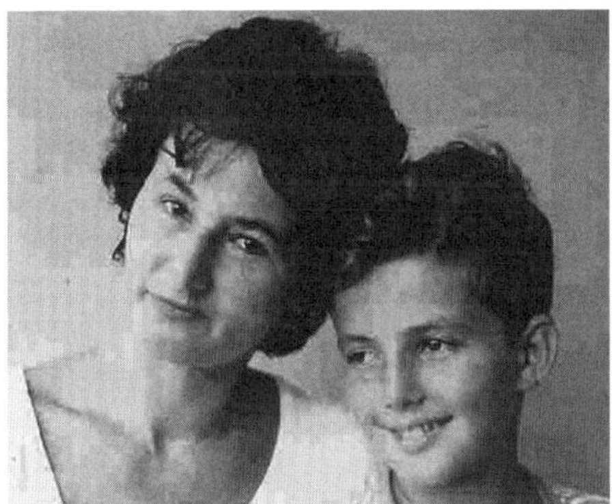

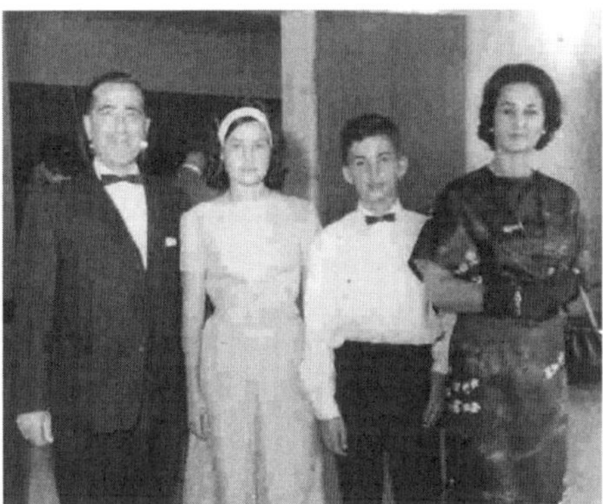

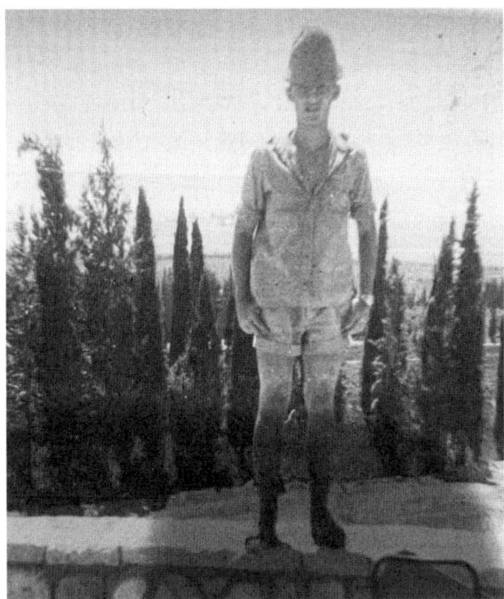

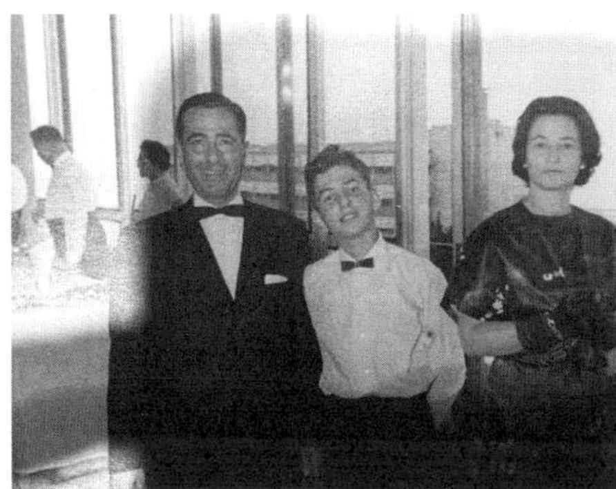

Three

Infantry

Even my sons turn narcoleptic whenever I start a sentence with "When I was in the infantry..." Therefore, I will not dwell long on that chapter in my life.

The truth is that I desperately wanted to be a paratrooper like my adored *kibbutznik* cousin Yossi, on whose heroism I tried to model myself. Immediately on arrival at the *BAKUM* (classification and screening base), I volunteered for the paratroopers. But I was rejected by their selection committee. I remember having been ushered into a large room where at least twelve officers, red paratrooper caps on their heads, were sitting behind a long table. They started bombing me with questions, but I was grossly intimidated and probably mumbled nonsense. I recall, however, one question they asked: "If we won't admit you to the paratroopers... what would be your second-choice unit? Where would you want to go?"

"Only the paratroopers. I must be a paratrooper!" I insisted.

It was the incorrect answer. Many years later, I met a military psychologist who used to attend such selection committees. "Your answer reflected immaturity, an inability to face reality," he said. "You should have listed another proper front-line unit as an alternative..."

It was a huge disappointment. My juvenile dreams – a red beret, red boots, silver wings on the chest, jumping from airplanes into the Sinai Desert sand – instantly evaporated. The fate of those rejected by the paratroopers, or the various elite commando units, was the famed Golani Brigade – the 'plain' infantry – a brigade well known for its rough life and the brutality of its 'low-life' soldiers. By low life, I mean that most of the riflemen were Sephardic Jews deriving from low socioeconomic strata (many from what was called then the "development towns"). The officers and NCOs were usually Ashkenazi Jews from the more educated classes. It was my first opportunity to mix and get familiar with the less privileged Israeli society. Young and naïve, I did not sense the simmering resentment that would eventually bubble up and tear the country apart.

I enlisted in 1968, just a year after the Six-Day War. By then, the War of Attrition with Israel's neighbors had already been smoldering. Thus, during the three years of my regular service, I would move with the 13th ("Gideon") Golani Battalion, company *gimmel* (C), from one front to another. So, we would spend a week of ambushes in the rain-soaked southern Lebanon, hunting for PLO infiltrators, followed with three months patrolling the border on the freezing Golan Heights; then six weeks trying to catch Palestinian 'terrorists' in the steamy Jordan valley; and three months in the bunkers at the hot Suez Canal – under constant heavy artillery fire. In between, there were summer maneuvers on the Golan Heights and winter maneuvers in the Judean Desert. Then, we went back to action, wherever it may be needed.

Dressed in thick camouflage uniforms (French army's surplus) we were constantly drenched in sweat during the sultry Mediterranean summers. In winter, on the Golan Heights, we froze in the water-clogged old Russian overcoats (confiscated from the Syrian army after the Six-Day War). We were relatively well fed on the front but during maneuvers we often went hungry. That was a young, spartan, lean army then, not the army of today that is overfed, over digitalised, high tech and immensely wasteful, spending fortunes on a single smart bomb massacring scores of innocent Palestinians.

Rather than telling war stories, let me offer a potpourri of memories that those years evoke.

I remember that we marched, walked, and ran a lot, so much so that my feet bled, and my legs and thighs hypertrophied disproportionately to the rest of my body.

I remember the red sun descending behind the Egyptian desert or rising on the snowy slopes of Mount Hermon.

I can still smell the lush spring vegetation on the banks of the Jordan River and feel the chilly wind blowing on the stony hills of Samaria. Those years brought the biblical landscapes into our senses and souls.

I remember searching Palestinian houses in occupied Gaza: the men assembled in the yard, the women and children squatting in the corner, looking at us with dark, frightened eyes, fresh pita bread on the table, the smell of urine and feces from the open latrines. (Already then, immature as I was, I started to realize that the occupation of another people is wrong – but in this memoir, I will stay away from non-medical politics as much as I can.)

I remember the eerie sensation of moving into the line of fire – crouching down deep in the troop carrier – driving along the long, sandy dike leading to the *Mezach* (the pier), a fortified perimeter opposite the Egyptian town of Suez, notorious for the Egyptian fire it received, and the number of casualties. There were deep shell craters all around, with loud bangs of artillery, acrid gunpowder in our nostrils, and our faces were pale and tight.

I remember a bullet-pierced road sign hand-written: "We looked death directly in its eyes, and death had looked away." We, as eighteen-year-old kids, suddenly realized that people were dying there.

I recall long months by the Suez Canal: constant bombardments, ambushes, patrols, direct hits. At sunrise, bodies of dead Egyptian commandos at the edge of our perimeter — like discarded small bags of potatoes dressed in yellowish uniforms — *are these our monstrous enemies?*

I remember a night patrol along the Suez Canal opposite the town Port Said and fragments of Russian-made 82mm mortar piercing my ass and face; Orli, the platoon leader, loading me onto his shoulders, running for shelter in the deep dunes, evacuation by an 'ambulance' tank, then a chopper, and finally a fixed-wing airplane — reaching a Tel Aviv hospital to undergo surgery.

I remember the late General Ezer Weizman, who would become the President of Israel years later, meeting us at the evacuation station in Bir Gifgafa. He squatted at my stretcher and asked: "What's your name, soldier? What would you like to do after the army?" "I'll be a doctor," I replied. I remember the weeks of recuperation at the hospital: the hands of young nurses, the unfulfilled, frustrated lust — for love and sex.

But the most vital awareness from these days, one that stayed with me, is the delight of being young, strong, fit, tanned, covered in sweat and dust, clad in oily fatigues, carrying a heavy infantry harness, a loaded Uzi in my hands, finger on the trigger, walking in front of my squad into the sinister night; that pleasurable bitter-sweet sensation down in the pit of my stomach, hoping, but afraid, to contact the enemy — and ready to die. Some may call it "militarism," but I, in retrospect, cherished this most.

Those years spent in open fields, bunkers, and deserts awoke in me the fondness of lilac dusks, violet sunsets, various smells of nature, and the hunger for love. And my first real love — or was it just a romance — did transpire during the last year of service. Her name was Jascia, a Jewish German medical student visiting Israel during Passover with her father; her aunt and my mother had bonded during the Second World War in Poland. I was at home on a brief vacation from my unit on the Golan Heights and immediately took an interest in this fresh-looking European beauty. She was fair, freckled, about my height, and well-curved; she dressed fashionably and smelled deliciously of expensive perfume.

On my first vacation day, I took my father's car and drove with Jascia to the Sea of Galilee. It was a fresh, windy spring day. I accessed the lake through a dirt road and the banana plantations south of Capernaum. I spread an old blanket on the beach pebbles, and we stretched out under the cool pale sun. She went into the water and dove but immediately ran out. "It's freezing," she said, lying down on the blanket, placing her wet body and face tightly against mine. Oh, the smell of the damp hair and the perfumed face! Next, our bodies united in an instant lust. She was my first. Our love glowed. We consumed it for a week until she flew home, and I returned to my unit. We continued exchanging love letters, but after a few months, her letters cooled off, gradually becoming formal and less frequent. However, I did not lose hope and fantasized about meeting her again, making her mine.

In August 1971, I was discharged from the army. It took place at the same military base near Tel Aviv, where I had joined the IDF precisely three years prior, where I was rejected by the paratroopers — a scar on my ego. I guess that the boy had changed a little during those years — becoming tougher, prone to taking risks, and used to uncertainties and chaos. Wilder.

* * * * *

Left: recruit, on the Golan Heights, 1968. Right: with best buddy Amikam Reshef, Jordan Valley, 1970.

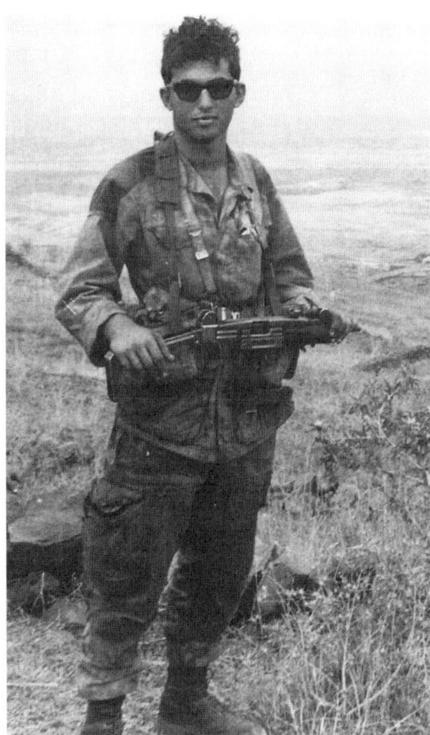

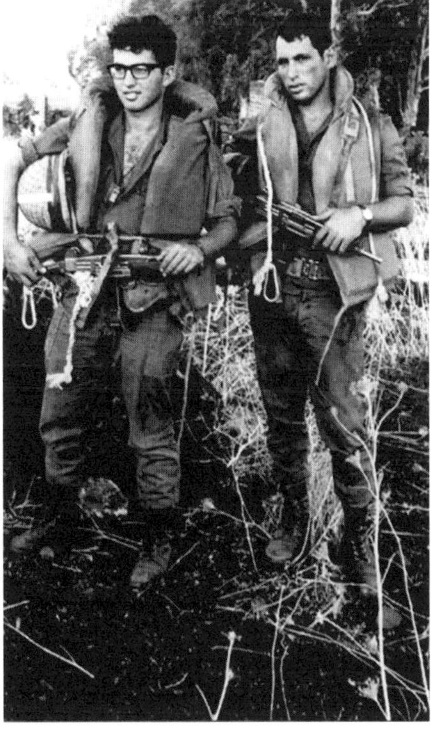

Four

Siena, Tuscany

Let us then leap forward to the summer of 1971, when I arrived in Italy. What I remember most is the first evening in Siena. The everlasting reddish twilight; how the slanted, gentle rays of the setting sun lit up the narrow alleys of Siena on that late summer's day, which to us, arriving from the Middle East, seemed to last forever. One always remembers the day of arrival; the following days tend to fade away.

Siena, Tuscany, Italy. It was late August 1971. My friend Eli Horovitz and I landed at Rome's Fiumicino Airport earlier that day. For both of us, discharged only a few weeks prior from three years of service in the infantry, it was like landing on the moon. In Rome, we boarded the train to Siena. We rode second-class in a compartment packed with Italian soldiers traveling from Sicily to Milan: dark, gesturing, sweating in the sweltering heat of the non-air-conditioned carriage, they appeared to us like Arabs. We offered them duty-free Marlboros, to which they helped themselves enthusiastically. In turn, they shared their bread, cheese, and wine with us. The Italian language we knew encompassed only *si*, *no*, and *grazie*, but it did not take long to establish friendly comradeship with those guys. It foreshadowed our relationships with the Italians during the next two years — what gentle, warm, welcoming, and non-xenophobic people they seemed to us!

Why were we going to Siena? To study medicine. Why Italy? Because only the 'brightest' had any prospect of getting into one of the three Israeli medical schools, each admitting fewer than a hundred students per year. To be admitted, one required top scores in the matriculation high school exams — ours were below average — and star performance in an elaborate set of psychometric tests and interviews. I did not even bother to apply. I took off to Italy along with many of those who were rejected.

Italian medical schools, from Bari in the south to Milan in the north, attracted international students, not only from Israel but also from the United States, Greece, and Arab countries. All that was required was a valid passport, evidence of high school graduation, and the ability to pay for tuition and living expenses. In Italy, there was no *numerus clausus*. Any university could admit as many students as it wished; the more it admitted, the more it profited. And so, an average first-year class at a medical school would include well over a thousand students. However, fewer than twenty percent of those who enrolled would eventually graduate — still too many for the overly congested Italian doctors' population. The dropouts occurred mainly during the first three years, and those who managed to progress to the clinical years tended to graduate, with many needing more than the minimum of six years to do so.

The academic program was 'liberal': attending lectures was not obligatory; even the clinical years were voluntary in that one was not required to have any contact with patients. The emphasis was on examinations: one had to pass a certain number of examinations listed in the curriculum, and that was it. One chose to sit before the examiners — all exams were oral and public — only when one felt prepared. Indeed, many students procrastinated.

We got off the train at Siena's provincial-looking railway station late afternoon. We chose that small, hilly, medieval Tuscan town and its ancient *Facoltà di Medicina e Chirurgia* over Bologna, which had been very popular among foreigners, or over Rome or Milan because someone at the Italian consulate in Haifa had marveled about how fantastic Siena is. And indeed, what we saw that first evening was magical: the narrow alleys leading to the Piazza del Campo lit by the fading Tuscan sun; elegant small antique shops, fancy shoe boutiques; well-dressed girls trotting hand in hand in trios on high heels, the click-click sound on the cobblestones echoing from the walls; restaurants with white tablecloths, candles flickering, waiters standing on the porch, folded white towels on their arms: "*Prego, signore...*" But could we afford it? And how would we order? After three years in the desert and trenches, we were like savages entering civilization.

We registered at the *Università*. The students' *mensa* was closed during the summer, but we could lunch and dine in one of the many trattorias which accepted the subsidized food coupons we received from the University (wine included!). In the trattorias we started to learn Italian: *bistecca di maiale, osso bucco...* We noted that the locals pronounce the "c" or "k" like "h," the "bucco" becoming "buho." We understood that *maiale* is pork, and because we had heard the words "*Madonna di maiale*" in the streets, we tried to order it in the trattoria, not realizing that the phrase was an extreme profanity.

We rented a flat near the medical school. I purchased a 1957 white Vespa 150cc, but a week later, when I gained confidence in riding it, a speeding Alfa Romeo forced me into a wall. I survived. The Vespa did not. The academic year still weeks away, we loitered around the cafés surrounding the renowned Piazza del Campo.

The local girls, attractive as they were, did not seem to care much about poorly dressed young *stranieri* (foreigners). Many American and European tourist girls frequented the piazza; some came to Siena for a summer course in Italian. I remember approaching an American, blond girl who sat alone, sipping a cappuccino, absorbed in an Italian dictionary. It was where I learned the phrase "fuck off," which the American uttered without lifting her head. A few minutes later, she was successfully picked up by an ugly Italian; her goal indeed being to learn Italian.

Rejected by the opposite sex, we kibitzed at the tables of the Israeli medical students who had arrived in Siena before us. We looked with great admiration at those who had passed the third-year examinations. Our respect for them grew when we heard that just recently, an Israeli student had ended his own life by jumping from a window after failing, for the fifth time, the exam in *anatomia*. The apparent leader of the veteran group — anorexic, poorly shaven, chain-smoking MS cigarettes, which he held between shaking, yellow-tipped fingers, told us gravely: "Listen, guys, if I was you, I would leave this cursed town as soon as possible. Examinations are impassable... forget about *anatomia*... I almost died... It is like studying Tel Aviv's phone directory by heart. You still have six weeks before the semester starts. Take my advice and go to Bologna."

* * * * *

I decided to abandon ship and leave Siena. But where should I go? I called my father in Haifa. "Look *Aba*, Siena isn't for me. Too difficult. I'll fail." A few days later, he called back.

"Son, I spoke with the Chief of Orthopedics in Munich; he'll help you get into their medical school. Leave your things in Siena and go to Munich; you can stay with the Schwartzs. I've already spoken to them. Who's Schwartz? He served with me during the war. No, he isn't a doctor. He was a *sanitar*, an orderly in my hospital. He married a Russian peasant when he was imprisoned in Siberia; I helped his wife and children. Now he works for the Voice of America, transmitting propaganda to the Russians. You'll need money, eh? Go to Appel's *apoteke* in Schwabing. Herr Appel will give you two thousand Deutschmarks — he owes me his life. Yes, during the war. Everything happened during that war."

* * * * *

Siena, 1971. Top: dining with Eli Landau (left) and Eli Horovitz. Bottom: in front of our flat. (Eli Landau graduated in Italy, became a cardiologist in Tel Aviv and a successful food writer and critique in Israel. He died prematurely of colon cancer. Eli Horovitz, who had served with me in Golani, graduated in Italy and became an anesthetist in Israel and in South Africa. I have never heard from either of them since our Italy days.)

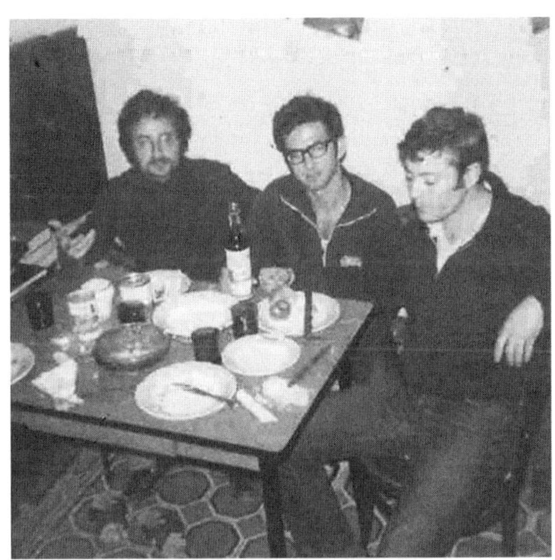

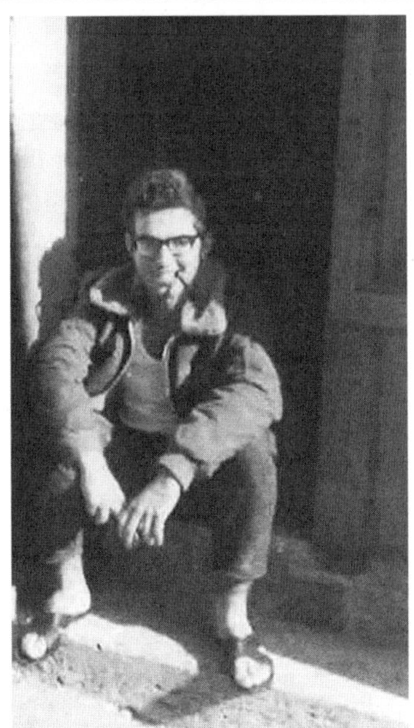

Five

The German affair

I took the night train to Munich. It was the beginning of October 1971, but winter had arrived early that year. Dawn found me in Austria, beyond the Brenner Pass: snowy alpine peaks, picturesque little villages, smoking chimneys on the rooftops of cute little wooden houses. It looked to me like a scene from *The Sound of Music*, or color illustrations from the Hebrew translation of a book by the Brothers Grimm that I had enjoyed as a child. It was the first time I had entered Germany. At the border, officers of the border police, clad in long black leather greatcoats, loudly entered our compartment. In guttural German, they ordered: *Alle Pässe bitte!*" I shuddered.

My Munich affair turned out to be a dead end. The Schwartzs allocated me a folding bed in the living room. Their two teenage daughters, covered with acne, spoke German, Russian, and French but no English. The pharmacist, Herr Appel, handed me the promised 2000 Deutchmarks adding, "We would have invited you to dinner, but we're leaving for Spain." At the medical school, they said that to register, I would have to complete a year of German language studies at the Goethe Institute, 2500 DM per month.

I burned my days walking up and down the endless Leopoldstrasse, freezing in my thin Israeli flight jacket. I gaped with interest at the appealing hookers around Schwabing but did not have the heart to spend 100 DM per half an hour. One night I overheard Mr. Schwartz whispering in Polish to his Russian wife: "When will *he* leave; how long will *he* be sleeping in our living room." I knew I had to move on. *Why not drop in on Jascia?* It was more than a year since our brief love affair in Israel. I knew that she was studying medicine at Aachen University.

Another night train, this time east to west across Germany, from Munich to Aachen, arriving at that medieval university town at five in the morning.

Light snow was falling; the air smelt of coal fire and freshly baked bread. From the *Bahnhof*, in my thin summer shoes, I sloshed in the dirty, already melting snow towards the student dormitories where, according to my address book, Jascia was residing. From the doorway, I rang Jascia's apartment. After a few rings, she replied in a sleepy voice, "Ja?"

"It's me, Moshe," I said.

"Who?"

"It's me, Moshe."

Silence. She must have been aware that I had gone to Italy to study medicine, and suddenly, I was knocking on her door at 6 o'clock in the morning.

"Oh, please come up." She stood at the top of the stairs, clad in a morning gown, her hair wild and face sleepy. We kissed. "What are you doing here?" she asked, "let me prepare some coffee." If my surprise visit was unwelcome, she was too well-mannered to show it. Sitting near her at the breakfast table, I could smell her unwashed body, the relics of that perfume I remembered so well – and I wanted her badly. I restrained myself.

We spent the rest of that day driving through the neighboring Netherlands in Jasica's tiny Fiat 850. We chatted and laughed like two old friends but maintained physical distance. We sat down for dinner in a cozy Indonesian restaurant in the evening. Under the dimmed light, I hugged Jascia, trying to draw her to me. She resisted. "What's wrong? What's the matter?" I asked. She said nothing and continued as if nothing happened. But the next day – I spent the night on a separate couch in her room – she told me it was all over. A few months after her vacation in Israel, she had met somebody older and "more mature." I realized there was no hope of reviving Jascia's love for me. My dream had been shattered. A melancholy descended on me. It would last a year or so.

I had to move on, away from Jascia, away from Germany. I called my father for instructions. He advised: "Son, you'll have to return to Italy. Why don't you try Bologna? But you'll need a car. Let me talk to David in Nuremberg." David, a stepson of my father's sister Erna, was only thirteen when the Allies liberated Sachsenhausen. In that concentration camp, he miraculously survived, slaving in a munition factory alongside his father (his mother and all siblings were all gassed). After the war, he remained in Germany, engaging in the business of selling carpets. So, I bid farewell to Jascia, who drove me to the station and – only now – hugged and kissed me warmly. I climbed on the train to Nuremberg where, in pouring rain, 'uncle' David – dark, balding, with a physique of a wrestler — his German wife (average looking blonde), and their two little well-behaved blonde kids were waiting for me at the *Bahnhof*. David's modest Opel station wagon delivered us to their small, unassumingly furnished flat.

The following day David loaded me into his Opel, and we were off to Schweinfurt, a smaller town in Bavaria, where he owned a carpet store. About one hour from Nuremberg, David suddenly left the *Autobahn*, stopping at a little village. "We'll stop for coffee with a friend," he explained. His Hebrew was atrophic; we communicated in a mixture of Polish, Yiddish, and German. We arrived at a driveway of a neat villa. He knocked on the door. His friend appeared: a tall and blond female in her late 50s, but remarkably well preserved; they hugged and kissed.

"Please meet my friend Elfriede," David introduced us. While coffee and *schtrudel* were served on golden-rimmed porcelain plates, I gazed around: spacious rooms, Persian carpets, and numerous artworks on the shelves and walls — like in an Italian museum. David's body language told me that Elfriede was more than just a friend and that he was the master of this house.

That same evening, in a Turkish restaurant, where the *Gastarbeiter* gathered to smoke and play *Shesh Besh*, over *shishlik* and *raki*, David told me his story: after the liberation of the camps, he had been a thin, skeleton-like teenager roaming the streets — "I was like a wild animal." She, in her late 20s, who had lost her husband on the Eastern Front, sheltered and fed him. She'd taught him German and manners and sent him to school. "I grew up in the camps… I was a beast... she brought me back to life… my wife doesn't know about her." The picture became clear: this middle-aged Jew was leading two separate lives. The first, the official one, with an ordinary German family; the second, the secret one, with his older rescuer and probably lover, to whom he had entrusted his fortune. As a kid who had survived the death camps, David knew better than to put all his cards on one table.

After dinner, David deposited me in his carpet store for the night; "I have business to attend to in Munich," he said, "I'll be back tomorrow." My bed for the night was a thick pile of handmade Tabriz rugs. I immediately collapsed into a deep sleep. Munich, Aachen, Nuremberg, David's tales, the bleak October landscapes, and weather — so alien to an Israeli kid — stirred up depressing dreams.

Suddenly loud bangs on the door: "*Polizei, aufmachen.*" I woke up from the dream covered with sweat: *Is this the Gestapo?*

* * * * *

I unlocked the door barefoot. Luckily, it was 1971, twenty-six years too late for the Gestapo, although the faces, the long leather greatcoats, and the coarse language could fit the picture.

I never learned to which branch of the police they belonged or what they wanted exactly. Did 'Uncle' David deal with smuggled carpets? Most probably. Did he evade tax? Very likely. Or did he use the carpet shop to cover up for trading drugs with his Turkish friends? Possible. At that moment, when I was shoved into the back seat of a black Mercedes, together with my only suitcase, I did not know that I would never meet David again.

The police station was neat, organized, and well-lighted. The police officers were grumpy and rigid in German fashion but not abusive. They asked for a passport once they discerned that the young man was a foreigner.

Their *führer* grabbed the navy blue hard-cover Israeli document in his chunky fingers: left, right, right, left — he turned the Hebrew document frustratingly; "*Scheisse,* where does it start and where does it end?" I helped him to the front page and produced my student ID from Siena. In primitive German I stated: "*Ich bin Israeli, ich studiere Medizin in Italien... jetzt Ferien, tourist...*" As to my association with Herr David, I explained that he was a distant family member.

Soon I found myself a free man, walking the wet streets. I staggered to the main post office and placed a collect call to Haifa.

My father laughed: "I knew that David is doing *Luftgeschäfte,* but now it appears he's in the *Unterwelt* as well... but don't worry about him, he's indestructible, now go and catch a train to Frankfurt, sit in the dining wagon and get yourself something good to eat. Uncle Georg will be waiting for you... if not he, somebody will."

* * * * *

We had never met, but the man waiting at Frankfurt-Hoechst *Bahnhof* identified me immediately. Thin, of average height, with short-cropped white hair, a well-trimmed mustache, and dressed in a light blue shirt, dark tie under a navy, blue-striped suit and matching trench coat, patent leather British shoes — 'Uncle' Georg looked like a respectable German industrialist. When he hugged and kissed me on my two cheeks, I noticed his deep blue eyes and the smell of aromatic aftershave.

"You look like your father... ach... your father and me, before the war, in Lemberg, we'd such a good time together... och, those Polish girls." While chatting to me in perfect Polish, the uncle walked us to his brand new Mercedes Benz 450SL. We drove off to Sulzbach along the damp *Autobahn.*

At home, over the years, I had heard much from my father about his maternal cousin Georg. Together with Georg they left their Galician hometown at the foot of the Carpathian Mountains to study medicine in Prague. A year later, Georg switched to architecture but never graduated; instead, he excelled in womanizing. He was an officer in the shattered Polish Army when the Germans invaded Poland.

With his pure Aryan look, he had acquired a false Polish Catholic identity and joined the Polish Merchant Navy. Thus, he was saved from his family's fate — turning into ash. After the war, Georg married a Polish woman, had kids, and continued touring the world as a ship's purser. In 1963, while his ship docked in Hamburg, he developed acute appendicitis and was hospitalized. After the operation, Georg decided enough was enough and would not return to his Polish wife across the Iron Curtain. It took him a few days to charm a Jesuit hospital nun — a young virgin that could have been his daughter.

Along with the marriage arrived German citizenship and a new identity of a *Volksdeutscher*; a false architect diploma was relatively easy to arrange. Next, the charismatic polyglot joined a large German contracting company. It made a career of importing workers from Turkey and North Africa. Eventually, he retired with the ex-nun, who gave him a set of blond twins, Kaya and Kayus, in a great suburban house built on money fleeced from the company by the builders he had imported from Turkey.

Sulzbach proved an affluent suburb on the edge of Frankfurt, and Uncle Georg's mansion was grand indeed. Israel in those years was a Spartan-like country, and I had seen only in American movies the spacious, carpeted rooms, numerous bathrooms, and color TV. I found the 'new' aunt-ex-nun Mathilde pleasant enough and hospitable, but not somebody I would have advised to leave the monastery. Since then, I have come across a broad spectrum of German women: however attractive, well-mannered, proper, and engaging they appear on the outside, there is a detectable hardness and rigidity in their inner structure, as if they had swallowed a long broom. Of course, there were not a few exceptions…

The next day, in the afternoon, after a few phone calls from the uncle, a shabby-looking, pockmarked Turk showed up at the driveway with a Volkswagen Beetle 1200. The cream-colored exterior looked in good repair; as to the car's condition, the Turk declared: "It's a 1959 model, but the engine is new, and the roof is retractable." The uncle handed out a few bills and proudly announced, "This is your new car." *How generous*, I thought. Later I learned that the uncle immediately wrote to my father asking to be reimbursed 600 DM ($172 in 1991) for the car. He hid the car in the garage so the respectable neighbors would not see such a wreck on his property.

Finally, after a few weeks, my first German expedition ended. Driving southbound on the *Autobahn* in my 'new' Volkswagen — the first car I owned — I was elated by the reassuring *pukpukpuk* racket coming from the rear of this reliable "people's car." On the outskirts of Darmstadt, I picked up a hitchhiker who was a Scottish student traveling to Italy. Then the window wipers packed up. There was only one solution to combat the shower of mud splashed by the road-crazy Germans bypassing us at 180km per hour: the Scot had to pay for his ride by becoming a human wiper. Every few minutes, I manually retracted the roof through which the Scot used a rag to achieve some visibility. For his gallant service, I treated the Scot, who seemed even more impoverished than I, to a meal of sausage stewed with onions, cabbage, and a few beers.

We crossed the Alps at St. Gotthard. At that time, the Gotthard Tunnel served only the railways; the cars had to take the steep, climbing, tortuous Alpine Pass, followed by numerous downward bends towards Tessin and Italy. Ice-clear alpine air, snow-covered peaks, deep blue lakes, magnificent villas on the cliffs; further down below the tree line, the aroma of fresh hay, cows grazing with heavy bells around their necks... this was my first encounter with the thrilling beauty of Switzerland. Late that evening, the Scot requested to be dropped off in Como, Italy. In a semi-deserted lakeside restaurant, we celebrated the last moments of our short-term friendship, wolfing down a plate of spaghetti Bolognese and sharing a bottle of cheap wine. I remember he was a nice lad; for some reason, I recall where and what we ate, but not his name or how he looked.

I continued alone southwards, along the *Autostrada del Sole*. Towards morning, around Florence, I turned into the winding road leading to Siena. The Beetle lacked a car radio, but I had a transistor tuned to Radio Luxemburg; however, the best music to my ears was the constant clicking of my new 'limousine.' What a lovely car! I loved it. As I approached Siena, I noticed how the bright dawn illuminated the ancient city's walls. Simultaneously, I smelled the black, dense smoke emerging from the rear of my car.

* * * * *

Left: Jascia (1970) (she became an ophthalmologist in Dusseldorf, married to a dentist, mother to a son). Right: in my 'new' Beetle, crossing the Swiss Alps to Italy (1971).

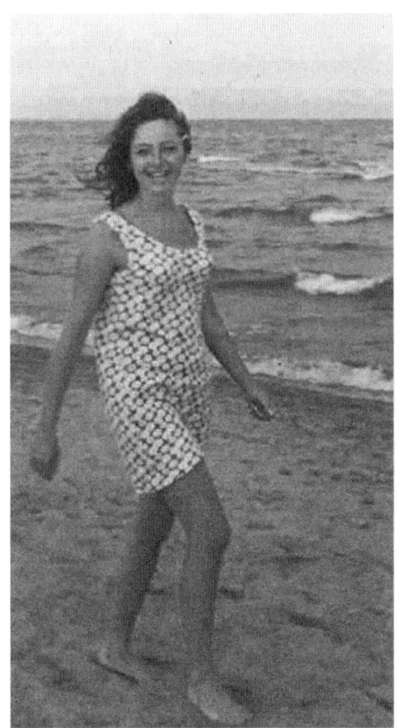

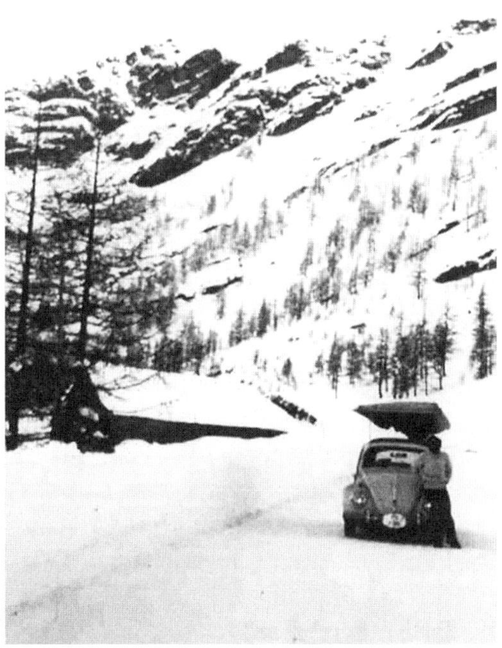

Six

Modena — the first examination

The Beetle's engine had to be replaced. It cost me the equivalent of two months of sustenance allowance. I received from my father 150 US dollars each month (it would be about $964 today). I still remember the exchange rate of those days: I got 620 Italian lira per dollar – almost a 100,000 lira per month. I could live comfortably on that. That is if I would not squander it on misadventures with cars.

On a rainy autumn day, I loaded the Beetle with all my possessions, the mattress on the round roof, and headed northward to Bologna – the site of the oldest university in the Western World. In 1971, Bologna was so popular among students that its medical faculty refused to accept my transfer from Siena, and it was also impossible to obtain any accommodation in that town. After two weeks of sleepless nights among snoring, drug-using 'tourists' in the youth hostel on the outskirts of that beautiful town, sustained by cheap pasta at workmen eateries, I decided to migrate further north, on the Via Emilia – built by the Romans in 109 BC – to Modena.

Modena is a mid-size medieval town famous for its Maserati and Ferrari cars, Balsamic vinegar, arcaded sidewalks, sparkling Lambrusco wines, Luciano Pavarotti, mortadella, and beautiful blonde girls with small sharp or slightly hooked noses. But on that gray, early November day, I knew nothing about Modena and its delights; I only wanted a roof over my head and to start studying.

At the students' admission office, I met another Israeli, Jochanan – who eventually became Chief of Anesthesia in Jerusalem. Together we rented a two-room, one-shower complex at the *Casa dello Studente*, just above the *mensa*. Our neighbors were mainly from the south of Italy, collectively termed by the stuck-up northerners as *studenti meridionali*, and a bunch of Arabs: Palestinians, Syrians, and the rest of the Levant. In the corridor and the *mensa*, we attempted to exchange words with 'the enemy' – these were the years after the Six-Day War and before the 1973 October War. Some greeted us with a smile; others looked away, not wanting any contact with the murderous Zionists.

Three months after arriving in Modena, we planned another day trip to the lakeside town of Lugano, just across the Swiss border, to stock up on cheap chocolate and gas coupons. Car gas was costly in Italy. Hence, to promote tourism, foreigners entering Italy, driving cars with foreign license plates (my Beetle had the Zoll German license plate allocated to cars bought by tourists in Germany), could buy discounted Italian gas coupons before crossing the border. It was illegal for us students residing in Italy to do so, but we took the risk. We would drive across the Swiss border and buy the maximal allowance of gas coupons at a Swiss Bank; back in Modena, we would sell half of the coupons to owners of gas stations, sharing and pocketing the difference — around $150 per trip. But that January morning, when we descended to the parking lot, my beloved Beetle was not there; it was gone, and so was my passport. I called the Israeli Consulate in Milano and was told: "You idiot. Who would be so stupid to leave an Israeli passport in his car… with all these Arabs hovering around. Now one is entering Israel with his picture on your passport and a bomb in his pocket…" The car was never found. Right up until the summer break, I walked and studied.

Finally, I started attending lectures in the vast theater. More than 500 students were in our class; this was considered a small class — in Bologna, they had a thousand first-year students. Of course, the lectures were in Italian, and I understood absolutely nothing. So, while everybody was taking notes frantically, I had the chance to study my new colleagues. More than half were locals, northern Italians from Modena, and its vicinity: eighteen-year-old kids, fresh from high school. I was struck by how well dressed they were, according to the prevailing fashion: tight bell-shaped trousers, superb Italian leather shoes, fancy shirts — very narrow at the waist — camel hair overcoats reaching down to the floor.

There were numerous girls among the students. Lovely girls, invariably slender and, already in the early morning, dressed to kill: high heels, miniskirts, full makeup. The rest of the class consisted of the much less extravagant *meridionali* and us — a tiny group of *stranieri*. Each morning, while we would schlep ourselves in the deep, wet snow, the locals would arrive in their constantly polished cars — Italians love their cars — that ranged from the tiny Fiat Cinquecento, Fiat 127 or 128, to Lancia, Alfa Romeo, and even Ferrari. At lunch break, the *meridionali* and we would slog back to the *mensa* for a plate of hot pasta, whereas the locals would speed off home to dine with mama or papa, or to one of the fancy restaurants in *centrocitta*. It was when I was first exposed to the feeling of being poor and a stranger.

After a few weeks of attending lectures that I did not understand and several futile attempts to pick up one of those leggy princesses — the only 'success' was cute Simonetta M. (the one name I remember), who, during lunch, agreed to walk with me around the *duomo*; she allowed me to buy her a *gelato*, but in the evening was 'busy' — I decided to skip lectures altogether.

My brain was dry — not that it was disused, but it had never been properly used. During the preceding three years in the army, my highest intellectual activity, beyond that of studying navigation and manuals of Claymore mines, involved reading old *Playboy* magazines in dark, dusty bunkers, or at night, to candlelight, in tiny field tents. The only literary book I read during those years was *Fanny Hill*… and here I was sitting with vast volumes of *Biologia, Histologia, Biochemia,* and *Physiologia*.

I started with the first book. Using an Italian-Hebrew dictionary, I translated it word by word. In red ink, I entered the Hebrew translation above the Italian. When the meaning did not make sense, I used the Italian-English dictionary and often had to open the English-Hebrew dictionary when I did not understand the English term. I could increase the pace when the book was filled with red Hebrew characters because many words became familiar. In parallel, I listened to the Italian radio and chatted with the *meridionali* at the *mensa*. When I finished with the *Biologia* book, I started to 'paint' the *Histologia* book in red. At night, I paced up and down my tiny room, citing long paragraphs from these books aloud. I could not speak Italian, but I could talk biology and histology in Italian. Even today, I can quote whole sections from these two books. In mid-year, when the course of *Biochemia* commenced, I started attending the lectures: I did not have to take notes because I already knew the book by heart.

* * * * *

The examination period began in May. As I mentioned, this was a totally free system: you could take all four first-year examinations or none. You could continue to be a first-year student forever. You had a small book called a *libretto* in which the exams you passed or failed, and their scores, were registered; once you passed all the numerous required examinations, you became a *dottore*. You were a medical doctor!

The examinations were public. They were conducted in a lecture theater before a committee of three professors in front of a large, frenzied crowd of spectators. The seats were packed with students awaiting their turn – many of them who had failed previously, now preparing for a re-examination, hoping to learn how not to fail or to enjoy the fiasco of others. The minimum passing score was 18; the top score was 30. Those who did even better received *trenta cum laude* (30 plus).

The first exam I took was in *Biologia*. The long roster posted on the doors of the medical school announced that I would be walking up to the guillotine on the first day of the examination period – which would last a few weeks. The chief examiner was *Professore* Cognetti, an elderly gentleman with protruding ears, known for his super-nervousness and short temper; and – worst of all – an alleged dislike of *stranieri*.

At the *mensa*, my left-leaning *meridionali* buddies jested merrily at me, sliding their forefingers across their necks, and adding, "Cognetti... *fascista*." They predicted my imminent slaughter. Two days before the exam, I stopped studying. What for? I have no chance. I should return to Israel and join a kibbutz. I got a haircut and purchased a tight Italian shirt in the open market, where everything was discounted. Finally, in desperation, I bought my first bottle of whiskey in the supermarket (I believe it was White Horse blended Scotch). The bottle was half-empty on the morning of my looming execution.

* * * * *

Morning, 9 o'clock. The arena is filling up with the gladiators on their way to glory or death. There is a huge audience ready to watch the blood bath.

Jochanan and I sit together, pale and soaked in sweat. We watch how the ferocious Professor Cognetti eliminates Italian candidates who sing fluently in beautiful Italian — like Pavarotti. What about us? Would we be able to say anything meaningful in Italian? Abdullah — a mustached Jordanian we know from the *mensa* — who had already failed twice — is dismissed by Cognetti with a sarcastic comment: "Signore, why don't you go back to Jordan..." The Italian audience chuckles lightly — this is not the day of the *stranieri*... especially not when the chief examiner is known to have supported Mussolini, eh?

One more to go before me: Mihai, a Jewish Romanian from Bucharest. We know him from the synagogue, and Romanian is a Roman language; thus, Mihai sounds almost like an Italian. He boasted that he would only accept, in any subject, a score of 28 or more. But after fifteen minutes, we see the Romanian escaping from the auditorium, head hanging low, with a lowly "18" stamped in his *libretto*. Now it is my turn.

I stroll down the steep stairs toward the stage. My head is throbbing, my stomach aching — a nasty hangover. I sense the crowd in my back and see Cognetti wiping the sweat irritably from his forehead, looking impatiently at his watch.

I climb the elevated wooden podium and collapse on the hard wooden chair facing the three inquisitors. I focus my eyes on Cognetti's bald scalp and his fanning hairy ears. Without raising his head or showing any interest, he roars: "Signore Schein, please tell us about Mendel's Second Law of Genetics." Like all Italians, he pronounces the "Sch" as "sk", converting my name to SKAIN.

"*Si Professore, certo...*" I look in my mind at the relevant pages from the book, including my Hebrew translation, and start reciting. As I continue, the alleged *fascista* lifts his head, and I note his bright brown eyes gazing warmly at me. He nods his head repetitively, agreeing with each word and sentence. The answer to the second question brings a smile to his face.

The auditorium is dead silent in expectation: would he ask another question — the one for the *trenta cum laude* — the 30+? Cognetti nods to the young chic *professoressa* on his left; she, a parasitologist, inquires about some worm. I forget the creature's name, so I imitate, gesturing with my two hands, how it crawls. I hear loud laughter behind my back. Cognetti lifts his hand and orders *silencio*. He smiles at me and vigorously shakes my hand. And announces, "*trenta cum laude*." I climb up — nay, I fly up — to the doors where Jochanan is waiting. I treat him to a cappuccino and dolce at the nearby bar.

It was my first scholarly victory — no academic success would ever be as sweet. I did not realize that then, but that first *trenta cum laude* had given me a tremendous boost, the subconscious awareness that I can do it — I, the "high school retard," can excel. I doubt whether old Professor Cognetti — lying in his grave for many years — understood how crucial his appraisal had been to the future life of that obscure student from the Middle East.

I called my father. Satisfied with the unexpected triumph of his hitherto hindered son, he generously offered, "Well, son, why don't you get yourself another old car, perhaps get it from one of the graduating foreign students…" The following week I drove around in a beautiful red Volkswagen 1500, 1968; not another Beetle, but a round-bodied Berlina, with a rear engine and a substantial front boot.

* * * * *

What I remember most of the years in Italy is studying day and night. Studying anatomy during the second year — not on cadavers but from atlases and texts — was even more challenging. Dissection of corpses was not practiced in Italy then, for how could they provide enough cadavers for so many students? The computerized 'virtual body' animations were still many years away. So, what was left for us were some second-hand skeletons and massive anatomical tomes. I used the volumes by the Italian Giulio Chiarurgi, and the German Johannes Sobotta, although my friends swore that the series by the Frenchman Leo Testut were much better. Luckily, my father sent me a few expensive volumes by the American Frank Netter — his fantastic colorful illustrations facilitated the perception of the tridimensional view of the body's cavities. How we studied anatomy reminds me of Chekhov's short story, *Anyuta,* where the hero paces across his tiny room, mumbling to himself: "The right lung consists of three parts… Klotchkov raised his eyes to the ceiling, striving to visualize what he had just read. Unable to form a clear picture of it, he began feeling his upper ribs through his waistcoat." This is exactly how we used to study anatomy. After the first exam's *trenta,* I would not compromise for anything less.

I remember the chalky fogs that would engulf the Po Valley for days and nights, the wet chill penetrating our poorly dressed bones. I remember the cobblestone pavements in *centrocitta,* glistering in the rain. And the early spring bloom of the gardens in the *viali* surrounding the old town. I can still smell the scents emerging from dark, crowded *salumerias*: prosciutto, mortadella, salamini, and coppa hanging from the ceiling, and on the floor huge Parmesan cheeses — from the nearby Parma. Yes, I smelled all those delicacies but seldom consumed any of them. I breakfasted in my room: percolating coffee in one of those little Italian percolators placed on a hot plate, munching a white *panino* roll with some soft cheese. Lunch and dinner we ate routinely at the *mensa*, except on Sunday evenings when the *mensa* was closed and we would drive downtown to the same little pizzeria, always choosing a fat calzone washed down with a pint of draft Peroni beer. It was our only luxury.

I remember the small synagogue and its irritating rabbi. In that synagogue, we were discovered and adopted by Mr. Riegler and his family, who would regularly treat us to delicious Friday dinners at their small villa. Overfed with homemade pasta and fortified with *Lambrusco di Modena,* we listened to Zigi Riegler's story. He had been eighteen years old when World War II ended, the sole survivor of his Central European family. In 1946, he was going on foot through Italy towards the south, hoping to board one of the illegal ships sailing for British-ruled Palestine.

On the street in Modena, destitute, hungry, dressed in rags, he had met Lena — a corpulent Catholic Italian girl ten years older. Thus, his journey to Palestine was interrupted forever. Zigi had taken over the family's glue factory. Lena had given him two daughters while her mother — the diminutive *nonna* — commanded the kitchen; she cooked so well that by the time we met them, Lena was double the size of her skinny husband. She looked as if she were his mother. I remember Lena chain-smoking MS cigarettes and sipping *apperativi,* followed by her beloved Lambrusco, which was like water to her. At their table I learned that there is little pleasure in eating good food without wine. "*Bevi, bevi,*" (drink, drink) and "*mangi, mangi,*" (eat, eat) Lena would constantly command, heaping more tortellini on my plate. "You look like a *pulcino*" (a small chicken), she would scold me. What happened to them? The *nonna* broke her hip and died during my second year in Modena. Both Lena and Zigi passed away over the years. I've heard that their youngest daughter became the chess champion of Italy.

What about women? Local *studenti* did it in their small cars. Often at night, one could see bare legs sticking out of the retractable roofs of a tiny Fiat Cinquecento. The *meridionali* frequented the railway station where, for a few lire, aging toothless whores provided a relieving *boccino* (*bocca* means mouth). I didn't find such practice attractive.

I remember my first trip to Venice in the spring of 1971: Piazza San Marco at dusk with fading sunrays, a salty canal fragrance, doves fluttering above; couples walking hand in hand or sipping white vermouth at the cafes; fried seafood on the plates; orchestras playing Charles Aznavour's "*Que c'est triste Venise…*" (How sad Venice can be, it's too lonely to bear, when you have lost the love that you discovered there…"). So many beautiful women were around, and I needed one so badly.

* * * * *

Late June, after the examinations, most students would escape Modena and the sweltering Po Valley until the autumn. I flew back home to Haifa. Back then, Haifa had a young medical school that admitted a selective number of Israeli students from Italy directly into the fourth year. Encouraged by my unexpected success in Modena, my father tried to have me accepted into the second year in Haifa. An interview with the Dean was arranged. As scheduled, I arrived at the office of the Dean, who had also been known as one of Israel's greatest surgeons — the man who invented the central splenorenal shunt for portal hypertension. The lady at the reception said, "Professor Ehrlich would be late. Why don't you talk with Professor Bental, the Vice Dean?"

Behind the heavy desk in a dark room, shaded from July's dazzling sun, sat a large, dark, bald man who looked at me gravely. The great professor of neurology did not waste any moment on preliminary pleasantries with the lowly first-year student from Italy.

"So, your father thinks that you are ready to enter *our* medical school? What were your matriculation scores in math and physics? Sixty percent?" His face showed contempt. "And you think you'll be able to cope with *our* curriculum? Our medical school is affiliated with the *Technion* — one of the best technological institutes in the world; our goal, the reason for our existence, is to create physician-scientists. You, you won't have any chance at all to compete with our carefully selected students. You will be left behind. My advice: go back to Italy and try again for our fourth year 'Italian class,' or try in Tel Aviv, and [he shrugged] not everybody has to be a doctor. Now go in peace." I did not manage to utter a word.

In the corridor, on my way out, I stumbled upon an elderly gentleman. He stopped me: "You must be the young Schein, eh? Sorry to be late. My name is David Ehrlich." He led me into his spacious Dean's chancellery, and after learning what the neurologist had told me, he smiled kindly: "Oh, math, physics, doctor-scientists, they really believe in it. *Nu*... let them. I wanted to create a medical school in Haifa. We had to develop a few gimmicks to justify it, but you and I should not take it too seriously." With a fatherly tone, he continued: "Go back to Italy for another year, and I will admit you into the third year and don't worry about him," he pointed to the wall, "it is how some of them are."

I would return to Haifa's medical school, not a year later as planned, but eighteen years later — as a senior lecturer and department's deputy head. There I would meet the now retired and ailing nasty neurologist; I must admit that it gave me some satisfaction to talk to him as a surgeon to a patient, although I do not believe that he remembered our previous encounter. I do not think much about Haifa's medicine as a mecca of science; the opposite is true. However, that neurologist — he has since died — who implied that I was an idiot may have had some vision: in 2004, two professors of Haifa's medical school received the Nobel Prize for chemistry.

After a bright Israeli summer and many glorious days on the sandy beaches of the Red Sea along the Sinai Desert, I gloomily returned to Italy. My pessimism deepened when I found that my lovely red Volkswagen 1500 had become a wreck. Eli Landau, an Israeli student to whom I had left my car — he eventually became a cardiologist in Tel Aviv and a newspaper food columnist until his death (2012) — reported to me laconically:

"After I dropped you off at Bologna Airport, I returned to Modena. Suddenly, the front axle collapsed, and I rolled over. I am lucky to be alive..." Instead of offering compensation, he accused me of almost killing him. At a small garage where my wreck had been dumped, the mechanic said: "Your friend must've driven like a *pazzo* (crazy man). He crashed into a lamp post and rolled over; the *machina è finita*."

What should I do? I was expecting my parents' visit in a month or two, and I had promised to show them around Modena and Bologna. The sly Modenese *meccanico* devised a solution: "The body is *finito* whereas the engine, tires, and all other parts are in excellent shape."

He led me to his backyard, where an empty body of an older Volkswagen 1500 was rotting. "To merge the two will cost you 150 *dollari*, paint job, another fifty; we'll use your German Zoll license plates and documents, which obviously won't fit the hybrid's body number. But you are not going to show it to the police, eh? And for this body, you pay me $25 *dollari*, a total of 225, *va bene*, all right?"

I was driving the new azure white 'VW hybrid' two weeks later — a car that would have a tremendous impact on my life in the short- and long-term future.

* * * * *

Top: Modena, in front of the the *Casa dello Studente*, 1972. Bottom: Modena, studying on the roof with Jochanan, 1972.

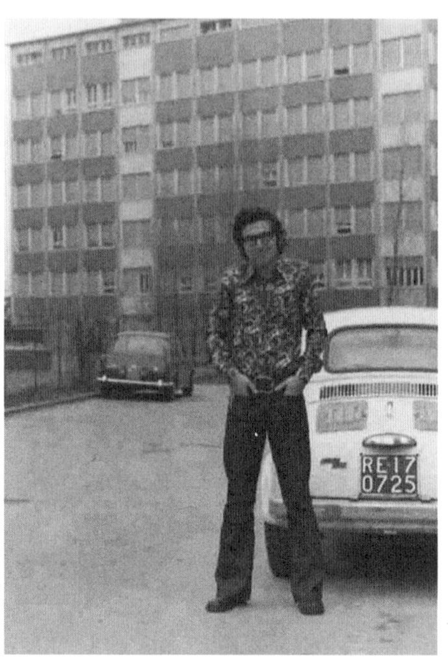

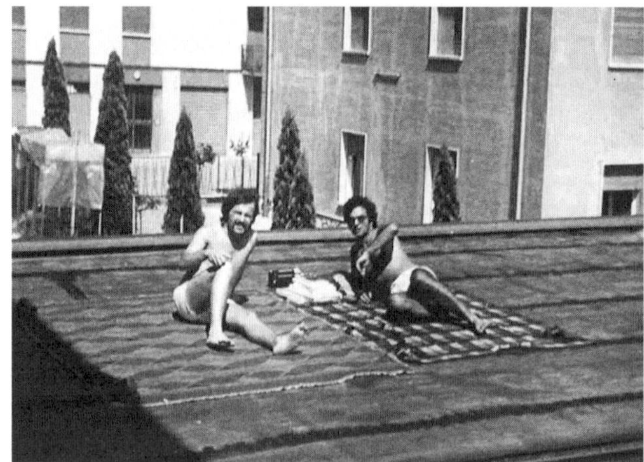

Seven

The enchanted summer

It was the summer of 1973. With the great examination in *anatomia* behind me and a few more *trentas* in my *libretto*, I believed I was entitled to a grand tour of Europe. I invited my best friend Amikam to join me from Israel. Amikam was a big and robust *kibbutznik* from the Jezreel Valley. We served together in the same Golani infantry company throughout basic and advanced training, the NCO course, and the "rifle company." After discharge, Amikam returned to his kibbutz, using his huge hands in the cattle barn and hunting for Scandinavian girls in the kibbutz's swimming pool. When I picked him up at Modena's railway station, Amikam looked like a kibbutz poster boy: tall, muscular, suntanned, in old shorts, a T-shirt, open-toe brown sandals, and a hundred-pound military kitbag on his shoulder. His eyes opened in awe — the farm boy encountering the marvels of Europe.

We had my 'new' Volkswagen, a military hiking tent, two old sleeping bags, a little portable gas cooker, a pan and pot, Swiss army knives, and two mess tins. Our money reserves were scarce, however. Our destination was Scandinavia. The plan was to live off the land: sleep in forests, open fields, or wherever somebody offered a free bed. Food? We knew how to survive on 2-3 dollars a day: hot soup, boiled eggs, fresh bread, basic cheese, and fruits, and whatever we could 'borrow' from the farms on the way. We were warned that Scandinavia was extremely expensive, but we had a few Danish girls' addresses, which filled us with optimism.

So, on a sunny late afternoon in June, we drove north, crossing the Dolomites into Austria. In Tyrol, we crawled into a vacant pig stall for the night, but three barking dogs and an angry farmer chased us away. In a south German forest, we were attacked by swarms of nasty, anti-Semitic biting flies. North of Hanover, another angry farmer aimed a hunting gun at us when we helped ourselves to his apple tree. We headed northbound towards Flensburg at the Danish border. After a week on the road, when we crossed the border into Jutland, we had already realized that Europe is not exactly the Sinai Desert or the Galilee, where you can fall asleep anywhere, where hospitable Bedouins would invite you into their tent for a cup of black-bitter coffee, a piece of pita bread smeared with olive oil and fresh *zaatar* (herb blend of thyme, oregano, marjoram or a combination of the three, along with other spices including sesame, sumac, cumin or coriander), and a few olives (or, some would say, stab you in your back…). We recognized that Europe was more civilized; hence, you had to have some money and pay for everything, even for erecting your tent on a camping site.

Denmark, however, proved to be a paradise. The most fascinating aspect of traveling is the realization of the marked differences between national characteristics. We crossed the border and drove a few miles through unchanged nature, but the first Danish town was so different from the last German one: smaller, cozier, and cleaner, homier and more relaxed. Suspicious and arrogant faces of "leave me alone" changed into inviting, sincere, and, yes, naïve smiles. We entered — disheveled, dirty, unwashed — into a small *kro* (pub), where we asked for coffee and some bread and butter. The blonde barmaid smiled and served us a large porcelain pot of freshly brewed coffee, bread, butter, and jam. When we wanted to pay, she refused our money: "This is a bar, and we only sell beer and liquor…" We looked at each other: so, these are the Danes, no wonder they were the only Europeans who managed to save almost *all* their Jews during the War.

We continued north: narrow lanes sheltered by trees winding across the flat and intensely green landscape. We saw well-fed cows, yellow-haired kids, and neat villages; the calm wind was blowing from the North Sea — like a picture postcard. We arrived at Skanderborg, a serene little lakeside town south of Aarhus. I still remember the address: Louisenlund 3 — a large wooden house on a lush garden leading to a boat landing; expansive Danish windows on all sides of the house to let in as much sun as possible. It smelled of flowers, freshly cut grass, and rotting lake plants. We found Karen sitting on the open porch: a book on her lap, a Carlsberg beer in her hand, and a filterless cigarette — she smoked Prince, a Danish equivalent to Gauloise — between her lips. That is how I remember her best.

Karen had spent a year as a volunteer in Amikam's kibbutz. During the previous summer, she joined Amikam and I on a tour of the Sinai Desert. At that time, she had a boyfriend in the kibbutz — we were "just friends." Now we had an address in Denmark… One would not describe Karen as a stunning beauty — she was not an exact copy of one of those electrifying Nordic amazons one noticed all around. Her hair was fair, she was slim but not too tall. One remembers best her large blue eyes, dry skin, and breath, which smelled pleasantly of cigarettes and whiskey. Karen's parents received us enthusiastically. Their house, and Karen's separate lake cottage, became our base for the entire summer — the last carefree summer of 1973.

Imagine a cool blue lake under a clear sunny sky, Danish pastries, cheese, and herring for breakfast; if Karen's father was around, Aalborg kummel schnapps was served alongside in frozen thumb glasses. For dinner we ate fried baby eel from the bottom of the lake and rice pudding. Throughout the days, we drank Carlsberg and Tuborg beers, which the

Danes drank like water, and French or Spanish table wines with dinner, and into the night; Janis Joplin screaming in the background; barbecues on the beach, and dinner parties in the open air, swimming under the moon — until the wee hours of the night. On weekends, we would explore the disco clubs in the neighboring towns of Horsens or Kolding: dark rooms packed with the most beautiful and friendly blonde girls who knew how to move their bodies. Days, weeks, months of sun, water, nature, food, drink, books — no worries — and a bed with Karen's warm body next to mine. It happened naturally, without much talking — she moved into my bed one night. Like in paradise.

At the end of the summer, we explored Sweden and Norway and returned to Jutland.

It was time to say goodbye. Being young, naïve, and penniless, it did not occur to me then that Karen's father — not a wealthy man but a humble home builder — had supported us for many weeks. I wonder what makes some people so generous and hospitable.

In memoirs, characters appear or disappear, and the narrator fails to divulge their fate. So let me tell you what became of the main characters in this episode. Amikam returned to Israel, left the kibbutz, studied medicine, and specialized in neurology. You could see him in the corridors of his hospital in Afula, dressed in a long black coat and a derby hat, his face covered by a thick black beard — the *kibbutznik* became an Orthodox-Hasidic Jew. And Karen? At some stage, we became quite fond of each other. Then she married, had a son, divorced, studied in Aarhus, and now, she lives happily, remarried to a university professor in Aalborg.

Ten years later, when on a prolonged study 'exile' in Leeds, UK, I decided to visit Karen in Aalborg. I took a night ferry to Jutland through a surprisingly calm North Sea. Karen hosted me in a modest rented bungalow at the edge of town, which she had moved into with her little son after her divorce. I was allocated to the son's room; the son moved in with his mother. On the first evening of my stay, Karen's boyfriend came over for dinner. I remember a tall blonde guy, serious looking, at least five years older than me. I learned he was a Swede, now pursuing an academic career (something in international economy) at the University of Aalborg. Despite the candlelight and plenty of booze, the atmosphere was tense, the conversation heavy. The Scandinavian academician did not appreciate my sudden appearance at his girlfriend's house. Who could blame him? After dinner, Karen drove with the boyfriend to his place, leaving me behind with her son.

The following day the boyfriend had to leave town for some lectures. That night, after her son had fallen asleep, Karen moved into my room. How nice to reunite with an old flame — mainly if the separation had been natural and entirely benign. We had a few days to engage in the charming illusion, as if we were an old married couple, realizing that at the end of the week, our 'reunion' would cease forever. On Monday, she drove me in her old black Volvo to the railway station; we sat silently holding hands at the station buffet. A freezing ocean wind blew outside.

"I hope I'm not pregnant," she said.

"You can't be. I was careful."

"But I'm worried."

I had a beer, she cried, and we held hands. I have not seen Karen since.

Many years later, around 2010, Karen Googled me and sent an e-mail. She was now happily married to that same Swede — currently a professor — working as a social worker. We continued a friendly but sporadic communication via e-mail until she wrote: "My husband discovered that I have been in touch with you. He demands that this stop. You will not be hearing from me again. Please do not write anymore. If you do, I will not reply. Do understand I cannot risk my marriage."

* * * * *

Let us return to the end of the enchanted summer of 1973.

We had to get back to Italy. From Jutland, we drove south, through Germany, entering the Netherlands. We planned to cross Germany, through Munich, towards the Brenner Pass, into Italy. However, the German policeman at the border looked at the car, examined the Zoll license plates, and exclaimed: "*Nein, nein,* your Zoll plates have expired. *Zollnummer ist gültig* only for a year. This car is no longer legal. You can't enter Germany."

We turned around and attempted another border crossing a few miles to the south. Here the border *Polizist* was even more pedantic, and he opened the hood and inspected the car's body number. "Oh, this car doesn't correspond to the plate number… this is illegal… criminal… you must leave the car here."

"And what about our luggage?" we pleaded.

He shrugged: "Take whatever you wish and go; however, this car stays here, and you won't be entering Germany. Be happy that we let you go. This crime deserves a jail sentence." He continued cursing and mumbling about gypsies, *beatniks,* and foreigners in general.

The car was all we had, and the money on us would not even buy a train ticket to Amsterdam. In desperation, we demanded to see the *commandant.* The latter — older, fatter, and more human — listened to our laments about being "poor medical students, somebody sold us this car, we didn't know…" He melted: "*Ja, gut,* OK, take your *Scheisswagen* and go wherever you want but stay away from *Deutschland, oder…*" We jumped into the blue-white car and sped away. But where to go?

Amikam consulted his address book. "There is a guy called Carl. It's in Schaffhausen."

"Where on earth is this? It sounds German. We're not allowed there."

"No, this is somewhere in Switzerland. Carl was a volunteer in our kibbutz a few years ago, he befriended my father, and they are still corresponding, exchanging stamps. Why don't we cross Switzerland and drop in on him for a day or two? From there to Italy shouldn't be too far…"

"Why not?"

We consulted the map and selected a route through rural Belgium, Luxembourg, and France. Two days later, we crossed the border to the western, French-speaking part of Switzerland; we continued eastwards toward the German-speaking region.

On a hot August morning, we crossed an old bridge on the Rhein River. On the right, we saw the Munot — Schaffhausen's medieval castle — nestled high among dense wine grapes on the ridge. We located Carl's address: it was a rustic three-story house. We opened the wooden gate and entered a well-groomed garden: flowers, strawberries, and a plum tree. It smelled of vegetation, and butterflies and bees hovered around. Amikam knocked on the door: it opened.

What I saw was a young girl, around seventeen years old. I immediately noticed her slim but muscular, tanned legs below a short, yellow summer dress. She wore high-heeled sandals. Her toes were painted red. I liked it. I also noted her long dark blonde hair tied around at the back. Her face was alluring and when she smiled and said, in accented English, "I'm sorry, but Carl and his wife are not at home, they left for the weekend, perhaps you can come back on Monday," I noticed that her right canine tooth was slightly askew. Before she closed the door in our faces, I rushed forward, "And you are?"

"I'm Heidi, Carl's sister."

* * * * *

Five days later, we were driving again in the blue-white Volkswagen, now from Schaffhausen to Zurich. But this time Amikam was in the back seat. In the front sat Heidi — not in the passenger seat but almost sharing the driver's seat with me — her body melting lovingly into mine. I dropped them off in Zurich: Amikam was to catch a train to Paris, then a flight to Israel; the teenage girl was to enroll in a nursing school in Zurich.

I continued south, towards the snowy Alps, which glittered far away, basking in the glorious summer sun. I felt intoxicated by that seventeen-year-old Swiss girl. I savored her yielding, unconditional surrender, her innocent and instant devotion. At the same time, my head was crowded with the events of that enchanting summer. The memories of that teenager would remain with a few images: dancing in a dim, wood-paneled Swiss tavern, a night picnic under a full moon reflected in the Rhein River, and, above all, her tender persona and blossoming beauty.

As I climbed the Alps and descended into Italy, my body continued to long for the Swiss girl's softness, but my mind planned forward: sell the car, ship the books, organize a flight ticket, and return home to Israel. A telegram from my father had reached me in Switzerland, announcing that my entry to the third year in Haifa's medical school had finally been secured.

* * * * *

Arriving in Modena I found it a deserted steaming inferno. I rented a small attic room from a *signora* where the unendurable heat and aggressive mosquitoes made sleep impossible. I started packing and driving boxes to the post office. Then, on the third day in town, I was stopped by a pair of *Carabinieri*: these were tall police officers mounted on shiny, powerful Moto Guzzi motorbikes — knee-level shiny black boots, black leather jackets, matching helmets — I always wondered why the *Carabinieri* looked like Mussolini's Blackshirts.

One of the cops dismounted and approached my car. *"Documenti per favore,"* he said.

I handed him my international driving license and the car documents. He held them near his nose, opened the car hood, looked in for a few minutes, and commanded: "Please follow me to the police station." I realized that my car was doomed. But what about me?

Interrogation: the room was full of smoke and unbearably hot, the air static below the noisy ceiling fans. For hours, I had to endure observing the thick index finger of the 'blackshirt' interrogator, hammering on his old typewriter at a rate of a word per minute: M...O...S...H...E...S...C... Finally, the cop said: "*Dottore* (in Italy, even a first-year medical student was addressed so), you can go home but never leave town. You will be summoned to court in a few weeks. Until then, please present every week, with your passport, at the office of the *Questura*. Your car has been confiscated." A friendly police officer drove me to my room with everything I could salvage from my car.

A few days later, I took a train to Milan, an Alitalia flight to Rome, and an El Al flight to Tel Aviv. Advice: if you wish to engage in criminal dealings with the police — do it in Italy! At least, this was the situation in the pre-digital era.

My Italian chapter was over. I could not predict that three months later, just after the 'surprise' of the Yom Kippur War, Heidi would appear in a yellow oilskin raincoat and matching yellow rubber boots — like a good old Swiss girl hiking across the border into the Black Forest — at our front door in Haifa.

* * * * *

Left: summer 1973, with Amikam in Copenhagen; with the 'new' VW in Norway. Right: Heidi in 1973.

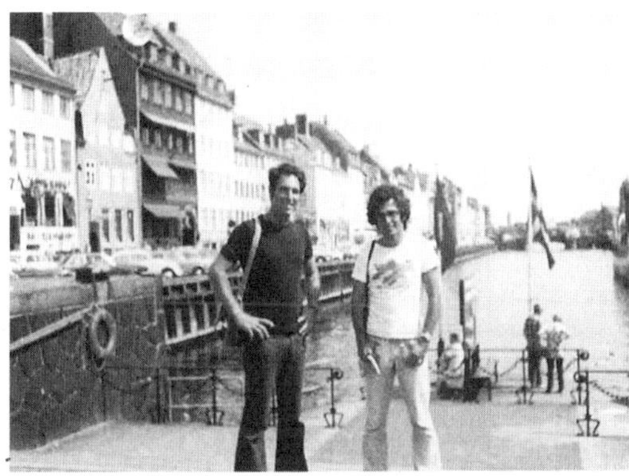

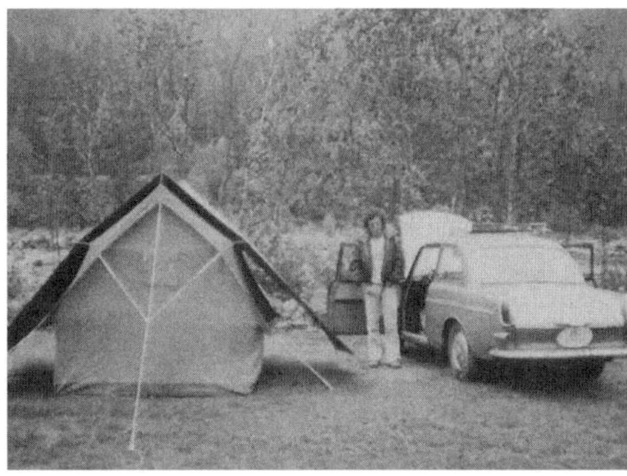

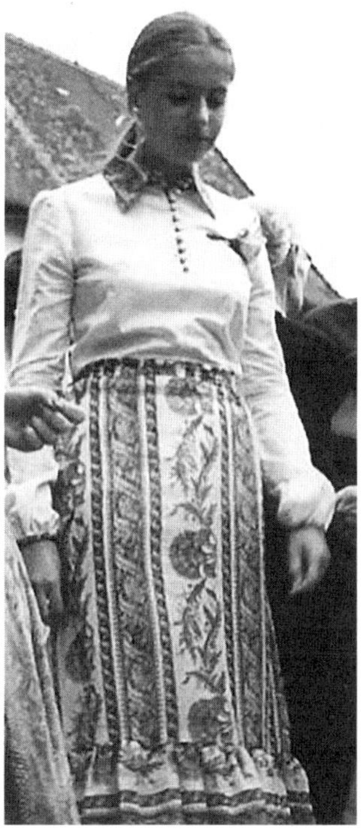

Eight

The Yom Kippur War

Haifa, October 6, 1973, Yom Kippur, the Day of Atonement. My mother wakes me up, "A call for you. It's Amikam, from the kibbutz." I look at the clock. Shit, so early. Just an hour ago, I went to bed after a night shift as a nursing aid, wiping shit off geriatric patients' asses in my father's hospital.

"Hell, Amikam, why so early on Yom Kippur, you atheist *kibbutznik*? Why don't you pray and fast instead?"

Amikam is not amused. "Listen, Schein, what's happening? Were you called up?"

"Called up? Where? Are you crazy? It's Yom Kippur. Let me sleep."

"I mean… called up to the Army, to *miluim*, the reserves. The entire kibbutz was summoned half an hour ago, me too; there are rumors that there'll be a war, or perhaps there's a war already."

"Look Amikam. I know nothing about it. Besides, I don't have an assigned reserve unit. I was studying in Italy, remember? Luckily, I don't have to participate in any silly reserve maneuvers."

"OK. We'll be in touch. I have to rush now." Amikam hangs up.

I go out to the balcony. From here, high on the slopes of Mount Carmel, Haifa's Bay seems relaxed under the morning's gentle autumn sun. It is a clear day. One can see the mountains of Galilee, with Mount Hermon watching from behind and above; to the north are the white cliffs of Rosh Hanikra — the 'Israeli Dover' — marking the Lebanese border; and far to the east, buried in a haze, are the trans-Jordanian heights. The downtown below is silent like a graveyard. It is always so on Yom Kippur, when the traffic and all urbane activities come to a complete standstill.

It is so quiet that I can hear the distant hum of the powerful missile boats returning to the port after a night patrol, leaving a foamy trail behind in the calm, blue sea. A taxi whines past in the street above our house. *A taxi on Yom Kippur?*

I stretch and wipe my eyes. What war? What nonsense? I look down toward the left corner of the port, where the navy boats are stationed. Nothing, no activity even there. Another taxi drives by. A bunch of neighbors in dark clothes, tennis shoes, *yarmulkes,* and prayer books in their hands shuffle toward the synagogue to resume their Yom Kippur prayers. I go to the kitchen, turn on the electric kettle and insert a slice of bread into the toaster. When was the last time that I fasted on Yom Kippur? I turn on the radio; nothing. On Yom Kippur, all Israeli radio stations are silent. I shift the dial to the BBC:

> "From the BBC World Service, London, the news at Seven Greenwich Mean Time. There are reports about an Egyptian and Syrian troop buildup on Israeli ceasefire lines on the Suez Canal and Golan Heights. Our correspondent in Tel Aviv reports about Israeli mobilization of reserves…"

The phone rings. It is my father calling from a hospital near Tel Aviv. A week ago, he developed a spontaneous pneumothorax and wanted to be treated there by his friend, a thoracic surgeon. "Son, they are evacuating all civilians from this hospital, making it 'military only.' It seems like a war is gathering, come and take me back to Haifa. Yes, I'm OK, and my chest tube is out. I've called my hospital already; they'll send Dr. Aginski with you, yes, just in case… please hurry up."

* * * * *

A few hours later, my father is already waiting at the Tel Hashomer Hospital — meticulously dressed, a suitcase in one hand, a cigarette in the other.

We immediately turn around towards Haifa. My father rides in the front passenger seat, Dr. Aginski — one of my father's assistants in the Department of Orthopedics — in the back. Now the coastal highway, deserted two hours earlier, is filling up with military and private cars — men rushing from synagogues to their military reserve units. I drive fast. We pass Hadera approaching Zichron Yaakov, 33km to go, and then suddenly: "I can't breathe," says my father, pointing with his right hand to his left thorax. The burning stub of his non-filter Kent is pinched between his fingers.

"I think it's the pneumothorax again," my father says.

I press the accelerator's pedal down to the floor, and my father's new Oldsmobile, Omega, 1973, groans and vibrates. The speedometer touches its ceiling; looking at how fast the road moves under us, I know we are traveling at least 160kph. This stretch of the coastal highway, at Haifa's northern outskirts, is as wide as an airstrip — it was built to serve as an emergency airstrip if and when military airports were destroyed. On this sunny October day, with the calm Mediterranean Sea on the left, the citrus and banana orchards, and the green hills of Mount Carmel on the right, it seems as if the Oldsmobile will soon take off and fly.

I see my father's gray face and sweat on his forehead. I know that this car cannot go faster. We are nearing Haifa. Deserted beaches appear and vanish on our left as if filmed from a helicopter. I overtake a northbound military convoy. In the mirror, I see Dr. Aginski glued to his seat, holding onto the seat belt straps, terrified by the speed and the car's maneuvers. He has a surgical kit, including a chest tube with which he could treat my father's redeveloping pneumothorax.

But he didn't. Now, more than fifty years later, I can guess – I could not then – what went through Aginski's mind during these minutes. He was probably thinking: should we stop and insert the chest tube at the roadside now? Or should we continue? In another fifteen minutes, we'll be in the hospital; will he survive until then? How long does it take to die with a tension pneumothorax? The last thing I need is to have my hospital director dying on me during the procedure…

My father was gasping and turning blue. We entered Haifa and started climbing the curving streets of the Carmel, leading to the hospital. We rushed him to the OR where the Chief of Surgery inserted a chest tube and immediately departed to join his military surgical team. I found my father in the recovery room, loudly groaning from pain: "It's so sore, I can't take it." He desperately squeezed my hand. My father never, never complained about anything, and now, his suffering felt like a knife striking my chest.

"He's just had a suppository for pain," said the recovery room nurse, listening to the radio at her desk. But my father pointed to his rectum: "It's not in… it fell out." I uncovered him, located the lost suppository, and with my index finger pushed it deeper into my father's rectum. "Deeper, deeper," he instructed me. This was the first time in my life that I had done such a thing, and to do it to one's father was traumatic.

His pain increased, and so did his suffering. I approached a young surgeon who entered the room: "He's in pain, help him, give him something, and do it now," I screamed.

"He has severe COPD, bad lung disease. I can't give him morphine. He'll stop breathing," the surgeon explained indifferently, as if lecturing medical students. I became violent and dragged him to my father's bed: "Just give him something to stop the pain or…"

That scenario, my father suffering, and the indifference of medical personnel, froze in my head. It comes up whenever I see patients' sufferings and their families in distress.

We wheeled my father to a room overlooking the sea. A red sun was descending rapidly into the Mediterranean. From the nurses' station, we heard a radio broadcasting a message from Prime Minister Golda Meir:

> "Citizens of Israel, shortly before 2 p.m. today, the armies of Egypt and Syria opened an offensive against Israel, launching a series of air, armored and artillery attacks in Sinai and on the Golan Heights. The Israel Defense Forces have entered the fight. They are beating back the

assault… our enemies had hoped to surprise the citizens of Israel on the Day of Atonement when so many of our people are fasting and worshipping in the synagogues. The aggressors thought that we would not be ready to fight back on this day. We were not caught by surprise…"

What now? I ran to our house just down the road from the hospital and called the office's contact number for reservists who study abroad. A male voice replied: "Just stay where you are and don't nag us with calls. We are busy enough. Wait for us to call you."

Oh sure, they'll call me when the Syrians start entering Haifa. A good car on empty roads could cover the distance from the Golan Heights to Haifa in one hour. I changed into my old infantry garb: shirt, trousers, and high boots. I packed my khaki canvas rucksack: shaving kit, toothbrush, soap, small towel, three pairs of underwear and socks, two books, a pipe, a pouch of Amphora Red, and a civilian pullover — nights may be cold up there in the north. What else? I grabbed a 50dL bottle of Johnnie Walker Red from my father's bar. Now, I thought, I am ready to go to war.

Back to the hospital. My father was sleeping, with my mother at his bedside. She looked up at me and understood immediately: "Where are you going? You don't have a unit, and what about him?" She pointed at my father snoring under an oxygen mask.

"He's fine for now, and I must go, and you know I can't just wait. I'll go north and look for Yossi's unit. Mama, you know that I must go."

She hugged me. "Be careful." I kissed my sleeping father and left. They had their own past wars, which had been much crueler than ours, and they had lost all their dear ones and could not afford to lose more. But I didn't think about that then. How rarely do we understand and consider our parents' feelings.

* * * * *

"Haifa at night" postcards show this beautiful mountain-coastal town with a panorama of lights. But that night, a total blackout was enforced on the entire country — Haifa was pitch-black. I raised my hand, and a car stopped: "Where can I take you soldier?" I hitchhiked in the eerie darkness northbound towards Akko, the ancient Crusaders' seaport town. Here, the junction of the roads leading to the Upper Galilee and the Golan Heights bustled with frantic activity. I saw three buses parked at the roadside, loaded with soldiers; the roofs were overloaded with bazookas and ammunition boxes. Beside the front bus, I recognized the dwarfish Erwin, previously my company commander in the Golani Brigade, now a major and a deputy battalion commander, shouting something into his radio. I approached him: "Hey, Erwin, would you take me with you?" He recognized me in the darkness: "We are packed like sardines, sorry, find yourself another *tramp* (ride)." He climbed into the bus. They drove away; many of these young Golani kids would never return. A few weeks later, the deceptively lackluster and uncharismatic Erwin would have to take over the command of his battalion and become one of the heroes of that war.

Another *Egged* bus stopped at the junction. We — there were many like me 'searching' for the war — rushed to climb on. I sat near an older guy. When he lit a cigarette, I saw a yellow mustache and a blue working shirt; he smelled of cow manure. The bus started the ascent towards Tzefat in the Upper Galilee.

"Guys, anyone here from Yossi Schein's armored reconnaissance battalion?" I uttered into the silent dimness of the bus.

"Oh, I'm with Yossi," whispered the farmer at my side, "we were almost killed at Jenin's junction in '67, and now we're going to eat shit again. I'm Micha, and who are you?" Of course, he did not use the term *shit* but the local equivalent *chara,* which sounds juicier.

"I'm Yossi's cousin."

"OK. Our gathering point is in the Pilon Camp, near Rosh Pinna. Just stick with me."

A cool wind blew from the direction of the Sea of Galilee when the bus dropped us off near the camp. From the road, we took the same climbing shortcut through the rocks that I remembered when my Golani Battalion had been stationed here. The eastern sky lit up intermittently, and a coarse rumble came from afar, like a series of thunder claps. From where we were, in a straight line, the Golan Heights was less than fifteen miles away. *Hell, are the Syrians so near?*

The camp was pitch dark. The headquarters were illuminated with oil torches, people rushing in and out, and phones ringing. In one of the rooms, I located Yossi, the reconnaissance battalion commander, who had arrived from his kibbutz just an hour before us. Next door, men were busy cleaning the personal weapons they had just been issued. The familiar smell of rifle cleaning mixture (oil and high-octane gas) reached my nose, and suddenly the past two years in Italy seemed to have never existed, and I was back home.

"*Shalom* Yossi," I said as I approached my beloved cousin. Years ago, I, the small boy who arrived from Poland, had adopted Yossi as my much older Israeli brother. He complied. Yossi, a farmer, a decorated hero who had fought in all wars — a salt of the earth character — had taught me to swim and to drive a tractor. He babysat me during long summers in his kibbutz. He had become my role model. However, I never managed to emulate his charming personality and ability to lead others by inner strength and personal example. I had never observed Yossi raising his voice, losing his temper, getting angry, or using anything but calm and pleasant language sprinkled with humor — always a smile on his face. His soldiers adored him. They were ready to follow him to hell. I remember one of them commenting to his buddies: "Yossi is *katan*, but his *katan* is huge." In Hebrew, *katan* means 'small' or 'short' but is often used as a synonym for penis. Obviously, in army jargon, a large penis reflects the machoism-heroism of its owner. Anyway, in Hebrew, it all sounds better…

Now Yossi — handsome, short, slim, athletic, and sunburned, with always laughing eyes — recognized me coming towards him in the dark room.

"Hey, what are you doing here? Aren't you supposed to be studying in Italy?" Others would add "what the fuck" to the "are you doing here," but not Yossi.

"Oh, I returned home a few weeks ago."

"How's Karl? I heard he was in the hospital?"

"Aba is OK. I just drove him back to Haifa. I don't have a unit, so I came looking for you."

Looking at his eyes, I noticed that he was not happy. I could read his mind: why did you come? I have enough on my plate, we are going to war, and now I'll have to ensure you'll return home alive. He forced a smile and shook my hand warmly: "We are to join the Division in the morning and move across the Jordan River. Not all our Zeldas arrived (a Zelda was what Israelis called the USA-made M-109 armored personal carrier). We'll have to squeeze in. Why don't you join Uri's company?" He pointed at a tall guy with captain ranks on his shoulders, "Uri, give this kid a ride on your Zelda, will you? He may think he's a doctor but he has many years to go. I hope he didn't forget his soldiering."

In the next room, an old officer registered me formally: Address? Blood group? Next of kin? Now I was entitled to be buried in a military cemetery. Next, I was issued with an Uzi (a submachine gun), a flak vest, ammunition, and a helmet. A field gas stove was burning in the yard where the cook served black coffee in metal mugs. Loaves of bread, margarine, and a container of jam were placed on a nearby table for everyone to help himself. After 'dinner,' I joined the crew of my Zelda; most of them were at least fifteen years older than me. We greased the vehicle's wheels, tightened its chains, installed the machine guns, and loaded boxes of ammunition, water Jerry cans, food rations, and personal belongings. Then we collapsed, exhausted, on the ground around our Zelda. The sky started to light up from the east, the side from which the thunder of war continued to sound throughout the night. I buried my face into the familiar granular and rocky earth, inhaling the exquisite fragrances of dry shrubs and herbs into my nostrils, and slept. Thirty minutes later, Yossi appeared and raised his voice — he did not know how to shout: "*Chevre* (guys), wake up and climb on your Zeldas. We'll re-assemble beyond the Jordan crossing. I'll speak to you then."

I laid myself down at the bottom of the grease-stained belly of the Zelda and dozed intermittently as the vehicle rocked like a ship on a stormy sea. Now the radio was tuned to the divisional frequency. We could listen to the conversations between the tank platoons already engaged in the fighting ten miles east of us, where the Golan slopes into the Jordan River.

I looked around my Zelda: everybody was asleep except Uri at the turret and the driver. The battle seemed so far away. Time to sleep. I trusted Yossi to guide and safeguard us.

* * * * *

Mid-November 1973. At the end of the eighteen-day-long Yom Kippur War, Yossi's reconnaissance battalion held a stretch of the ceasefire line at the western outskirts of Damascus. From our positions on the top of Tel Antar — one in a series of extinct thumb-like volcanoes that dot the Golan Heights — we could see on a clear night the lights of jetliners landing at Damascus' international airport. But the clear nights were few, and the Golan Heights welcomed us with its typical late autumn gloominess: endless masses of black and wet granite stones, ancient man-made terraces constructed with a limitless supply of boulders, lonely, stunted oak trees, isolated groups of tall eucalyptuses bending in the wind, and islands of Sabra cactuses — all nestling under low, dark clouds.

During the days, we patrolled the no man's land in our jeeps and Zeldas, exploring the recently conquered Syrian territory: abandoned fortifications and bunkers — this used to be the Syrian rear. We would come across a partially burned, rotting enemy corpse here and there. But what is embedded in my mind is this: deep in a secluded ravine, surrounded by a thicket of cactuses, a seemingly intact Israeli Centurion tank; inside — four rotting boys, their faces blackened and swollen with enormous putrefying blisters. What happened? How did they die? The stench was unbearable. I climbed up the walls of the ravine and vomited my breakfast.

I remember the abandoned Arab villages: little houses with small rooms; oriental carpets, beds, blankets, small iron cast stoves at the center, Arabic coffee pots, small glasses for Turkish coffee, *nargilas*, jars with balls of goats' cheese marinated in olive oil. Depressing. Abandoned cows, sheep, and goats roamed in the empty orchards. Each day we would slaughter one of them for an early evening feast of grilled meat.

At sunset, we would lock the gate of the perimeter. The lucky ones were billeted for the night in bunkers and trenches; others, including myself, spent the night in the belly of a Zelda, taking turns watching at its turret. The nights inside the metal skin of the Zelda were cold. We covered ourselves with as many blankets as we could get and stood to watch with our legs inside a sleeping bag. We drank hot tea and coffee from thermoses

— Russian troops would have warmed themselves with vodka; the British Army would have provided its line soldiers with rum or Scotch, but the Israeli Army of those days was mostly a bunch of teetotalers.

At midnight, before hitting his mattress, Yossi would walk around the perimeter chatting with those on watch. I remember a pitch-black night, rain pouring down incessantly, the fierce wind blowing, and sounds of explosions from far away — probably Syrian commandoes shooting at another perimeter. Suddenly I hear Yossi's voice from behind, "Hey, it's me." He climbs on the Zelda and sits near me at the turret; he puts a gloved hand on my wet poncho: "Listen, they've just radioed from the division command. Your father is not doing well. He's to undergo an operation. Tomorrow, at sunrise, we'll ship you down to Haifa..."

* * * * *

Left: cousin Yossi Schein (late 1950s). Right: winter 1973, with a buddy after the war on Mount Hermon.

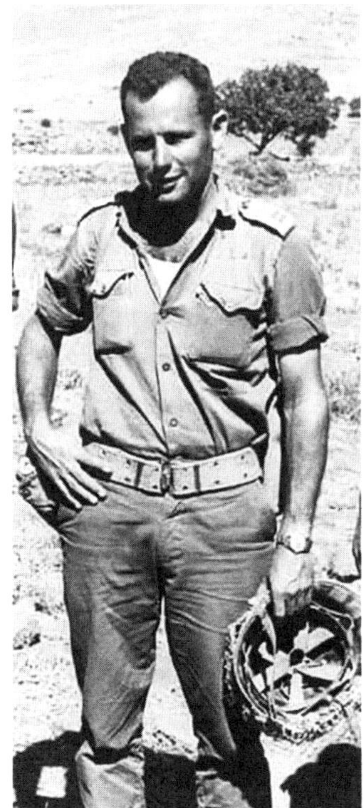

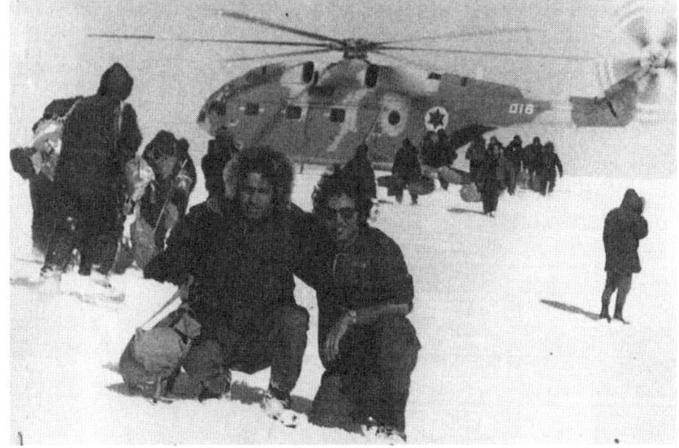

Nine

My father

A few weeks later (January 1974), after we buried my sixty-two-year-old father, I returned to my unit. By then, it had moved to occupy positions on the snowy summit of Mount Hermon.

On the northbound bus, I read a book by the poet Yehuda Amichai. This poem captured my attention:

"Four years my father fought that war of theirs,
And did not love or hate his enemies.
But I know he was forming me, even there,
Day by day, out of his tranquilities…

He gathered with his eyes the nameless dead.
The many dead for my sake unforsaken,
So that I should not die like them in dread,
But love them, seeing them as once he saw.
He filled his eyes with them. He was mistaken.
Like them, I must go out to meet my war."

I will share a digest of my father's story, which I carry like my private Bible. I have known my father for only twenty-three years, but, most probably, no one has influenced me so much — genetically, emotionally, and intellectually — as he did.

My father, Karl, was born in 1911 in Turka, a small town, 135km south-east from Lviv, in the region of Eastern Galicia, which then belonged to Austria until the Poles took over between the two world wars. Today it is a part of Ukraine. When Karl was five years old, his father, a poor charcoal burner, died, leaving a family prone to the hardships that struck the region during the First World War. Then, the young boy started attending the traditional Hebrew "*Cheder*," his only source of education until he was twelve.

During the 1920s, the financial situation of the family improved owing to the success of Karl's elder brother in business in Prague. This change in fortune allowed the teenager to enter a secular Polish high school from which he matriculated at seventeen.

In later years, my father would reflect on the humiliating poverty of those years: "One pair of shoes, a fish on Friday (I was the youngest, so I ended up with its tail…), and chicken (soup) served only on Sabbath." The first automobile appeared in Turka in 1925 and made a great impression on the boy, perhaps explaining why he would find so much pleasure in buying new cars in his later years.

In those days, because of the prevailing anti-Semitism gripping Polish academic institutions, the gates of medical schools were virtually closed to young Jews. Those who aspired to become physicians were forced westward to the universities of Central Europe and Italy. The young Karl chose Prague and, in 1929, entered the German language Charles University. In Prague, like many young Eastern Jews, he was attracted to the ideology of communism, perceiving it as an antidote to the miseries of anti-Semitism and poverty. He became an active member of the Communist Party and was arrested by the secret Czechoslovakian police after addressing a student gathering. In 1935, he received an M.D. degree and was immediately expelled from the country, which was then ruled by the anti-communist Masaryk. Karl returned to Poland and, until 1939, served as a house surgeon at the Jewish Hospital in the Polish town Lwów (Lemberg under the Austrians; today it is Lviv under the Ukrainians).

In 1939, the Germans invaded Poland, dividing it between themselves and Russia. In Lwów, which the Russians occupied, Karl advanced to the position of an assistant surgeon in Lwów's University Hospital. Most probably, his previous communist record saved him from liquidation or deportation to Siberia by the Russian secret police — a common fate awaiting the Polish intelligentsia. In 1941, when Hitler suddenly broke the treaty with Stalin and invaded Russia, Karl was recruited by the retreating Red Army. With the Germans approaching, Karl still managed to visit his hometown Turka and part with his mother, brothers, and sisters. It was their last family reunion. Soon, under German occupation, they, together with all Turka's Jews, would be deported and destroyed.

* * * * *

In 2003, I decided to visit the provinces of my father's youth in Galicia. Turka, two hours' drive south-east of Lviv, proved a tiny town spread out on a few hills at the foot of the Carpathian Mountains. Before the war, its population of eight thousand was half Jewish and half Ukrainian; now, it is only Ukrainian. I found the old cemetery, where generations of Scheins had been buried. The few of the remaining tombstones were unrecognizable. Nicolai Mihailovicz, the local chief surgeon, took me to the home of an old *babushka*. "She may be familiar with our prewar citizens," he suggested.

"Oh sure, the Schein family," the babushka exclaimed, "of course, I knew them. They lived just around the corner in that house," she pointed towards a small brown house. "Many left for Palestine before the war; the others, when the Germans came, were locked in our old factory, kept there until the transport, and then…" She shrugged her shoulders.

I stood under the hot sun, looking at my father's old family house. Almost sixty-three years ago, on a hot summer's day like this, my father came to this place to bid farewell to his mother and sisters before moving eastwards with the Russian Army. What do I feel now? Did I feel like a Palestinian visiting his old father's house in Jaffa, now occupied by Jews? No — not at all. The Palestinian would want his house back, to return 'home,' he would hate those who took away his home and fields — but I was left cold and unemotional. I celebrated the end of my visit in the best and only local restaurant, generously hosted by the local surgeon. The food was outstanding: beetroot-*borscht* soup mixed with fresh cream and savory meat dumplings; tender beef cooked in cream and fresh herbs — delicious. Nicolai Mihailovicz raised his tea glass, filled it to its rim with vodka, and toasted slyly: "To our Jews whom we miss so much!"

I was depressed by Lwów, now Lviv: the aging pianist playing Strauss' Waltzes at the deserted hotel's breakfast room; the old imperial buildings without their original masters; the beautiful Polish churches locked or turned into museums; the Jewish synagogues that became schools. I visited what was once the Jewish Hospital where my father had trained to be a surgeon — now some "institute," the Star of David still engraved on its turret.

After the hot day, Lviv was suddenly sponged down by a massive thunderstorm. In the light of the après rain twilight, the town appeared beautiful but bleak, like a museum. It had lost its soul because it had lost most of its original inhabitants — the Poles had been sent en masse westwards, and almost all of its hundred thousand Jews had been killed on the spot or at the nearby camp Belzec — including those who would have become my uncles, aunts, and cousins.

* * * * *

During the years 1941 to 1943, my father, leading a field hospital, retreated deep into Russia with the badly beaten Red Army. We know little about this period — *why didn't he ever write a memoir?!* — only a few pictures of female nurses/comrades/lovers and anecdotes he told years later remain. The hospital, poorly equipped and 'starved,' as was the rest of the Russian Army, was overwhelmed with wounded combatants. Giant white maggots swarmed in traumatic and postoperative wounds; they were considered beneficial — effectively debriding and cleansing pus and necrotic tissues. The operating tent was the only heated structure; surgeons collapsed and slept on and under the operating tables between operations. Without adequate food, recreational activity among surgeons and supporting staff centered on vodka and smoking. Genuine vodka was, however, scarce. One morning, three miles away from the advancing German tanks, my father found his entire team of drivers 'cold-dead' after consuming anti-freeze fluid mistaken as medical alcohol. Under enemy fire, the hospital retreated in a few vehicles, leaving most equipment behind. As real cigarettes were not available, the surgeons smoked *makhorka*. Years later, my father enjoyed demonstrating how *makhorka* was produced: a large piece of newspaper, or political pamphlet, is rolled into a cone, which is filled with cheap, coarse tobacco.

Heavy *makhorka* smoking undoubtedly initiated the severe chronic obstructive pulmonary disease he suffered later. During these years of lost battles and hopeless retreats, my father developed a compassion for the tragic fate of the Russian people. On occasion, years later, when the whiskey replaced the vodka, he would sing old Russian folk songs — his favorite was the Volga song — to the pleasure of his friends.

An immense volume of surgery on the front had made Karl a dexterous and swift war surgeon. He developed his technique to arrest torrential hemorrhage from gunshot wounds to the subclavian vessels — deep behind the clavicle. After extending the entry wound, he would insert the jaws of a large plaster of Paris 'cutter' around the head of the clavicle, instantly avulsing the sternoclavicular joint and the attached musculature. The exposed artery would then be ligated. During those harsh years, the practice of self-inflicted gunshot wounds to the extremities, mainly hands, was not uncommon among the front troops. Such attempts at self-mutilation to escape battle were punished with death by the military authorities. Each day, communist party military commissars, *politruks*, and army police would inspect the wounded, searching for near-range gunshot injuries to hands and feet. Offenders would be summarily executed. My father learned to identify such wounds at the receiving station: he would immediately amputate the injured part, saving the self-mutilator from a firing squad but risking his own life. Many years later, one of those amputees recognized my father in a Tel Aviv restaurant and fell on his neck.

In 1943, the winds of war started to change direction. My father was transferred to the *Armia Ludowa* — the newly assembled communist Polish Army; he became the Chief Surgeon of its First Army. He advanced westwards with the now victorious troops and, in 1945, entered Berlin with its occupying forces. I have a small snapshot of him from Berlin, sitting on the front stairs of a heavily damaged, charred monument and building. He had a green Soviet-type forage cap, a wide smile, a few medals on his tunic, the permanent cigarette in his right hand. How did he feel, sitting there, on a bright summer day, on the ruins of the Hitler regime that had destroyed his family? I always believed the photograph had been captured in front of the damaged *Reichstag* (the German parliament). However, after a visit to Berlin and studying old prewar albums, it became apparent that my father's picture was taken in front of the Kaiser Wilhelm Memorial, erected in 1897, severely damaged during the Battle for Berlin and destroyed in 1950 by the East German authorities.

In 1948, my father was the first post-war Polish surgeon to be sent to the West by the World Health Organization to "observe capitalistic medicine." Before leaving for the United States, the authorities demanded that he changed his name to a Polish-sounding one. Thus, Schein had become Szaniewicz. Nine years later, in Israel, the original "Schein" returned. During his American tour, my mother and baby sister Sylvia — I was yet to be born — were left behind as 'hostages,' ensuring my father's eventual return from the 'corrupting west.' My father spent one year in the USA, practicing orthopedics under Dr. Leo Meyer in New York, followed by a stint at the Mayo Clinic in Rochester. Karl was impressed with America and its medicine. He learned English rapidly; it became another language he mastered after Polish, German, Russian, Czech, Ukrainian, Latin, Hebrew, and Yiddish. He also became familiar with American culture and brought back with him to Poland a collection of Paul Robeson's records; Robeson was considered politically acceptable by the communist authorities.

On his return to Poland in 1949, my father was posted to the Island of Wolin on the Baltic Sea. Here he directed a 3500-bed 'clandestine' military hospital assembled to receive the communist casualties of the Greek Civil War being fought at that time. The emphasis was on delayed reconstructive surgery of war injuries. The encounter with American medicine was a turning point in the career of the now thirty-seven-year-old surgeon. He ceased being the classic "I do it all" general surgeon of the prewar and war eras and devoted himself to orthopedics. The knowledge gained during WW II and in Wolin was now channeled into a stream of publications and books on trauma and war surgery. In 1951, after I joined the family, my father was nominated to head the Department of Orthopedic and Traumatology at Łódź's University Hospital. He became a Professor of Military Surgery at the local medical school. As his authority regarding war surgery increased in the Eastern Bloc, he was called to advise the North Koreans, then fighting the Korean War, on organizing their frontline medical services. In 1953, he became the Chief Surgeon of the Polish Army. Around that time, Stalin died, and information about the crimes of his hideous regime started to leak. Old friends who had 'disappeared' began returning from the Siberian camps with tales about the fate of friends who did not make it. For my father, this period represented the end of the 'political awakening' process. In 1954, he resigned from the Army and took leadership of the Orthopedic Department in a Warsaw Municipal Hospital.

In 1956, Gomułka, the Secretary of the Polish Communist Party, who had come to power to replace the hitherto Stalinist regime, opened the gates of Poland so that the tiny percentage of Jewish Poles who had survived the Holocaust could emigrate. It was then that we left for Israel. My father would never express a desire to see Poland or Russia again.

My father's first job in Haifa was as an outpatient clinic surgeon, treating minor injuries. He, who was driven in a chauffeured car for years, began commuting to work on a public bus and was frustrated by the lack of operative activity. However, after a year in Israel, he became the Head of Orthopedics at Haifa's Municipal 'Rothschild' Hospital. He rapidly upgraded his almost-forgotten Hebrew; as his charismatic qualities began shining through, he was nominated as the Director of his hospital. In that position, the old traits of the war surgeon came through; my father fought for cost-effectiveness against reckless spending and extravagance. His hospital was the last one to introduce disposable needles and suture material; he continued to use re-sterilized needles, never understanding why others did not enjoy threading the thread through the needle's eye.

My father was not an 'easy' boss. He did not lose the volatile surgeon-like temper of WW II. Twenty-one years after his death, an operating room orderly recalled: "Initially, we were scared of him. When things went wrong, he yelled and cursed at us. He shouted at his doctors too. But when the storm subsided, he shared jokes with us over tea. He even knew the floor sweepers by their name." Another retired OR nurse said: "He established his own OR rules, which would not be acceptable today. During long operations, he would periodically stick his head through the OR doors to puff on a lit cigarette, held by his favorite nurse… only he was allowed to do so."

When my father was fifty-three, he suffered his first myocardial infarction. High blood pressure was diagnosed and treated as "essential hypertension." In 1967, during the long waiting period before the Six-Day War, my father prepared his hospital for war. The stress of those days took its toll, and he was hospitalized for severe exhaustion. In the next war, the War of Attrition, fought between 1968 and 1970 on Israel's four borders, my father was only indirectly involved through me. Because of his poor health, my mother and I tried to alleviate his anxieties. When I used to call him from the bombed trenches on the Suez Canal, I would claim that I was calling from the relatively calm frontline on the Jordan River. But when one day, returning home on leave, I took off my infantry boots, and a hefty dose of Sinai Desert sand spilled on the Persian rug, my father looked at me and smiled: he knew that one did not bring sand from the Jordan Valley. In

1969, when I was evacuated to the rear with mortar shrapnel injuries, he was not satisfied with the initial care of the wound. He demanded a more radical re-excision of devitalized tissues.

My father spent the Yom Kippur War undergoing prolonged tube thoracostomy drainage in a ward congested with combat casualties. A persistent pleural leak failed to seal even after the installation of a pleural irritant. Eventually, an infection (empyema) ensued, and an operation, a thoracotomy, was recommended by Dr. David Adler, an ex-South African thoracic surgeon. A few days before the operation, Dr. Adler invited my mother and I to his villa on Mount Carmel to discuss the operative plan with us. I remember that I — a junior medical student — did not understand much of what he tried to explain. I trusted him. I had seen him, the great Chief of Thoracic Surgery, pushing my father's wheelchair in the hospital corridors to the radiology department, and I knew he was a *mensch*.

On the morning of the operation, on a sunny January 1974 day, my father shaved carefully and applied aftershave lotion to his face; he then hugged and kissed, on both cheeks, Russian manner, all his friends who lined up to wish him farewell, including the surgeon who was going to operate. Next, he hugged and kissed my mother, sister, and I. Then he was wheeled into the operation that he would not survive. Postoperatively, he developed persistent hypotension — the last time I saw him lying with an endotracheal tube sticking out of his mouth, his face unshaven and sunken. He died the following day. An autopsy was performed. Twenty years later, I met in Haifa the thoracic surgeon, now over eighty years old, who had operated on my father. "Didn't you know," he asked, "that the autopsy of your father disclosed a large pheochromocytoma (a hormone-producing tumor of the adrenal gland) which was probably the cause of his hypertension, accelerated atherosclerosis and, finally, the unexplained irreversible postoperative shock?"

And the 'best' physicians in town always looked after him, I thought.

A new clinic building in my father's hospital in Haifa was dedicated to his name. Years later, the memorial plaque was removed during renovations, never to be returned.

Later, even the name of the Rothschild Hospital was changed to honor an American Jewish foundation (Bnei Zion), and the affiliated Aba Khoushy Medical School was renamed after a wealthy Jewish donor (Rappaport).

* * * * *

What kind of person was my father?

He was thirty-nine years old when I was born, and I was twenty-three when I lost him — we did not have enough time to bond and become friends. He was elusive, remote, warm, and loving at the same time. He was moody and volatile, opinionated and a non-conformist — the latter traits, including impatience and arrogance, I probably inherited from him. My father was short but handsome; at social events, the women gathering around him claimed he resembled Humphrey Bogart. He enjoyed the company of women and had a few affairs, to my mother's distress. But what I remember most are his hands: often I look at my own hands, and I see his: smallish, soft, agile — surgeon's hands. I remember the ever-present remains of the plaster of Paris around the base of his nails. He would come silently behind my desk and gently pat my head, as I do now to my sons. I would freeze, anxious that he would notice that I was reading a trashy novel instead of studying for school.

The day before my father went for his last operation, I was notified that the Hadassah Medical School in Jerusalem had accepted me as a second-year student. After the war, they decided to accommodate a small number of 'deserving' students from Italy, those who had fought in the war. I noticed the pride in my father's eyes: finally, the kid made it! The problematic son will study in the best medical school in the Middle East — not in Haifa — he did not have too much respect for his local colleagues. I remember that last encounter at his bedside on the eve of his final operation. He did not speak much — why didn't he leave me with any final message, be it verbal or written, some instructions on how to proceed with my life? He did not leave behind a bunch of letters, a diary, or a memoir: such a waste of an eventful and dramatic life! "Hold my hand, son," he said and kept silent, thinking — thinking about what? And I held his hand that was now weak and emaciated.

And then he left the scene and abandoned me, the one who grew up in his tall shadow, to struggle on my own in his footsteps. I always missed the opportunity to grow up as a surgeon while he aged — to benefit from his advice and guidance. And I miss his hands.

* * * * *

Top: Karl Schein, during WW II, early 1940s. Middle: with Levi Eshkol, Prime Minister of Israel, Haifa, 1965. Bottom: with an 'unknown' English orthopedic surgeon, touring hospitals in the UK, in the summer of 1973. Perhaps this was his last picture.

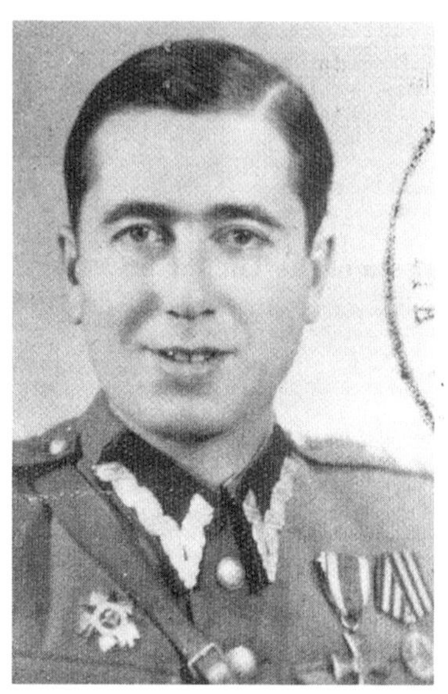

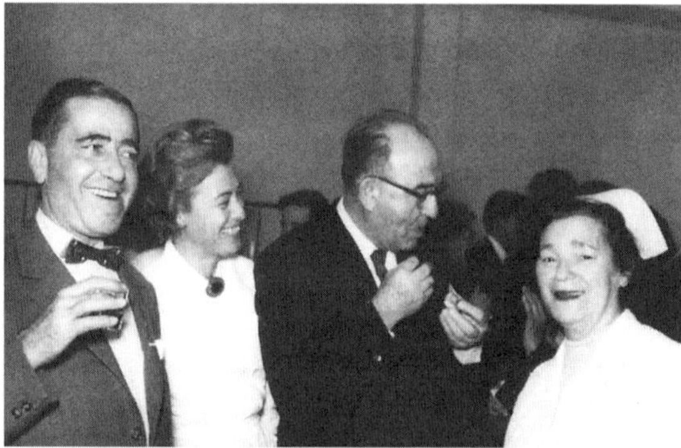

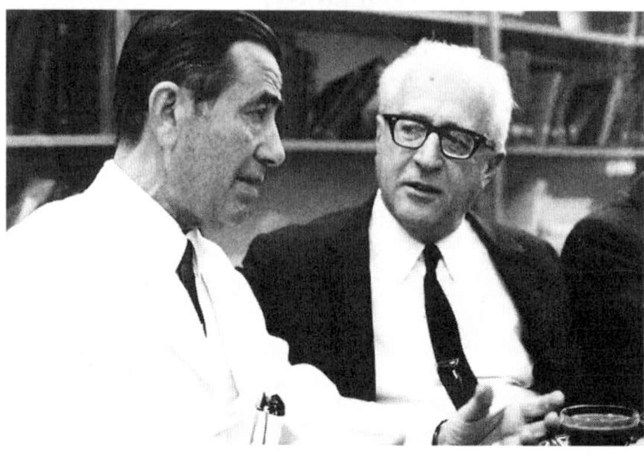

Ten

The medical school in Jerusalem

May 1974. Six months after the end of the Yom Kippur War, our reserve unit was released from active service. I headed to Jerusalem to join the second-year class at the Hadassah Hebrew University Medical School. Since the curriculum in Italy did not correspond to the one in Jerusalem, I had to repeat the second year, which was ending anyway.

I remember arriving in Jerusalem in my new cream-colored Volkswagen Beetle that my mother bought for me after selling my father's Oldsmobile – I could not afford the maintenance of a large American car.

A typical late spring *chamsin* pushed hot air and sand from the Judean Desert as I arrived at the Medical Center at Ein Karem. After registration at the students' office, I climbed the stairs to the dissecting rooms of the anatomy department, where I found the second-year class crowding, in small groups, around multiple cadavers. The smell of corpses preserved in formaldehyde was overwhelming. Having already passed anatomy in Italy, I was released from the anatomy classes. However, in Italy, we had studied anatomy from books – not on cadavers. Now I wanted to just 'dissect a little.'

"Shalom guys, I'm Moshe, a new student. Would you accept me into your dissecting group?" I politely approached three boys and two girls. They were busy poking their gloved hands into the pale-gray, turgid tissues of the formalin-soaked body of what was once a tiny, shriveled female.

"You must be one of the Italian guys, eh? You see, there are already five of us here," said a bespectacled girl, "and anyway, we heard that you Italians don't have to repeat anatomy."

So now I'm an Italian. I tried another group but again, "Look, there is no space around the cadaver, didn't you already study anatomy in Italy?"

The formalin stunk and burned my eyes. I decided that I had had enough of this. A week later, this anatomy class became internationally renowned: a few students bet on who would dare to eat a piece of a cadaver – they really ate it! Only a tiny bit, but this leaked into the local media and then to newspapers abroad, with headlines like: "Medical students in Jerusalem eat a cadaver." The three poor students were expelled. Did they go to Italy?

So, from now on, and during the forthcoming four and a half years, we, the few students admitted from Italy, were known as the "Italians." The other students, many of them young kids entering medical school before active army service (destined to serve as military doctors), could not forgive the fact that we were not admitted to this 'Ivy League' school on merit — like they were — based on academic excellence. Consequently, we 'Italians' formed our small group; we considered ourselves more mature and worldly; after all, we spoke Italian and enjoyed red wine.

During one of the first lectures in microbiology, I bonded with Avi Rubinstein, a smiling, chubby 'Italian,' with a knitted *yarmulke* on his head, who would become my lifelong brother. Later Avi trained as a neurosurgeon, clashed with the 'system,' studied law, and presently is a leading malpractice lawyer in Israel. Together with Avi and Jochanan, who had followed me from Modena, we formed a jolly 'Italian triumvirate.' Life was good to us in Jerusalem, benefiting from years of relative political calm — the first *Intifada* was still to come. As frequently as possible, we would roam the narrow alleys of the Arab bazaar in the Old City, always searching for the perfect hummus. Abu Shukri's old dive was the indisputable mecca of hummus. I remember watching the old Abu Shukri sitting on a low stool, a fez on his head, patiently crushing the cooked chickpeas with a wooden muddler. With our stomachs distended with hummus, we would stop at the nearby Jaffar's *Knafeh* joint to savor a slice of his legendary sweet-cheesy Palestinian delicacy. The afternoon would end with a Turkish coffee and a *nargila* in a little café near Nablus Gate. On weekends, we would often descend from Kiriat Yovel, cross a deep valley, enter the West Bank, and climb the slopes towards Beit Jala and Beit Lechem. Among the rocks and pine trees stands the Cremisan Monastery — famous for its wines. The winemaker, a Sardinian monk, would chat with us excitedly in Italian and let us help ourselves to the superb (and cheap) red wine. With our rucksacks full of bottles, we would retire for a picnic under the fragrant pines, on one of the sun-warmed rocks, and nap until sober.

Most medical students in Jerusalem sustained themselves working as part-time nurse aids in one of the city's hospitals. For a year, usually on weekends, I wiped the buttocks of incontinent patients at the geriatric department of the old Shaare Zedek Hospital. At some point, I realized that I was entitled to a four-year student stipend generously provided by the Defense Ministry to 'military invalids'; so now the Russian-made piece of shrapnel lodged in my ass proved valuable. The pay more than covered the rent for the flat that we shared and changed each year, the car maintenance, food, and drink, and the long magic weekends along the quaint shores of the Red Sea in the Sinai Desert. Tuition was covered separately.

For additional pocket money, we used to donate sperm. This is how it worked: Dr. Danny W. — then a young gynecologist, later a leading international authority on infertility (deceased in 2013) — would page me: "Moshe, come down and give me a dose." I would run down to the gynecology clinic, where the gynecologist handed me a small bottle. I would lock myself in the public toilet in front of the patients' waiting room. No *Playboys*, no *Penthouses*… but at that age, imagination sufficed, and after a minute or two, I would walk through the waiting room — the bottle in my hand, my face hot and sweaty — where the recipients were waiting for my 'dose.'

None of those women recognized that I might be the future father of their offspring. I would hand the bottle to Danny W. and pocket a large banknote. I did it for two years. I wonder how many kids I have in Israel today. They would have to be almost fifty years old now.

* * * * *

But most of the time, I studied, and I did it seriously. I maintained the habits gained in Italy: to read entire textbooks in English rather than the abbreviated, locally produced Hebrew 'lecture notes,' or distilled Hebrew versions of textbooks which often contained horrendous errors. I read each book only once, filling it with footnotes, then moved on. So while rotating through internal medicine, I finished *Harrison's Principles of Internal Medicine*, went over *Lange's Current Medical Diagnosis & Treatment*, learned by heart *The Washington Manual of Medical Therapeutics*, and finally mastered the subspecialty books such as *Hurst's the Heart Manual of Cardiology*. I tried to develop a practical and rational-based approach to common problems.

The first examination we took in Jerusalem was in microbiology. A week later, when the results appeared on the announcements' board, the class was scandalized: Jochanan got the second-highest score of 89% — just behind me at 91%. How could these stupid 'Italians' have received such scores when at least ten of the Israelis had failed? Surely there must have been some foul play. Somebody spread a rumor that Jochanan's mother, a Deputy Dean for Education, fed us with an early copy of the examination questionnaire. Fortunately, the scandal died quickly — we continued to do very well, although we never became too popular in the class.

Looking back through the eyes of one who has since taught many medical students, I recognize the image of the arrogant 'smart ass' which I must have presented to those around me: well-read and knowledgeable but opinionated, argumentative, and challenging — especially to the house staff. Already then, I became medically cynical and rebellious. During the pediatric rotation, I refused to draw the morning blood for the numerous investigations (this was the students' task) which were repeatedly ordered by the house staff. I objected to the unnecessary bloodletting. While rotating in the department led by the god of internal medicine (the almighty Professor Marcel Elyakim), I hung up in the residents' room an aphorism by Sir William Osler: "The greater the ignorance, the greater the dogmatism." This enraged the residents, who tore it down. Thus, I had begun a long career, which my future enemies would define as that of a 'problem maker.'

What was the origin of such defiance, the challenge of established order, attacking 'holy cows,' accompanied with sheer *chutzpah* against superiors, that gradually would permeate my evolving medical personality? Was it a continuation, in different garments, of my disruptive behavior in the elementary school, where teachers had considered me impossible — an 'impaired' child? Was the former pattern a sublimation of a desire of an immigrant kid to be noticed? Was the latter designed as an attempt of revenge against the 'system' — whatever it was or would be: *you thought that I'm a retard — now I will show you!*

* * * * *

I fell in love with surgery in the first week of my first surgical rotation at the end of the fourth year.

The notion that surgery was my destiny was embedded in me early on: my father's stories, his 'shop talk' with his friends, the bloodstains I had noticed on his underwear following a bloody operation — the desire to enter the ranks of this exclusive brotherhood. But would the real stuff appeal to me? I did not know — until 'my' first case on the second night of the rotation.

A young boy underwent an appendectomy for acute appendicitis. I was allowed to scrub in to assist the chief resident Ayalon (later a big shot professor near Tel Aviv), who in turn assisted the junior resident Aner (later a vascular surgeon in Jerusalem). I loved every minute — how skillfully and boldly these fabulous self-assured young men navigated within the abdomen and knew what to do inside.

Two days later, during evening rounds with Dr. Charuzim, the attending surgeon on call, an intern beckoned us to the boy's room: "The post-appendectomy kid has dropped his blood pressure, he's in shock…" We rushed to the kid's room; he was lying anxious, pale, sweating, and groaning with pain.

We looked at Dr. Charuzim: tall, dark, square-faced, arrogant, charismatic — considered by all a 'top knife' and a leading local Don Juan — what will he do now? Dr. Charuzim approached the kid and exposed the distended abdomen; he touched it, and the kid shrieked with pain — *peritoneal signs!* No muscle moved in Dr. Charuzim's stony face when he ordered: "Nurse, bring me a syringe and a size 14 needle!"

Without uttering a word, Dr. Charuzim drove the needle into the kid's abdomen and sucked on the syringe, ignoring the poor boy's laments. Then, like a hunter raising the severed head of a lion, like a fisherman demonstrating a trophy bass, or an Indian showing off the scalp of his enemy — Dr. Charuzim lifted the syringe high up in the air for us to see — it was full of dark blood.

"Take him back to the OR, now… I said now! The kid's bleeding into his abdo." Dr. Charuzim dropped the syringe into the waste bin and left the room without a word.

Lord, how that 'magician' impressed me! No ultrasound, no X-rays, no scans, no blood tests — only surgical judgment and skill. No prolonged meetings, grinding water, but instant decisions about life and death. Now I knew I wanted to be like Dr. Charuzim — a real surgeon and a great one, a lifesaving hero.

Later I would understand that the kid had suffered a banal and preventable complication, a complication I would never encounter again: a poorly placed ligature had slipped off his appendicular artery. Luckily the kid survived. As for the 'magician,' Dr. Charuzim, he became Chief of Surgery at a southern university and a guru of bariatric surgery.

But the surgeon who impressed me most in Jerusalem was the head of the surgical department, Professor Nathan J. Saltz, considered the father of modern Israeli surgery. I first saw him during the weekly departmental morbidity and mortality meeting: a bespectacled, medium size, older man (he was in his early sixties then), chairing the stormy meeting with great authority. Surprisingly, the meeting was conducted in English — with his New York-accented English; all others struggled with their Hebrew-accented English. I observed a hearing aid protruding from the professor's ear; he would cup his ear when listening.

Later I was told that he had served four years as a US Army battalion surgeon during World War II in North Africa and northern Italy; apparently, he had lost his hearing during combat. The professor would listen to the presentations, ask relevant questions, and prompt a lively debate. Finally, he would pronounce the judgment — like a supreme court judge. The orderly academic discussion, the discipline, it was so unlike what I was used to seeing in Israel — where everyone spoke over each other. I was impressed.

Each Tuesday of our rotation, Nathan Saltz would take our group of students (there were six of us) for an hour-long teaching session. Those few hours were the best teaching I ever had. I remember this: we sit in a small room, Saltz asks, "Who wants to present a case?" I volunteer a case of acute appendicitis. Saltz repeatedly interrupts me with "Why? Why the pain? What is the mechanism of the pain? Why the tenderness? What is the mechanism? Why did the appendicitis develop? Why does the appendix perforate? Why? Why? Why?" He spoke little; he wanted me to come up with all the answers. If I could not, he would ask the others. At the end of the hour, we knew more about acute appendicitis than the textbook could teach us. He forced us to think rather than listen. It was perfect.

Two years later, I returned to Saltz's department, now as an intern. During a night call, I argued with one of the surgical residents. He commanded me to do something (I do not remember what it was); I thought his decision was nonsense and told him "Fuck off, do it yourself." Next morning, I was summoned to see the boss. I knocked on the door and entered Saltz's spacious office; he was sitting behind the desk. He did not ask me to sit down. He conducted the procedure as if this were a military field tribunal, in English of course.

"So, Dr. Schein, did you tell my resident to fuck off?"

"Yes Sir, I did." I started giving him the story. He raised his hand and stopped me. "Listen my young friend," Saltz said, "during your future career, you will meet many people who are not as smart as you, who actually are much stupider than you. You will have to learn how to deal with them. And now go back to work." I noticed a faint smile on his face, perhaps a tiny wink.

Professor Nathan Saltz died in Jerusalem in 2003. He was ninety-one years old.

* * * * *

During the summer of 1977, between the fifth and sixth year of medical school, I took two elective surgical rotations overseas: one in cardiothoracic surgery, in the Montefiore Medical Center in the Bronx, New York, to be followed by general surgery at the Kantonsspital Winterthur in Switzerland.

It was to be my first visit to the USA. My American cousin Harold Bernanke helped arrange the cardiothoracic rotation in his hospital. He was an internist-cardiologist, admitting patients to the Montefiore Hospital, hence on friendly terms with the heart surgeons. Heidi's father (Heidi was now my 'official' girlfriend) offered to sponsor my flight, and I predicted that Harold would contribute towards my survival in New York City.

I took a cheap charter flight from Zurich to JFK. Unexpectedly, it had to stop over for a few hours in Newfoundland for refueling. This screwed up my internal time clock, so when we landed in New York I was completely disorientated. I took a cab to the northern Bronx, draining my limited cash reserves of perhaps 250 US dollars. It was dark, and the streets were empty when the black cabbie dropped me off at the main entrance of the huge, sprawling medical center. I schlepped an immense-bulging suitcase — during those days, suitcases had no wheels. I entered the building and started to roam the long, gray, vacant corridors. I was looking for someone to ask the way to the hospital's administration offices. I finally located a black security man but could hardly understand what he was saying. It would take me a few weeks to comprehend spoken American English. At last, I collapsed on a wooden bench outside the locked doors of the admin offices. I saw a fat black lady sweeping the corridor. She told me: "Man, what are you doin' here, it's 5 a.m., it's Saturday…"

But luckily, someone opened the office at 9 a.m., and I got a key to a hospital dorm room and coupons for the hospital cafeteria. I dragged myself to the dormitories through the endless passages and tunnels, each color-coded and named after some donors, and dropped off my things in the large but old-fashioned room — it must have been one of the hospital call rooms. I walked back to search for the hospital's cafeteria. I placed myself on a high stool at the counter. A huge black man dressed all in white placed a coffee mug in front of me. He looked at me with a question mark.

"A bagel and two eggs, please," I said.

"Howd'yawanit Sir?" the giant asked.

Hah. It was beyond me. The giant repeated himself a few times, each time slower, as if talking to a retard.

At last, a young black man in a white gown who sat on my right intervened: "Sir, he wants to know how you want your egg, sunny side up, whatever…"

It was beyond me as well: all I knew was a hardboiled egg, or fried egg, or scrambled. "Fried both sides," I said, and the young man translated to the giant. The bagel was superb. The coffee was weak. I looked around: *this is the USA, like in the movies*.

On Monday, I was introduced to the cardiothoracic team. It consisted of three full-time attending surgeons, two fellows working day and night, and two physician assistants. Most of the time I spent in the operating room — assisting the surgeons; the cases consisted of coronary artery bypasses, lung cancers, or artificial cardiac valves.

The fellows performed the operations under the supervision of the attending surgeons. I was the second assistant. The head of the department ignored me most of the time, but his deputy, Dr. Lari Attai, who had originated from Tehran, was very kind. He would explain things to me during the operation and let me suture the vein-harvesting incisions in the leg. Occasionally he would leave early and tell the fellow, "Teach Moshe how to close the chest." It made me very happy.

I made the point to learn about pre and postoperative care, especially fluids and electrolyte balance. To do so, I started to shadow one of the physician assistants day and night. His name was Doug Condit; I guess he was a few years older than me — a white guy from rural Colorado, who had served as a corpsman with the Marines in Vietnam. Doug 'adopted' me. Not only did he allow me to follow him throughout his busy working days, tolerating my nagging questions, but on some weekends, he would drive me around in his Nissan sports car to the seashores of Long Island. We would nap for hours on the hot sand, sipping beer. I felt some sadness in him, but did not inquire. I do not think there was any woman in his life then.

The cardiothoracic section had a vibrant social life. Over the six weeks I spent with them, there were many dinners at restaurants or the attending surgeons' houses to which I was invited. I was impressed with Dr. Attai's house in Westchester — it was a mansion. Even the doorknobs were lined with gold. I understood that American surgeons were very rich… at least a few.

A sweltering heatwave engulfed New York City that summer. On July 13, lightning struck, leading to a massive blackout that plunged the city into darkness. Looting and arson broke out, a thousand fires were reported, and thousands of stores were damaged or ransacked. The city was depressed and violent, and its streets were considered unsafe. I was warned to avoid the subways at night and on weekends. However, on Friday evenings, I would leave the Bronx, taking the shabby and desolate subway to Manhattan, to spend the weekend with my cousin Harold. He lived in an upscale apartment block — uniformed door and elevator attendants, a new Volvo in the basement garage — on the eastside, 88th York Avenue. Harold was then around fifty years old: medium built, dark hair, a little Clarke Gable-like pencil mustache. People commented that Harold looked like an Italian movie star.

He was well dressed — in his closets, I saw a vast collection of expensive suits and fancy shirts. Harold liked women. I remember riding the elevator with him: a beautiful young woman entered and stood near Harold. I cannot forget how he virtually sniffed-inhaled her — greedily taking in her perfume and whatever it represented into his lungs. He never married, exchanging partners, some for a long term, others for a short term, a few repeatedly. His single-bedroom apartment was sophistically furnished and decorated but a little neglected. The kitchen was essentially unused, and a high pile of old dusty medical journals covered the dining room table. I slept on the couch in the living room. On Sundays, Harold would linger in his bed with the Sunday *New York Times*, later dumping the pile of paper on my couch to read. It was then that I became addicted to this newspaper. He would hand me a bill of 100 bucks and say: "Go get yourself some bagels and coffee, my kitchen is empty." He would take me out occasionally for a quick dinner. Afterwards, he would go, I suspected, to one of his girlfriends. "Sorry Moshe," he would say, "I can't provide you with a woman. Just go and have some fun." I would receive from him another bill and wander the long streets of Manhattan until midnight. At the end of the rotation, I flew back to Switzerland. Who would guess that sixteen years later, I would return to live and work in the USA.

Harold passed away in 2017 at the age of eighty-eight.

Six months before his death, we visited him in his old apartment on York Avenue. He had been suffering repeated mini strokes and developed dementia. The full-time nurse who was now living with him opened the door. We found Harold sitting on 'my' old couch, clean, well dressed but shriveled. The remnants of the same old smile, the leftovers of the same sardonic sense of humor were still there, but he spoke gibberish. He doesn't recognize us, I thought. I strolled around the apartment. Everything looked the same as precisely forty years ago. We stood up to leave. I shook Harold's hand; Heidi hugged and kissed him. Exiting the door, we heard his weak voice, "Heidi, come here." She did, and then he asked, "Where is Moshe?" He recognized her but not me. In his will, he left a generous sum of money specifically to Heidi — not to me. He loved women!

* * * * *

In Switzerland, I immediately started with the general surgery rotation in the Kantonsspital Winterthur Hospital. I was allocated a room in the elegant nurses' dormitories, but I rarely stayed there. I preferred to lodge in Heidi's parents' house in Schaffhausen, which was only forty minutes away by train. I found the large surgical department organized according to the classical Germanic structure — running according to a rigid Teutonic chain of command and discipline. I received a printed nametag on my white coat. It said, *Unterassistent* (under assistant) *Schein*.

The assistants were the residents, so we students were the *unter*... The title of a qualified surgeon was *Oberarzt*; those higher up were called *Leitender Arzt*; at the top of the pyramid was the almighty leader — the *Chefarzt*. I was somehow disturbed by the sound bites of *unter* and *ober* that reminded me of the SS ranks of *Untersturmführer* and *Obersturmführer*.

We, the *unter* assistants, were required to clerk new patients admitted for surgery or presenting in the emergency room. One had to take a complete history, perform a physical examination, and document everything in writing. It being Switzerland, the documentation had to be neat, so handwriting was not allowed — it had to be immediately typed on dedicated hospital paper.

Heavy black typewriters were available throughout the hospital. The problem was that my German language skills were rudimentary, and I never learned German formally. Whatever I knew were the bits and pieces passively embedded in my brain, listening to my parents who would chatter in German when the topic was not suitable for the kids. That dormant language came to life after I met Heidi and started visiting Switzerland. However, my grammar usage was appalling and my experience with the written language was non-existent — I wrote German phonetically as if I were writing English. The fact that most patients used the Swiss-German dialect did not add to the clarity of the final product. I suspect that the doctors and nurses who read the documents produced by me had a good laugh.

Each morning, when I arrived to the operating room, I would consult the large blackboard on the wall for the schedule of planned operations. On one of the days, the first operation was listed as *Revision anus praeter*.

Anus praeter. What is that? I had never heard that term. I entered the almost vacant staff room. I saw the *Chefarzt* sitting in the corner, drinking coffee, a newspaper in his hand. I had been introduced to him briefly on my first day but had yet to have the chance to interact with him. I approached him, "*Guten morgen*." He looked at me over his glasses and nodded his head. "Can I ask you a question," I continued with my broken German, "What does *anus praeter* mean?"

The *Chefarzt* threw the newspaper on the table, his face reddening, "What? You don't know what *anus praeter* stands for. How is it possible?"

"Sorry, but I don't know what that term means… I just saw it on the blackboard, listed as your first operation… I would like to assist you, if possible…"

"But this is an international term. It is Latin, for God's sake, Latin. How could you not know it?" Now the head surgeon was screaming at me.

"In our medical school all such terms are taught in English, English books, you know, no Latin."

But for the *Chefarzt* the conversation was over. He stood up, picked up his reading glasses from the table, and left the room. I think I heard him muttering to himself, *Dummkopf*, idiot.

What's wrong with him? I was thinking. Perhaps a lowly student should avoid approaching the big boss directly? Was I too casual, not calling him *Herr Chefarzt*? The culture here is different, I thought, unlike the one I had been used to in Israel and just recently experienced in New York.

After the *Chefarzt* left the room, a young surgeon who must have been sitting in the other corner commented with a smile: "The boss can be a little grumpy in the morning. And by the way, *anus praetus* means — a colostomy. The boss is going to reverse a colostomy this morning. Revision *anus praetus*. Now you know."

Another operation that I remember involved the repair of an abdominal aortic aneurysm. In Europe, in those days, vascular surgery was performed by general surgeons. The operating surgeon was the deputy *Chefarzt*, Dr. Marti. He was a short, dark, taciturn man in his fifties. I was told that he was a Colonel in the Swiss Army. The first assistant was a senior *Oberarzt*, the second was an *Assistent*. Luckily, they let me, the lowly *Unterassistent*, to scrub in. The procedure progressed smoothly. Marti operated like a Swiss watch. Hardly a word was spoken, that is until I asked a question. I do not recall what I asked, only that it was directed to Dr. Marti. He stopped operating. He dropped the instrument from his hand and hissed at the senior *Oberarzt, wa hett er gseit?* (what did he say, in Swiss German). The *Oberarzt* repeated my question. Marti replied, murmuring something under his mask. The senior *Oberarzt* then addressed the *Assistent*, also in Swiss German: *saeged Sie im, er soell waered de Operation d'Schnoerre halte*. The *Assistent* turned to me and conveyed in 'high German' the message, meaning: "Tell him to keep his mouth shut during the operation." I already understood Swiss German and 'high German.' Now I was taught the meaning of Germanic hierarchy.

But the operation which was the most deeply embedded in my mind was a routine, elective right hemicolectomy — resection of the right side of the colon for a cancerous lesion. It was 'routine,' but how wonderful. The operating surgeon was a senior *Oberarzt*. Shamefully I forgot his name. He must have been in his early 60s, a tall corpulent German. I never heard him talking Swiss German, only 'high German' with a Bavarian accent. He used to limp badly, hobbling on an above-knee prosthesis. It has been rumored that he had lost his leg on the Eastern Front during WW II.

The operation proceeded as a video clip played fast forward. "*Messer*," he shouted, and the knife landed in his hand within a second. Ten seconds later, the abdomen was wide open — a single slice through the skin, fat, fascia, and peritoneum — like a virtuoso butcher working on a slaughtered pig. I saw his hands moving rapidly, exploring the abdomen, eviscerating the intestines, packing it away. He lifted the right colon with his left hand and started dividing the mesentery with the right. "*Los, los, los*," ("come on"), he shouted at the scrub nurse while the artery clamps were flying from her to his right hand, which clamped and divided the mesentery in a piecemeal fashion. *Plop*. The resected colon landed in the metal dish a few minutes later. "*Ligatur*," he screamed, and a roll of thread landed in his hand to tie the divided vessels. "*Anastomose*," he declared; he sutured the edges of the divided colon, in two layers. Like a Singer electric sewing machine, I thought. "*Faden… Bauch schliessen*" (thread, abdominal closure) — with a heavy thread threaded through the eye of a giant needle, the fat Bavarian closed the abdomen. Now, with the last knot being tied, he barked at the first assistant: "*Hautnähen*!" (meaning skin — stitch the skin). He turned around, dropped the bloody gloves, accepted a towel from the scrub nurse to dry his sweaty face, and left the room. I looked at the clock on the wall: twenty minutes skin to skin. All that time, no word had been spoken except the *los* and *schnell* and the huffing and puffing of the corpulent surgeon. This is how he did it on the Russian-German front, I told myself. *Los, schnell* — the Ruskies are coming. This is probably how my late father used to operate. Since that day, I have never observed such a virtuoso-like surgical performance. Now, I think, go and compare this with our new generation of 'modern' surgeons playing with their robot for long hours, as if time doesn't matter…

For some reason, the gruff old German was quite friendly to me. He was the only member of the senior staff who engaged me in personal conversation. "We have to have you for dinner…" he mentioned a few times. It never materialized. Yesterday (while working on this paragraph) I contacted a friend who currently works in the Winterthur surgical department, asking him to find out the name of the old, limping German surgeon who had worked there some forty-three years ago. "No one has heard about such an individual" was the reply.

I was not surprised. It reminded me of an aphorism: "Every surgeon should have a pet dog. When he retires from the hospital, he should leave his dog on the floor of the department he served because when he returns, the only one who will recognize him will be his dog." I will never forget that maestro.

By the end of the first month in Winterthur, I heard that the surgical ICU was short of nurses. I decided to offer my services. I introduced myself to the head nurse as a fifth-year medical student with extensive experience of moonlighting as a nurse. "*Ya ya*," she said, "can you start tomorrow evening, the night shift?"

The night shift started at 11 o'clock and lasted eight hours. I was allocated two critically ill patients. My job was to measure their vital signs, administer medications, suck out their endotracheal tubes, and change their positions. A cycle of the above procedures was required each hour. By the end of the hour, I had to start again. Not a second was left to look around and chat to one of the cute blonde nurses. The shift-leader nurse — blonde but not so cute — was watching like a hawk behind my back.

I must have performed reasonably because they continued scheduling me for 2-3 night shifts each week. More than a month later, one night, I was allocated an intubated postoperative patient. I do not recall what operation he had had, only that there was a drain coming from his chest — constantly draining large amounts of blood. I shared my concern with the shift leader. "Please call the doctor," I suggested.

She shrugged her shoulders and ignored me. An hour later, I emptied another half-liter of blood from the collecting container. "He's bleeding, call the doctor…," I pleaded. "It's 5 o'clock, the doctors will be rounding soon…" I left the patient, walked across the corridor, and dragged the sleepy ICU doctor on call out of bed. He was an anesthetist who spoke with a heavy Persian accent.

I do not remember what he did and how this case turned out, only that the next day the head nurse approached me and said that what I did was unacceptable. I broke the chain of command, "Only the shift leader can decide to summon the doctor on call." My career as a Swiss ICU nurse was terminated. But my clerkship was ending anyway, and by then, I had earned a few thousand Swiss Francs.

Never had I had so much money in my pockets.

At the end of the summer, I returned to Jerusalem. I knew I did not want to become a cardiac surgeon, sewing coronary arteries all day. And I had developed an aversion to Germanic-type medicine.

There was no doubt in my mind: I would be a general surgeon but first I had to finish medical school.

* * * * *

With Avi Rubinstein at the Old City of Jerusalem (1975).

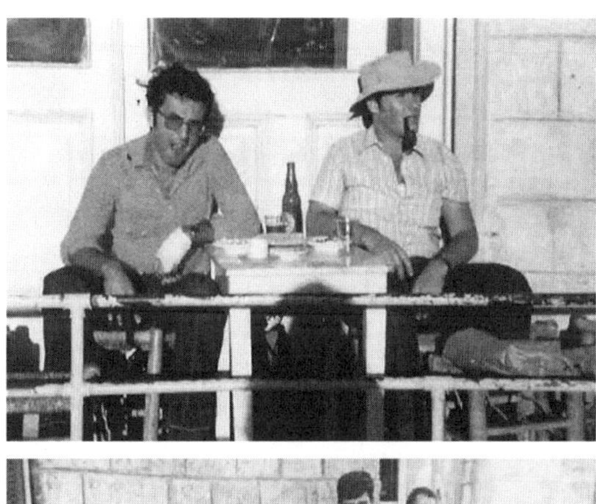

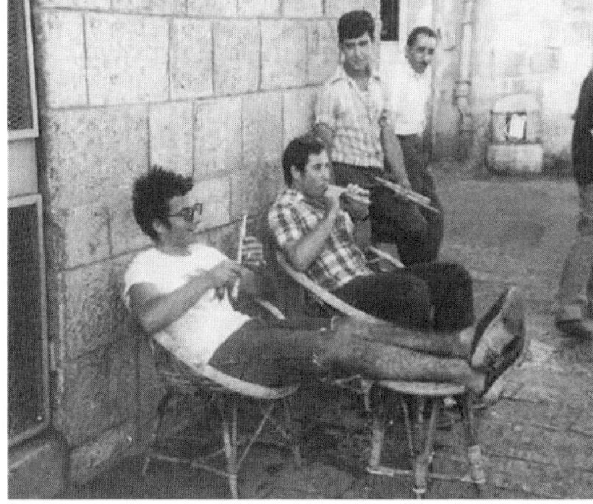

Top: Ein Karem, Jerusalem. In front of the medical school (1976). From left to right: Yochanan Schiffman, Yossi Berger, Moshe, Avi Rubinstein. Middle: Heidi on one of her frequent visits to Israel (1974). Bottom: cousin Harold Bernanke, M.D. RIP.

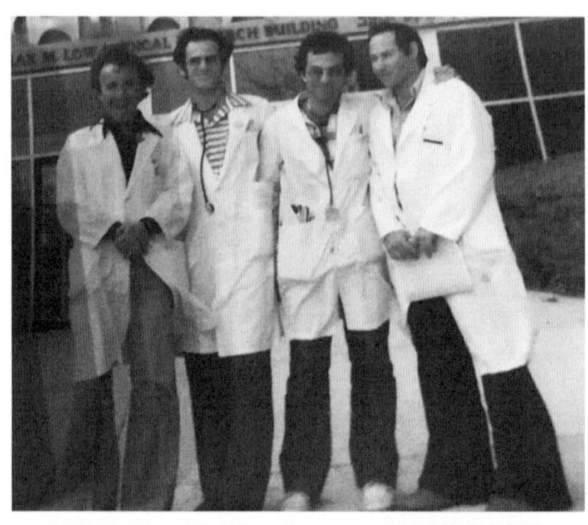

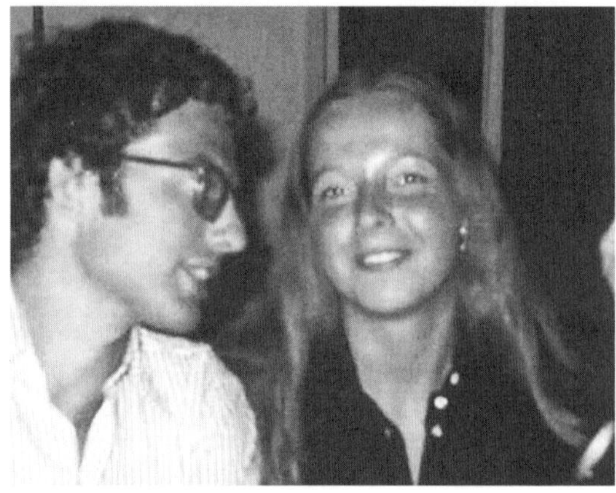

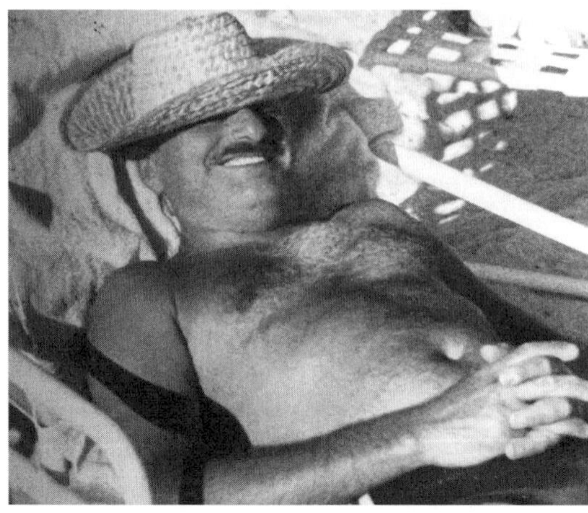

Eleven

Internship in Jerusalem

In the summer of 1978, after a couple of months of intensive studying, we took our final examinations: written and oral, in each clinical subject. I scored best in internal medicine and worst in surgery. I suspect the examiners were irritated with the many therapeutic options I offered; I did not know how dogmatic surgeons could be.

Next came a year of the mandatory rotating internship required before obtaining the M.D. degree, and I elected to do it at the Hadassah University Hospitals in Jerusalem. Heidi decided to join me. She drove her blue Opel Kadett from Switzerland to Venice. Israeli security men dismantled her car when she embarked on the Greek ship to Piraeus and Haifa, suspecting her of being a left-wing terrorist. But what was Heidi doing until then?

During my medical school years, Heidi lived in Switzerland, studying at a nursing school in Zurich. Our romance had simmered on a small fire, boiling up a few times a year when we met for extended vacations, particularly in Switzerland. In between, we led separate lives. We both enjoyed, privately, from time to time, some tasty fruit picked up along the way. However, deep inside, we perceived, but never spoke about it, that eventually, we would be united. At some stage, my mother had sent envoys to me with this message: "Why do you need this *shiksa*? Aren't there enough good-looking Jewish Israeli girls?" Yet eventually, she came to terms with the prospective daughter-in-law, who, in turn, attempted to convert to Judaism. She studied the Hebrew language and Jewish Laws but failed the examination in front of a panel of the Orthodox Rabbinical Court in Haifa. "Come back in a year," the old rabbis told her. I had discouraged Heidi from trying again. Whether she was (or will be) a Jewess or not — was not an issue for me.

In Jerusalem, we rented a tiny damp flat on Rechov Herzog. It was a converted storeroom with a rusty metal gate in the basement of a dilapidated apartment building, and it opened to a neglected, rat-infested back garden. The single small room represented our bedroom, dining room, lounge, and study. The kitchenette could accommodate one person at a time or a mattress for an overnight guest. The tiny bathroom constantly flooded when the shower was used. Heidi started working at a hospital for mentally disabled children while I began my internship.

Equipped with a solid fund of knowledge and a swollen ego, I enthusiastically plunged into the role of being a doctor. On the first day of the internship, I walked the corridors of Hadassah Hospital with my chest over-inflated, hoping that everybody would notice the freshly embroidered, in red, "Dr. M. Schein" on my new white coat.

I started to cherish the ability to make independent, crucial decisions, the pleasure of alleviating suffering, and the occasional glory associated with saving lives. The three months in internal medicine were delightful: while the senior residents spent the nights in the emergency room, we interns were responsible for the floors. During an average night, I had to admit and treat at least ten patients: the usual mix of older people with pneumonia, cardiac failure, and complex comorbidities.

I remember the satisfaction of solving problems — how *Harrison's Principles of Internal Medicine* and *The Washington Manual of Medical Therapeutics*, so well memorized, easily applied to those patients. In my pockets, I permanently carried three fully loaded syringes: morphine, lasix (a diuretic), and aminophylline (a bronchodilator), using them liberally. I learned how a small dose of intravenous morphine alleviates all kinds of suffering — especially pulmonary edema. In my chest pocket, I carried an IntraCath (a catheter used for insertion into large central veins). It was a potentially deadly device: a large 14-gauge needle was placed into the vein, the rigid catheter threaded through the needle, which was then retracted and fixed onto the skin with a plastic device called by us "*Sefer Torah*" — book of Torah). I aggressively, and much too often, popped those lines into the subclavian veins of anyone I judged may benefit from it: the early symptoms of *funktionslust* — a disease from which later I would be cured.

* * * * *

Here is a case scenario that stays fresh in my mind.

Early one morning, after a heavy night, I admit a middle-aged man with chest pain and a large left pleural effusion — fluid accumulation in the thoracic cavity. Listening to his heart with the stethoscope, I hear a loud rhythmic crunching sound — like the sound of crumpled paper. I insert a needle through his chest wall into his effusion, removing two liters of bloodstained fluid. I do not forget to send it also for estimation of amylase. In my admitting note, I enter: "Homan's sign, probably Boerhaave's syndrome (spontaneous perforation of the esophagus). Will need a contrast esophageal study."

An hour later, Professor Marcel Elyakim — the Director of Medicine, a tall bald man with a huge forehead, considered *the* national guru of medicine — arrives for his weekly grand rounds. His rounds are grand indeed: he walks like a pontiff in Rome for four long hours — solemn and never smiling —

followed by a massive crowd of disciples, admirers, and ardent believers. The patients are presented to the master by residents — we interns are never allowed to open our mouths not to irritate the great man.

The long procession arrives at my patient's bed within an hour or so. After the resident who saw the patient in the emergency room eloquently recites the case history, according to a specific formula advocated by the Director, the latter places his *Littmann* stethoscope on the patient's chest, closes his eyes, concentrates by contracting his forehead muscles, and listens.

Deep silence in the room. An old man in an adjacent bed moans *"oi vei"* but is immediately hushed down by the head nurse. The professor unplugs the stethoscope from his ears, scratches his forehead, looks down at his congregation, and declares: "Acute pericarditis. Probably infective. Start antibiotics and wait for cultures. If proven viral, he may need steroids." We move to the next bed. God has spoken.

As always, between the male and female sections of the ward, the professor and senior staff retire for tea and sandwiches of cream cheese and sardines while we juniors hurry to continue with scut work.

I call the lab for results: the amylase levels in my patient's pleural fluid are sky-high. *Bingo*. I am sure this is Boerhaave's syndrome — perforation of the esophagus with the amylase deriving from the patient's saliva. I rush to the responsible resident: "Ethan, this is Boerhaave's. I was right! He needs a contrast study. He has a hole in the esophagus. We must rush. Any delay will kill him…"

"Stop blabbering, Schein. The professor said it is pericarditis." The resident shrugs his shoulders and rejoins the rounds.

A few hours later, the patient's blood pressure drops. Repeated chest X-rays show air in the mediastinum. A Gastrografin contrast study demonstrates an esophageal leak — Boerhaave's syndrome. The five professors of surgery who are summoned to discuss how to treat this rare entity decide to drain the esophageal hole through a posterior thoracic approach. When the patient survives after a stormy hospitalization of three months, a special medical-surgical symposium is conducted to discuss this fantastic success story.

The case was subsequently published in the *Israeli Journal of Medical Sciences*. Of course, I was not made a co-author. It was my early introduction to medical-surgical academics and how decisions are often reached — adding to my slowly growing skepticism and cynicism.

* * * * *

In Jerusalem, Heidi and I lived an almost parallel life. I worked day and night and had no social life, which forced her to find her own friends and activities about which I knew little, and it was better so. One afternoon I returned to our damp 'dump' after a thirty-six-hour shift to find a scribble on a tiny piece of paper: "I flew to Switzerland and will be back in two weeks. Heidi."

It was then when I met Alina — not a little affair but something that could have influenced the future. It was the first day of my rotation through the general intensive care unit when I noticed her stooped over one of the patients. Tall, slim, dark shiny hair, high cheekbones, well-made face — her sex appeal shone through the nurse uniform.

"Oh, good morning. I guess you're the new intern. I am Alina." She spoke BBC English with a slight lisp. I noted her small white teeth, the deep blue eyes and inhaled her perfume. She must be one of the new British ICU nurses, I thought. At that time, the Hadassah Hospital needed more trained intensive care nurses and had to import them from London.

"Who is she?" I asked a junior resident during a coffee break.

"Oh, forget her. She's a princess. Three months here, and nobody has managed to come near her, including all the professors. She's untouchable, believe me… no chance."

The following day Alina was helping me to turn the patient on his side so I could examine his buttocks. "Alina. This is not an English name?" I asked.

"No, no. It's Polish. My father's Polish, Mom's Ukrainian. I was born in England, the Midlands, you know." Now I understood the origin of this wild Slavic face. She turned me on.

"You speak Polish?" I asked and said something in that language. She straightened herself to her full height, smiled charmingly, and spoke back in perfect Polish. Not a trace of Anglo-Saxon contamination.

On that day, just before she ended her shift, I gathered confidence. "Would you come for dinner with me tomorrow night?" I asked.

"Of course." It was the Polish language! I knew it — it caught her.

During dinner at a Chinese restaurant, the Anglo-Polish beauty was rather formal. Later, at the cozy Jan's Tea House in Ein Kerem — Persian carpets, candle lights, classical music — she said, "Please come nearer," and wrapped her long arms around me. Stormy weeks, which turned into months, followed — Heidi returned, and I was cheating on her — in our flat, in the cold alleys of the Old City, and in Alina's room, where the walls were covered with icons, for she was an ardent Catholic. What impressed me was that she would shout "Holy Maria" in Polish when reaching climax.

I enjoyed the occasions when her night duties in the ICU overlapped with mine. At four in the morning, I would retire to the adjacent doctor's duty room for a brief nap. She would then take her thirty-minute tea break and quietly crawl into my bed… this was the nearest I ever came to the TV stereotype of the horny young doctor.

I had to decide. Heidi suddenly announced that she was pregnant and started to talk about the need to get married before our child was born. So, I made the decision, a good decision. No, here I am, embellishing the story. The truth is that it was Alina who sensed in what direction the affair was developing and abruptly stopped seeing me. In hindsight, she made the right decision.

Over the years, Alina kept me updated about her whereabouts. She left England for Cambodia, where she worked with injured refugee kids. She moved on to Lebanon and spent the 1980 war in a cellar of a Beirut hospital — shelled by the invading Israelis. In Beirut, she met and married an elderly, divorced Swiss UN administrator with whom she moved to Geneva. After divorcing him, she worked in a hospital in Geneva, converted to Judaism, and married a banker — a Moroccan-Swiss Jew. In 1993, she suddenly appeared with her new husband in our house in Haifa. She was in her last month of pregnancy. We managed to catch a minute or two alone in the kitchen, away from our respective spouses; we did not say much but just looked at each other and smiled. The last I heard from her, she was in Geneva, divorced again, with two dark Moroccan-looking sons. The orthodox Catholic girl is now a devoted orthodox Jewess. No more "Holy Maria."

* * * * *

Toward the end of the internship, I started to think about the next step that — I had no doubt — would be a surgical residency. I had to be a general surgeon and nothing else. The question was, where?

In Israel in those years, as it still is today, there was no organized system for applying and matching to residency programs. Instead, every applicant had to negotiate his position directly with the individual department. There were usually two or three surgical departments in a hospital, each of 20-30 beds, each selecting and accepting its residents separately — no more than one per year. To be chosen, you had to form a 'personal bond' with your department of choice. For example, do an elective clerkship during the final year at medical school, try to serve as an intern for a few months, and help the boss do a study (e.g., kill a few mice for him). In brief — bury your nose up their asses.

As the above-listed methodologies were not part of my armamentarium, I did not even bother trying to enter any surgical residency in Israel. Training abroad was something that I had thought about for years. The foreign fields always seemed greener to me than those at home. I memorized the names of the surgeons who had written all the surgical books I hungrily consumed and the exotic places where they practiced. I believed that the surgical training they provide was probably outstanding — wasn't Professor Saltz a product of American Surgery — not the dogmatic slavery I saw around? It was how I perceived it in my immature medical mind. I was also adventurous, with a constant *wanderlust*; besides, I knew Heidi would follow me anywhere.

Toward the end of the internship, I got offers from three residencies: Buffalo, New York, Vancouver, and Johannesburg. The Canadians even asked what size uniform I would need. A difficult choice: Buffalo so cold and bleak; Vancouver charming but so far away; and Johannesburg? At that time, many ex-South African professors were on our medical school faculty; all seemed so knowledgeable, astute, and polite — the kind of British colonial politeness, unlike the harshness of their Israeli counterparts. I asked for their advice that was unvarying: "Go to South Africa, Schein: good teaching, superb weather, cushy life, and man, you will cut… they'll send you to Baragwanath Hospital, and you will be sick and tired of cutting." They were speaking about cutting humans, of course — mainly blacks.

I sometimes wonder what would have happened if I had chosen the third option — Buffalo General Hospital. The hospital's Chief of Surgery was John H. Siegel (1932-2014), a famous surgical researcher and pioneer in critical care and trauma. I was related to John, as he was the brother-in-law of one of my cousins. My professional trajectory, let alone the course of my family's life, would most likely be completely different. But we decided: we're going to South Africa. I imagine that had my father been alive, he would have convinced me to go to Buffalo.

* * * * *

Heidi in Corsica (1975-6).

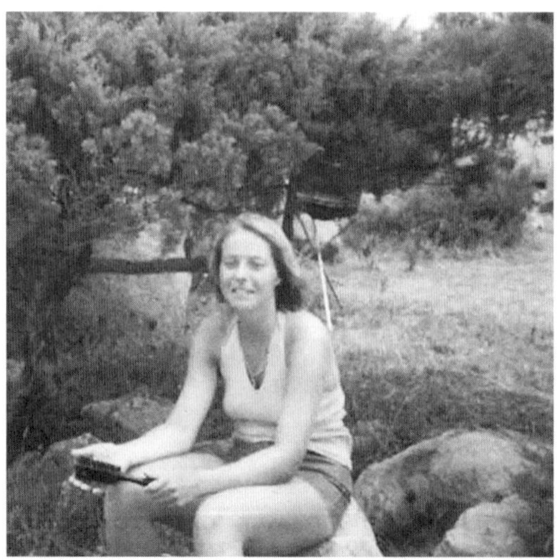

Heidi, 1975-6. Top: Sinai Desert. Bottom: Haifa.

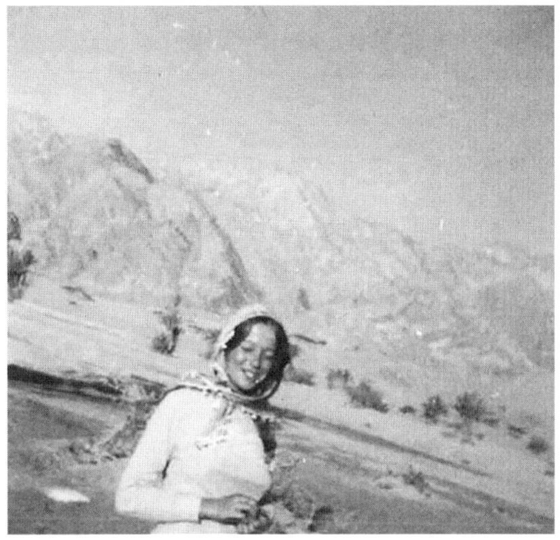

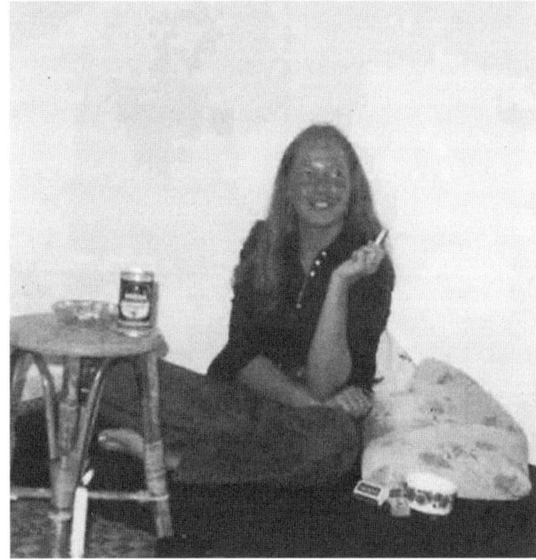

Twelve

The wedding

Well into her seventh month of pregnancy, Heidi resigned from her job at the children's nursing home in Jerusalem and returned to Schaffhausen, where she wished to deliver our child. But first, we had to be married. I planned to finish the internship, get the M.D. diploma, and only then join Heidi in Switzerland. In addition, I had to return Heidi's Swiss-licensed car to Switzerland. I intended to sail from Haifa to Ancona, Italy, and from there to drive to Schaffhausen. The boat would arrive in Ancona on April 10, 1980; the wedding was arranged for the next day, April 11.

It was a medium-sized Greek ferry that rocked violently in the choppy early spring Mediterranean Sea. The human cargo, mainly Italians returning after a pilgrimage to the Holy Land, was continuously seasick. The food in the cafeteria was appalling. I survived on bread, feta cheese sprinkled with olive oil, lettuce, and black olives, washed down with cheap bitter retsina wine. In the bar, I came across a bespectacled German archeology student — Bettina was her name. She was petite and swarthy, and proved to be a pleasant companion — a social intellectual companion; nothing else. I was on my way to get married.

After two and a half days, in the late morning on April 7, the ship arrived at the Port of Piraeus, dropping anchor for the day. Bettina disembarked to continue to Athens. I joined her for a day trip. The ship was to sail off towards Italy that night at 11 p.m. We took the train to Athens. After days of bread and cheese on board, we feasted on tzatziki and lamb kebab, and lots of ouzo.

Slightly tipsy, we climbed together on the steep path toward the Acropolis. The twilight was turning violet. A cold wind blew from the sea; the city gleamed far below. Finally, we reached the Acropolis, which was deserted, with not a human in sight. We stood there wordless, shivering in the breeze. Below us, the sea of lights was astounding.

We ran down to Athens, said goodbye, and I rushed to the train heading back to Piraeus. I looked at my watch — 9 p.m., time for a last good supper before the ship departed.

Near the gates to the port, I saw a decent looking taverna. I entered: a few locals were drinking ouzo and nibbling on pickles and fried calamari. In the corner, I noticed giant lobsters swimming in a large glass tank. I had never tasted a lobster before. *Let me try it once. Why not?*

The waiter addressed me in Greek.

"A lobster, please, and a liter of retsina," I replied.

"What size lobster?"

"The biggest, this one," I pointed toward a monster at the bottom of the tank. I did not have any idea how much it would be. I had a few drachma notes and a bunch of 100 dollar notes in my pocket. *It should be enough.*

I labored through the giant lobster. The meat was white and tough — not the taste of heaven I thought it would be. The retsina, however, was better than the brand served on the ship.

Ten p.m. "Waiter, the bill, please." I do not remember how much the bill was, but then it seemed astronomic — at least 125 US dollars. Was the giant imported from Maine?

"Sorry, no dollars, only drachmas," objected the waiter.

"No drachmas, only dollars. Ship leaving just now," I hoped he would understand basic English. I handed him two 100 dollar bills and asked for change, "in dollars, please." My watch showed 10.25 p.m. I must go now. Another waiter rushed to a neighboring store to get me the change — in drachmas.

Only when I stood up, I noticed how drunk I was — the liter of mild retsina had gone down like spiced juice. But it was all gone now. I stumbled toward the port's gate, presented my ship permit and passport to the sentry, and rushed towards the pier. It was dark and deserted. My watch indicated 10.45 p.m. "Fucking Greeks" I shouted to the black sea and starless night. Don't these idiots count their passengers?

I wandered through the deserted port, looking for an open office; they were all closed. My mind was foggy, but I had my passport and a few hundred dollars. And I knew that my best bet was Athens airport.

Back in Piraeus's train station, I noticed the clock on the wall: 00.15 a.m. My watch indicated, however, 11.15 p.m. *Fuck, this is a different time zone.*

* * * * *

April 8, 1980. Early morning at Athens International Airport.

I purchased a ticket to Rome. After an uncomfortable day in that congested and scruffy airport, the departure of my flight was announced. More troubles at the security check: "Sir, where's your luggage?"

"I don't have any."

"Not even hand luggage?

"No, it's all on the ship."

"Which ship?" And so on… until I almost missed that flight too. Remember, these were the days when airliners were often targeted by Palestinian terrorists, especially the ones taking off from Athens.

We landed at Fiumicino, Rome, late in the evening. At passport control, I suddenly remembered the discord with the Italian Police in Modena six years ago — do they have any record of it? But the unshaven *poliziotto* gazed at me without interest and motioned me through: *Va bene*.

It was a rainy, smoggy morning in Rome. I took a bus to Rome's railway station to find out that there were no trains. "There's a *sciopero generale*," a taxi driver explained. Anyone who has lived in Italy knows the meaning of this term, which so often inflicts this charming country: "a general strike."

"But are the buses running?"

"Some… private buses… may run."

"OK, take me to the central bus station."

What followed, to cut the story short, was a tortuous journey of about 230km, on multiple buses, westwards, across the Italian peninsula.

On April 10, at 3 a.m., the rain stopped when I arrived at the ancient port of Ancona. The night was clear, and I saw my lost ship tied to the pier just off a long seaside avenue. The passengers had already disembarked and driven away. The tired crew was unloading some cargo. I clambered on the jetty and approached the first officer, who started a rapid verbal barrage: "Signore, where did you disappear? Greek police are looking for you, Italian police as well, your luggage is at the police station. The car? We didn't have the keys. We had to break a window. The battery was flat. We dragged it to the police station. Anyway, good to see you alive."

I waited until the *meccanico* opened his garage, fixed a flat tire, recharged the battery — the window would have to wait — and collected my baggage at the police station. After paying the mechanic, I was left with just enough money for the gas and tolls of the *autostrade*. Forget about any food stops.

It was 2 a.m. the next day when I parked the Opel near Heidi's parents' house in Schaffhausen, Ungarbühlstrasse 61. I found everybody sleepless and tense: where did the groom disappear? After a bath, shave, and breakfast, we rushed to town to get me a dark suit (the first one I had ever owned). The trousers were too long, but a few in-folding pins had to do the job for immediately we had to attend a civil wedding at the City Hall. It was conducted in Swiss German by the *Stadt* Secretary, Herr Uelinger. He lectured us for forty-five minutes. I was too tired to concentrate much on his preaching uttered in the local Swiss dialect. I only thought: *this better be a good marriage after such a saga.*

Should I include such banal snapshots of our wedding and how I arrived at it in a memoir? Isn't it like forcing on guests a slide show of one's last vacation in Paris? But be that as it may, the wedding party, lasting from early afternoon until after midnight, was a typical German-Swiss affair. There was a cruise on the Rhein River under a pale, cool pre-spring sun; champagne and tiny sandwiches with air-cured, thinly cut alpine beef; a stop at a riverside church for a non-religious ceremony — trying to satisfy the Swiss relatives. (I suppose that not all of them were ecstatic watching a Swiss girl marry a foreigner in her last month of pregnancy — not just a foreigner but a Jew.) Finally, the dinner was held at a *landstube*: wooden walls, long wooden tables, flowers; the food being mixed salad, creamed fresh mushroom soup, a roast of veal with potato croquettes and asparagus, fruit salad, ice cream, and cookies; drinks included one-liter carafes of Schaffhausen red landwine, coffee, *kirschwasser*, and Williams Pear Schnapps.

It is where and when a tribute should be paid to Heidi's parents, my in-laws, Berta and Karl. Both are dead now. Berta died of Alzheimer's disease at the age of seventy-nine, and Karl passed away at the age of ninety-two. Both were humble, hardworking Swiss citizens. They belonged to the older generation but welcomed change. They were conservative and liberal at the same time. They were of modest means but very generous. They, small-town people who rarely traveled abroad, had immediately and warmly accepted me into their family as if I was one of them. I could not have wished for better in-laws!

* * * * *

> "That fall, the snow came very late. We lived in a brown wooden house in the pine trees on the side of the mountain and at night there was frost so that there was thin ice over the water in the two pitchers on the dresser in the morning... The pine wood crackled and sparked and then the fire roared in the stove... we could see the lake and the mountain across the lake on the French side. There was snow on the tops of the mountains and the lake was a gray steel-blue."

These are Hemingway's words from *A Farewell to Arms*. It was when Lieutenant Henry, an American volunteer ambulance driver, and his pregnant lover Catherine Barkley, a British nurse, desert WW I in Italy to the calm Swiss Alps. Here, in a farmhouse above Montreux, the young couple awaited the arrival of their baby while enjoying the rustic alpine atmosphere.

Our situation was like Henry and Catherine's, except it was early spring. So, after the wedding, not expecting the baby's arrival for a month, we retired to the Bernese Alps — to Adelboden, where Heidi's family used to spend summer vacations at the Bärtschi family farmhouse. The two-storied wooden house was glued to the slopes high above the village, just below the upper forest line. The wood-paneled guest section included two tiny bedrooms, a kitchen, and a lounge. It was plain: low ceiling, no phone, no TV, a large porcelain tiled stove burning in the corner. Herr and Frau Bärtschi, and their minimally retarded son Goeddel, lived below, next to the barn, alongside a few pigs and a cow.

Even at these heights, the snow started to melt, turning heavy, wet, and dirty. Yet, the almost 3000-meter Albishorn, behind the house, and the majestic 3244-meter Wildstrubel and its glacier, in front — mountains we used to climb during the summers with Heidi's father Karl — stood white as ever, glistening in the sun. At night we slept on hard straw-filled mattresses under soft eiderdowns, the windows wide open. And through the windows, the moonlit Alps were invading the room with the smell of fresh pine, rotting grass, and wood fire mixed with the aroma of the fermenting hay and hogs in the barn. During the days, we did what we always did in the Alps, the same thing everyone does — hiking and resting in the inns. And the inns were dark, warm, and smoky, with their peculiar alpine inn aroma consisting of fresh cheese, spilled wine, evaporating schnapps, and *stumpen* — the cheap coarse cigars smoked by the mountain people. Coming out of the inn, the cold air would sharply invade our lungs, and the rush of mountain streams and cow bells would ring loudly in our ears.

Back to *A Farewell to Arms*, let Hemingway describe what happened one night, a week into our stay in the mountains:

> "One morning I awoke about three o'clock hearing Catherine stirring in the bed.
>
> "Are you all right, Cat?"
>
> "I've been having some pains, darling."
>
> "Regularly?"
>
> "No, not very."
>
> "If you have them at all regularly we'll go to the hospital."

It was how it was with us but with two differences: first, Heidi never called me "darling." Second, I asked her: "Aren't these just Braxton Hicks contractions, a false alarm?" Yet, like Hemingway's couple, we acted immediately. They called for a taxi and drove down to Montreux; we decided to drive back to Schaffhausen, four hours away. It snowed heavily that night; with Herr Bärtschi, I needed an hour to clear the steep path from the farmstead to the main road.

While Hemingway's Catherine lost her son at birth and later died of postpartum hemorrhage, our story had a happier end. When we reached the foot of the Alps around the Thunersee, Heidi's pains subsided; it was indeed a false alarm. Our first son Omri was born two weeks later, exactly thirty days after the wedding.

The morning after he was born — aren't all births taking place at night? — I returned to my in-law's home to sleep. (If you read *A Farewell to Arms*, you perhaps would remember that Lieutenant Henry did not sleep after his Catherine lost their son; he went into a café, had ham and eggs served in a round dish, and, to "cool his mouth… drank several beers." After having another beer, Lieutenant Henry returned to the hospital to learn that Catherine had suffered a lethal hemorrhage.)

In those days, the mandatory policy in Switzerland was to keep the mother and offspring in the hospital for an entire week. However, a day after delivery, Heidi asked to be taken to town for *kaffee und kuchen*. The nurses reported the crime to the *Herr Direktor* of Gynecology and Obstetrics. I was summoned to the Director's office. The latter, a distinguished-looking man in his mid-60s, addressed me severely. He said: "*sehr geehrter Herr Kollege*, you, now a young physician, surely understand how important complete rest is to the physical and emotional wellbeing of the mother and her baby." "*Ja, Ja,*" I responded, but the following day I took Heidi and our newborn son home against vigorous protests by the nurses. A week later, we flew to Israel.

* * * * *

Top: our wedding in Schaffhausen, 1980. Sitting with eight-month pregnant Heidi. Standing from left: Carl, Heidi's brother, Karl, Heidi's father, my mom, Heidi's mother Berta, Carl's wife (now ex) Eva, their daughter Christina. Bottom: with Heidi and friends at the wedding.

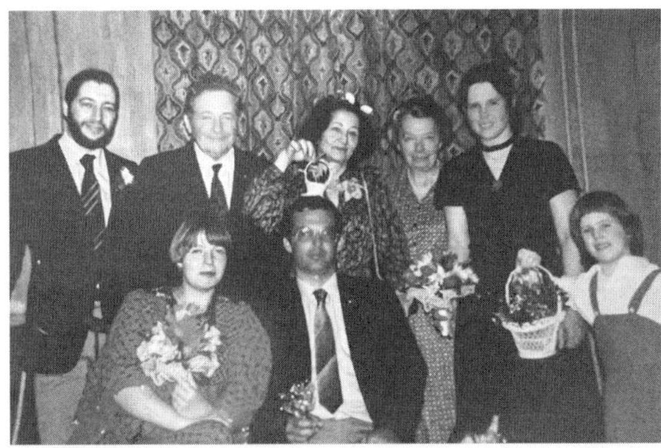

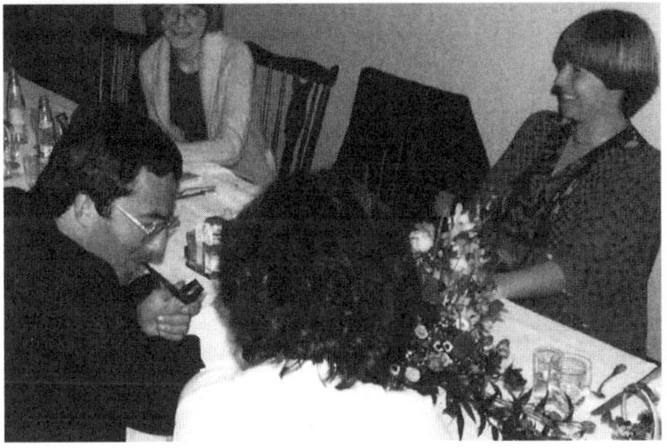

The Bärtschi family house, Adelboden, Switzerland.

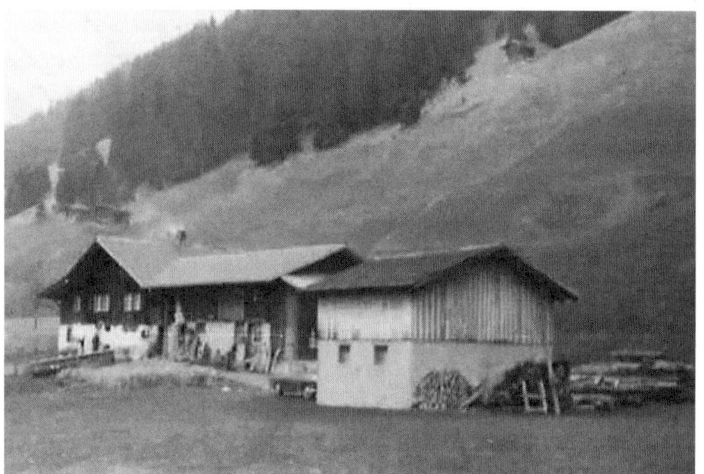

Thirteen

Going to Africa

Late May 1980. A scorching *chamisn* day. With the ten-day-old, incessantly crying baby, Omri, we landed at Tel Aviv's airport. My friend Bubi D. picked us up with his ancient air-conditionless Subaru; its radiator started boiling on the way to Haifa. What do I recall from these six weeks of the stopover in Israel before we continued to South Africa?

First, there was Omri's 'Brit' (circumcision), which was uneventful.

Second, I had to obtain a formal M.D. degree that, in turn, depended on the approval of my M.D. thesis by the appropriate university committee. The subject of my thesis was "The surgical management of esophageal varices at the Hadassah University Hospital: 1970-1980." It was a retrospective study, a review of patients' charts; for Israeli surgeons to perform a prospective trial was unheard of. I chose to write my thesis under the tutelage of Professor Arie Durst, a handsome, charismatic, and immensely successful 'top knife' – one who operated on prime ministers and top-notch rabbis. However, doing so created a huge problem for me as the professor was always unavailable. I would stop at the OR a few times a week and ask: "Professor, when can I show you my thesis?"

"Oh, Schein, why don't you come back and wait for me here in the OR tonight at nine? We'll drive home, have dinner and speak," he would say, smiling. He would always smile and 'agree' with you. It was his secret weapon – probably one of the reasons he became the most popular consultant for a second opinion in the country. When consulted on surgical disasters, he would never admonish with, "You were wrong" or "I would have done this differently." Instead, he would say, "You had bad luck, you did whatever you could, and now I suggest you do this…" I should have learned this approach from him…

But when 9 p.m. arrived, the professor would start an emergency renal transplant or assist another surgeon in a reoperation for some complication. Eventually, one night – during my internship – my luck struck, and at 10 p.m., I was sitting in the professor's spacious BMW on the way to his home. A modest dinner of what tasted like reheated chicken schnitzel and rice, both extremely dry, was served in the kitchen by the professor's wife. A little pale and fragile-looking child, I think it was a boy, climbed on the professor's knees. A few years later, I heard the child died from some rare immune disorder. After dinner, the professor settled in his reclining chair, shook off his shoes, and commanded: "Come on, Schein, read me your thesis!"

"Where should I begin?"

"Ah, read everything from the beginning. I am listening," while the professor closed his eyes. I started at page 1, and there were 120 to go; on page 3, he lightly snored. I stopped.

"Schein, go on, I am listening." Then the phone rang, and it rang again and again until midnight.

It was when people would call the professor asking for *"protekzia,"* which in local slang means "a plea for help" — a member of the *Knesset* calling to ask for 'help' about his cousin who had suffered a postoperative complication in Tel Aviv or the Chief Rabbi of Haifa begging for *protekzia* for his brother in Brooklyn. The professor would listen carefully to all such pleas, always agreeing to help: "My friend, let me see what I can do about this. Please call tomorrow after 10 p.m."

Finally, after midnight the Chairman said: "Schein, you write well... why don't you just show me the results."

"Sure. The overall mortality in patients who underwent a portocaval shunt was 90%."

"What!? Are you sure? Was it that bad?"

At that time, I did not realize that many surgeons did not know their own 'real' results, and most even didn't attempt to know — or did not want to know.

It was 1 a.m., and I knew the professor had five private cases lined up the following morning. "OK, Schein," he said," I have to believe that you reviewed the charts carefully. You could, of course, exclude patients who were almost dead before the operation, um, and this would cut the mortality to 75%, which would look better. Eh? You know how sick these patients are. It may make your thesis publishable in a journal."

I did not know then that Durst had been an eight-year-old boy when the Germans invaded his hometown Lvov (now Lviv — the town my father left simultaneously with the retreating Russian army). I did not know that he hid from the Nazis for four years with his mother in Warsaw (the town I left in 1957). Later he would publish a book *A Childhood in the Shadow of the Holocaust.* I bet that Durst knew nothing about me as well. He never inquired. How often we know nothing about our superiors, our residents, our students, our colleagues.

So now, before leaving Israel, I had to get my thesis approved by the Chairman of the Thesis Committee, (Associate) Professor P. (now deceased). He was the Director of Surgery in a smaller hospital near Tel Aviv. Two hours late for my appointment, the professor appeared in his green scrubs, tore off his facemask into the rubbish bin, and grumbled to his secretary: "It was a difficult Nissen," referring to an anti-reflux gastric procedure. Then to me: "You're Schein? Are you *oleh chadash*? (a new immigrant to Israel), from Russia?"

"No, Sir, I arrived from Poland exactly twenty-three years and three months ago."

"Well, I read your thesis," he pointed to his littered desk, "and I must tell you it is unreadable. Can't you write Hebrew? You may need some help from a professional translator."

"But, Professor, writing essays was my strongest skill in high school. There is little time left as I have to leave next week for South Africa to start a surgical residency."

"South Africa? Why South Africa? Who has heard about South Africa? I did my fellowship in New York, Brooklyn. We go to America, and in American medicine we trust. Anyway, I will approve your thesis, although it is hard to believe the high mortality, much too high, our results are better, of course, and Schein, if and when you decide to come back, you have to improve your written Hebrew."

Later in my career, I would encounter many 'surgical scholars' who would not tolerate any text unless written in heavy local medical jargon — to them, the correct written language. Years later, in Brooklyn, I wrote a biographical piece about Rudolf Nissen, the great German surgeon, a half-Jew, who immigrated to Brooklyn via Turkey and ended his career as the Chief of Surgery in Basel, Switzerland. A retired Jewish surgeon who had worked under Nissen at the old Jewish Hospital in Brooklyn told me a little about Nissen as a person; for this, I acknowledged him in the footnote and politely sent him the final draft of the manuscript. He wrote back: "Your manuscript is illegible; this is simply not the English language. It shows that you are a foreigner without any literary English skills. If you choose to submit this for publication, and I wouldn't, please do not cite me and remove my name. I would be ashamed to be associated with such a poor product." I complied with his request and had the manuscript accepted and published by the *Journal of the American College of Surgeons*. A month after it appeared, I received a letter from Tom Starzl, the father of hepatic transplant surgery and the most published surgeon ever. He wrote: "I wish to thank you for your piece about Rudolf Nissen… it was the best surgical historical article I ever read."

Regrettably, many reviewers for American medical journals and their editors — less a problem with their British counterparts — believe that medical English should be heavy, formal, and repetitive, using short sentences followed by periods. Semicolons and hyphens are taboo. Then one wonders why these journals are so dull to read.

* * * * *

My last task in Israel, before leaving for South Africa, was grimmer. Late at night, my sister Sylvia called: "Come up immediately. I'm bleeding." I woke up slowly. "Bleeding, bleeding from where? What's the problem?"

"Just come now!" She hung up. My sister was thirty-three years old then — not married but pregnant.

It was a planned pregnancy. Sylvia wanted the child and wished to be a mother. When I arrived in her cozy flat on Mount Carmel, I found her sitting on the toilet with a four-month-old male fetus — my first and last nephew — between her legs. My sister liked to knit; I found a piece of heavy wool with which I tied the cord and divided it with a kitchen knife. Then I took her to the hospital.

The events of that gruesome night were never raised between my sister and I.

Twenty-four years later, after she was found dead, lying on the carpet in that same flat on Mount Carmel, I searched through her diaries — she did not mention that night. But in another diary volume, she lamented her unborn son. (Much more about Sylvia the reader will find in Chapter 49.)

On July the first, 1980, the three of us (Heidi, I and little Omri) boarded an El Al flight to Johannesburg — a total unknown.

* * * * *

Omri's Brit, Haifa.

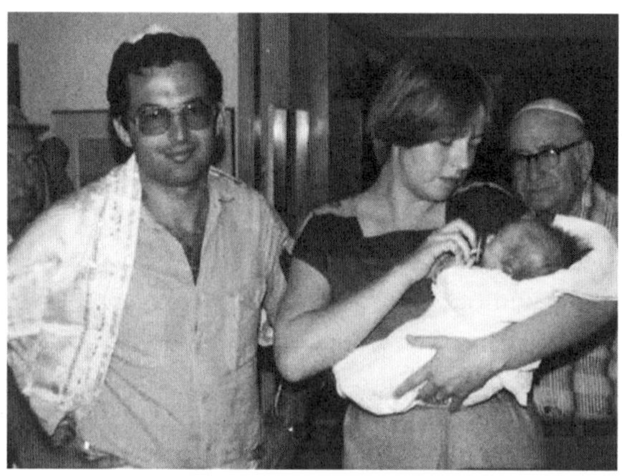

Fourteen

Early days in Johannesburg

July 1980. We landed in Johannesburg on a typical, chilly, sunny, Transvaal winter day.

Irrespective of how thorough your prior research and planning are — it was rudimental in our case — whenever you move to new places, the novel location will always be the unknown. Things will never turn out as planned. All we knew was that South Africa was a large, exotic, prosperous country; that the surgical training was excellent, and life was reasonably affordable and comfortable. Yes, we had heard about Apartheid but did not understand much about what it meant. The Israeli media maintained a favorable attitude towards the Apartheid regime, which supported Israel. It was 1980 — twenty years after the massacre of blacks at Sharpeville near Johannesburg, which signified the start of the blacks' struggle against Apartheid. We knew nothing about the struggle and continued to learn little in the following years, mainly because of the disinformation blackout enforced by the white semi-dictatorial regime. In fact, many whites in South Africa knew the bitter truth. But they had the desire to know while we — the newcomers, busy with our own little lives — elected to be blind. We were not unlike the privileged Russians enjoying a good life in Stalin's Moscow, who chose not to know who was being carried away in the windowless black buses driven across the town at night.

When we arrived in Johannesburg, a South African rand bought three US dollars — ten years later, when we left, you could buy one US dollar for six rands. We came with no money and left with no more than we came with, except two additional sons — Yariv and Dan — and a few good new friends and fond memories. And I left with a specialty — this is where I grew to be a surgeon and where I enjoyed the craft the most.

Being a surgeon after leaving South Africa would never be such 'great fun' anymore.

* * * * *

I press again on the replay button of what Gore Vidal called the "ancient tapes of memory." What do I see? I see an early morning in Johannesburg's Jan Smuts Airport with its shabby and depressingly crowded arrival hall. There are three separate lines for passport control: one — short and moving fast, is for white South Africans; the second — short and not moving at all, is for non-white South Africans — short because only a few non-whites can afford an airplane trip abroad; it is so slow because traveling non-whites are suspected as enemies of the State; the third line is ours. Its tail starts on the tarmac — it is for tourists (visas are necessary) and immigrants like us. Finally, two hours later, we arrive at the desk of a uniformed official: blond mustache, red face, barking impolitely in heavily accented, guttural English — this was the first Afrikaner we had ever met.

Quickly we would learn that all positions in public service branches are in the hands of the Afrikaners. In simple terms — the Afrikaners controlled everything — they had the power. The previously colonial British were allowed to lead the financial sector and to live like kings while the majority, the blacks, provided the muscle power for everything. The 'colored' people existed somewhere within a gray zone in between — more dark than light, I would say. The Indians and Chinese were considered a few steps above the blacks but still non-whites. Paradoxically, the few Japanese who arrived in the country were labeled as 'honorary whites' as Japanese business was appreciated. Finally, minorities like the Portuguese (who had escaped from the wars zones of Angola and Mozambique and excelled in producing and selling vegetables) and the Jews (who had arrived from the Baltic countries at the turn of the century and excelled in academics and making and selling money) were considered whites and left to prosper — as long as they acquiesced to the ruling regime.

Yuval, an Israeli friend of mine from medical school, who had arrived a few months before to train in orthopedics (he would become an ophthalmologist), drove us to his tiny flat at the staff residence of the Johannesburg Hospital, high on the Parktown Ridge. I remember waking up the following day, opening the window, and looking out: a frosty breeze blew in my face (July is the coldest month in the Transvaal), down below the total flatness of the (strictly 'white') northern suburbs came into view, spreading to the horizon and beyond Pretoria. The sun was already out, and the sky was cloudless; soon, the frost would disappear, and a pleasantly mild, dry winter day would last until sunset. No town can match Johannesburg's weather. In winter, it is sunny and dry — it never rains. Summer days are pleasantly warm but not humid, with almost daily afternoon showers. The vista of the northern suburbs from the window was brown, but the entire town would become a giant, colorful, lush garden during spring and summer.

Our first urgent task was to buy a car as the public transportation in Johannesburg was — is? — as rudimentary as it is in rural USA or Los Angeles; the few bus lines carried "non-white" signs.

"My South African cousin does business with Ronny Bass. He's a leading car dealer in Jo'burg. He'll give you a good deal," promised my friend Yuval.

That afternoon I was taken to Ronny Bass' car dealership on the highway to Soweto. The famous car dealer received us in a small room at the back of his showroom. A dark man in a dark suit was munching on a sandwich behind dark sunglasses in a dark room. "So, doc, you need a car, eh? How much you wanna spend? I've got a bunch of beautiful Mazda 323s. What? 8000 rands? No Mazda for this… tell you what, Abe here will show ya what you need. Abe, show doc the yellow Citroen, will ya? Doc, we give VIP treatment to our Israeli brothers. Nice to meet you." Back to his sandwich.

Abe, an aging Jew with a large nose, showed me the yellow Citroen GS, 1200cc, 1973. "Wanna drive this baby? See how she goes up and down. No one makes suspension like Citroen. Drives like Queen Mary. Ya know the ship?"

After a brief, nearly suicidal drive on the busy highway — suicidal because this was the first time I had to drive a car with a steering wheel on the right — I purchased the car. It turned out to be the worst vehicle I ever had, spending as much time in car shops as on the road. One night, a few months later, it died on us while crossing a flooded low bridge during a cloudburst. Heidi and I swam out to safety, but the car was done. From that night, it entered the family history as the "yellow submarine."

Here could be an opportunity to reflect on the ambivalent relationships between the Jews of the diaspora and their Israeli brethren — arriving to live among them. In this respect, I found that South African Jews are no different from American ones — yes, I know I am generalizing. Both entities are fond of Israelis as long as they protect and plow the Holy Land; oh sure — they are very welcome to come and visit but not to stay. Who likes poor and uneducated relatives to come and stay over? In South Africa, the children, and grandchildren of impoverished Jewish immigrants (mainly from Lithuania) wrapped themselves in an Anglo-Saxon veil. Their Yiddish-speaking grandparents had peddled old garments across the Transvaal. Whereas they, who had adopted a pseudo-British accent, now belonged to country clubs that tolerated *kikes*. They seemed to look down on us, who lacked what they perceived as Anglo-Saxon culture. I found many of them condescending.

* * * * *

My formal training program was to begin in January and follow a five-year curriculum. A year as a rotating SHO (senior house office), a year as a junior registrar (resident) in one of the affiliated 'non-white' hospitals, and finally, three years on the prestigious "Myburgh's circuit" in the giant 'new' Johannesburg (JHB) Hospital — its main corridor almost a kilometer long and as wide as the Fifth Avenue in New York — which (obviously) was reserved for whites only.

Professor Johannes Albertus Myburgh, "Bert" to his friends, was the Chairman of Surgery. He led an academic department that stretched across five affiliated hospitals and included numerous clinically independent subspecialties and surgical units. Myburgh, or "the Prof" as he was known, had grown up on a farm in the Orange Free State; he had been a Rhode Scholar in Oxford, trained in surgery in Cape Town, and had inherited the Johannesburg's chair from the great Professor D.J. du Plessis ("Dupp"). A tall man, square-faced, silver-haired, well built — he took part at the Melbourne Olympic Games as a runner — Myburgh looked like Cary Grant.

Myburgh was a solid surgeon and an academic genius. With all these qualities, it took him about fifteen years to destroy one of the best surgical departments in the world. During his reign, he also killed at least a thousand baboons in his elegant laboratory, where he attempted to prove, in vain, that total lymphoid irradiation is the optimal modality to induce immunosuppression after transplant surgery. Myburgh spoke English like an Oxford don and Afrikaans like an Afrikaner farm boy. But a Free State farm boy, he would always remain. I cannot forget this image: an afternoon interview in his spacious office; the almighty chairman behind his mahogany desk, talking to me and simultaneously, very carefully, clipping the nails of his long brown fingers with a large nail clipper fixed to a key chain. I was mesmerized, particularly by how he created a small mountain of nail clippings on his desk and how elegantly he managed to discard it into the ashtray, where one of his regular cigarettes was burning. More about Myburgh later. Now back to our first week in Johannesburg.

Until January, I was assigned to a few SHO jobs. The first was at the trauma unit of the Johannesburg Hospital. The trauma boss was Mr. Hymie Green, a South African Jew in his fifties. I presented myself before Hymie the day after arrival. He cheerfully pressed my hand: "*Shalom* Moshe, you will enjoy it here. You know, I fought with the *Haganah* in your War of Independence. I was only seventeen but volunteered, fought until '49, then returned to South Africa. Later I tried to practice in Israel but couldn't take the *chara*... I still know all the good words in Hebrew. You were right to come here — we'll train you well. By the way, do you have a place to stay? Not yet. Come and stay with me, yes, come with your wife and baby. I'm divorced, and the house is large. I'll pick you up tomorrow afternoon. The day after tomorrow, you will be on your first trauma call at night."

"With whom will I be taking the call?" I asked.

"What do you mean with whom? You'll be alone. You are here to learn surgery, right? Do you have a car? Good. What? Ronnie Bass, Citroen? *Oi vei.*"

Thus, we settled down in Hymie's spacious suburban house. His black maid — house servants were the norm — prepared a dinner of lamb chops; Hymie provided a five-liter box of chilled white Cape wine. I had never seen boxed wine before. I remember how it tasted. Delicious.

The next evening, at 6 o'clock, I presented myself in a shirt, tie, and white coat, as instructed, at the trauma section of the casualty department (ER) of the JHB Hospital. Hymie did not prove a talkative person, but from whatever instructions I retrieved from him, I learned that during the night, I — a first-year surgical trainee on his first day — would be responsible for the receiving area. "Oh, nothing to worry about. Our trauma nurses are superb, and you can always summon help from the general surgical team on call."

I remember two distinct incidents from that first night of my surgical training.

The first: Hymie calls around 10 p.m.: "Moshe, *ata beseder*?" (Are you OK? in Hebrew) and then: "Aren't you worried?"

"Well, of course, I'm worried. You know, being alone."

"No, I don't mean that. Aren't you worried about your beautiful young wife, um, alone with me?"

"Of course not." I did not understand what he meant. Was he kidding? I don't know, but I remember Hymie as a good man, although a little peculiar and talking in riddles.

The second incident: after midnight, the paramedics unloaded an injured man onto a stretcher in the trauma room. I clearly remember this scene: a huge young man, a biker, clad in black leather overalls and boots. His yellow hair is saturated in sweat, blood, and vomited gastric contents — his pink face — now rapidly turning blue — moist, and unshaven.

A cloud of evaporated alcohol hangs about the man who is combative, impossible to restrain. From time to time, he groans a faint "fuck man" (the "man" in Afrikaans sounds like *maan*); these are to be his last words. I examine him while the nurses insert an IV line and a urinary catheter and restrain his limbs. "Doctor, he's struggling for air. You'll have to intubate him" (transcutaneous oximeters were unavailable in those days).

"OK, get me a size nine tube. Give 10mg valium, please."

"Doctor, valium won't touch him. We use pentothal here."

"Whatever, just let's put the tube in."

Surely, you can guess what happened. It is so predictable that there is no need to finish the story. Pentothal (a paralyzing muscle agent) is given, and the drunk biker stops breathing, but I can't insert the tube — I simply can't visualize his vocal cords — so deep down in his fat bull neck. We continue bagging him, but his airway is clogged, and he is turning bluer. "Get the surgical team. He needs a tracheostomy," I scream.

"Doctor, they're all in the operating theatre, scrubbed."

I look at the monitor, where the complexes on the ECG are slow, slower, and sporadic.

Blind transnasal intubation? I still have to learn how to perform it.

Tracheostomy? I never did — in fact, never saw — one. Finally: a flat line.

So, they undressed, cleaned, wrapped, and rolled him away. *First call, first fuck up, first casualty* — on my personal learning curve.

Six o'clock the next morning. Hymie is strolling through the receiving area, a cup of coffee in his hand and a morning newspaper folded under his arm. He is examining the night logbook. "A biker, hum? Multi-trauma, difficult intubation. Yep, I know. You did well, Moshe. Now go home to sleep. Your young wife is waiting… and, hmm, I told Heidi to start looking for accommodation, Hymie's Hotel will accommodate you for two weeks only."

Yes, I was troubled about the night's events. I was faintly disturbed by the casual attitude of the system. *But this is how things are,* I thought. *I learned some lessons, and I will learn more tomorrow.* And soon, hopefully, I will be like one of these senior residents: navy blue college tie on their white shirts, who already call themselves Mister — those who know about everything and can do anything.

Much later, I would perceive that in any society where life is cheaper for some, it must be cheap for most.

* * * * *

After a brief stay with Hymie, whose house we were pressed to leave, we rented a bedroom at Helen's house in the northern suburbs. Helen was a shriveled, octogenarian, Jewish widow living alone in a spacious house, now in disrepair, but its prior glory evident. The terms included using the kitchen and living rooms, furnished as they were in the 1940s, and the vast neglected garden.

The house was surrounded by well-kept mansions with Mercedes and Jaguars in the driveways; the usual squads of maids, cooks, and gardeners loitering at the gates. This is what I recall of Helen's house: the musty, stale odors of decay, mildew, and cat urine; the yellow, brown dry grass on which, under the warm mid-winter sun, I played with little Omri, drank Lion beer, or napped after the night shifts at the trauma unit. I also recall Helen's abdominal aortic aneurysm, which I failed to diagnose. One night she knocked on our bedroom door and whined in her South African-Jewish-English accent: "Doctor, I have severe back pain."

I woke up, examined her, including the abdomen, and concluded: "You must have strained your back. Here, take these pills." A month later, she collapsed and died. The autopsy showed a ruptured aneurysm — an aneurysm that I had missed. Suddenly, the house filled up with members of the family whom we had never seen before. The possessions were divided — we got Helen's ancient cat, Louise. A "For sale" sign appeared at the gate. After three months in Jo'burg, we had to look for yet another accommodation.

Our next domicile was a rented tiny, rustic two-bedroom bungalow in the remote, modest but lush suburb of Ferndale, just at the northern edge of town. An acre of garden separated us from the property's main, ugly, and shabby, converted farmhouse, owned by the South African writer Wessel Ebersohn. Wessel, then in his mid-40s, was a very tall and handsome man with a white beard. He talked softly, in good English but with a marked Cape Afrikaans accent. He seemed shy, and his blue eyes expressed consideration and kindness. He had been raised in the Cape, never completed any formal education, and had worked for many years as a postal clerk in rural Transvaal. There he had met his wife Miriam — a short, well-built, small-town Afrikaner girl. I did not realize it then, but Wessel had published his first novel *A Lonely Place to Die*, only a year earlier. It immediately became an internationally acclaimed political anti-apartheid thriller. Although not aware of his literary success (the humble man never mentioned his books to me), I perceived that Wessel belonged to that tiny group of liberal whites — mostly English-speaking whites and Jews — the anti-apartheid activists.

A small crumbling shed stood on the lower confines of the Ebersohns' acreage, well below the swimming pool (which we were never invited to use) and our cottage, where the summer rains drained into a small stream. This was the servants' quarters for the Ebersohns' domestic *kaffirs*: Trafina, a middle-aged maid, and her son Moses, the gardener. Like any Johannesburg servants' hut, their hut also served their brothers, sisters, cousins, friends, and guests. That there was an entire black community living a parallel, shadowy, and subversive life within the white-only suburbs — using servants' back gates and lanes — we would learn, gradually, later. But what we saw then was a dirty little room without heating and sanitation, like a pig stall.

We soon noted that the liberal anti-apartheid Ebersohns treated their servants — the term "domestics" was preferable — not much differently as one would treat house dogs; that is dogs who are not allowed to sleep inside the house. Heidi, who spent hours in their house, observed the superciliousness which Miriam and her grown-up kids — not Wessel himself — reserved for the blacks. "They use two different voices," Heidi observed, "one, gentle, polite, considerate. The other, harsh, brief, impatient, used to approach the blacks." The servants never ate what their masters ate, but received inferior *kaffir* rations. The food pantry at the Ebersohns was permanently locked with a key — "ag, they steal, they always steal," Miriam explained.

Then there was Moses, the gardener. One morning I heard baby Omri giggling hysterically in his baby seat on the porch. I saw a short, thin young black guy grimacing behind the garden fence, baring his teeth like an ape, trying to entertain the baby. If I could write a novel about South Africa, I would choose Moses as the main character. Do you want to see Moses? Just read J.M. Coetzee's *Life and Times of Michael K.* Like Michael K., Moses was a disfigured and fatherless gardener, a simpleton — his mind was 'dull' and not quick. But behind this facade was a person who could not harm a fly.

Despite his sudden literary fame, Wessel was struggling financially — always looking for new sources of income, including a publishing business he established with his wife in their house. Heidi, now pregnant, was hired to help and spent the days in their office. One morning — naturally, I learned about this much later — Wessel approached Heidi from behind, put his hands on her bulging tummy, and confessed that he was attracted to her. I do not know what happened then, but within a month, we were told to look for another accommodation because their "daughter wishes to move into the cottage with her prospective bridegroom." It must have been Miriam's idea. Most probably, she realized that her husband had developed a crush on Heidi.

We relocated to a small, old stone house in Hurst Hill. It was a purely Afrikaans-speaking working-class suburb on the western edge of town. Rent was cheap, as a slum of 'colored people' was just across the main road. A few weeks after we moved in, I returned home unexpectedly early, after a heavy night, to find Wessel sitting with Heidi in the kitchen, drinking tea. "Oh, I just dropped by to check whether you settled in," he said. And then he left, and we never saw him again. He published a few more books, including *Closed Circle* (1992). On Google, I see that today Wessel is publishing and writing for commercial periodicals of financial interest.

A month after we moved to Hurst Hill, Trafina showed up at our garden gate, with Moses tailing behind, with a vast box balanced on his sweating head.

"Madame," she told Heidi, "We were fired. Madame Miriam said we stole food. I only took some leftovers for Moses. We were hungry." So now, a year after arriving in South Africa, we had our own servants, sorry, "domestics."

* * * * *

Top: the young Professor Johannes Albertus Myburgh (1928-2010). Middle left: first days in Johannesburg with little Omri. Middle right: Heidi with Omri and newborn Yariv in Hurst Hill. Bottom right: Trafina with Omri and baby Yariv in Ferndale.

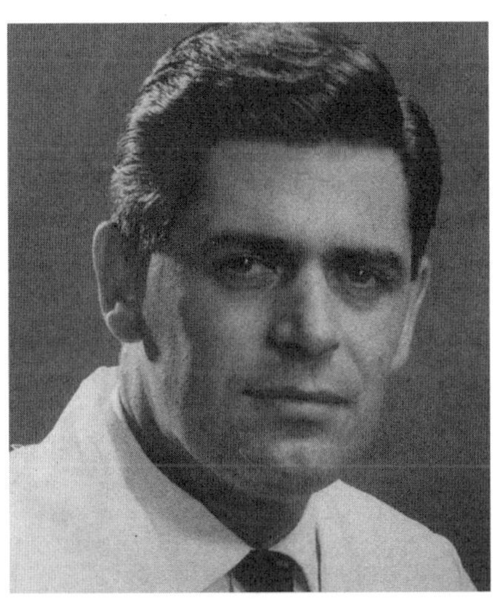

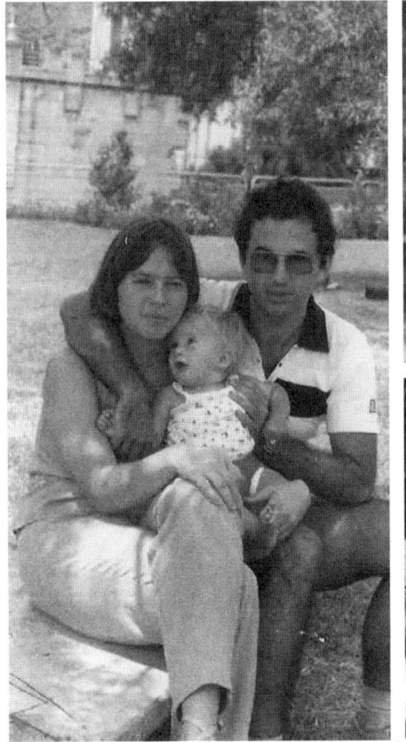

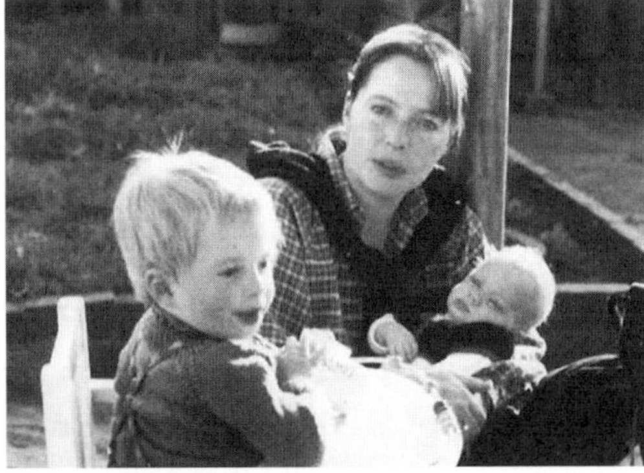

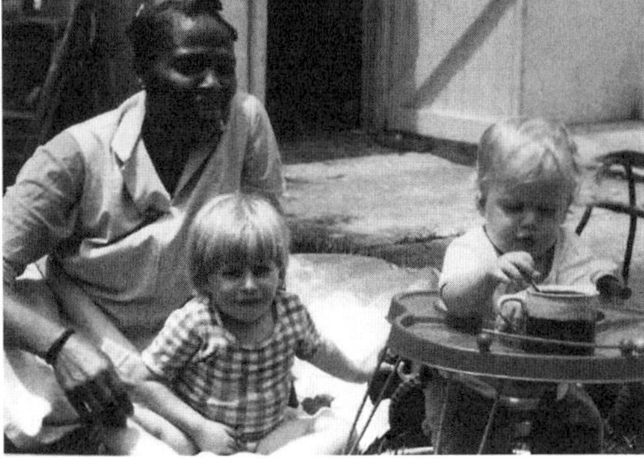

Fifteen

Senior House Officer

In October 1980, I was assigned to the Coronation Hospital. It was a teaching hospital serving the 'non-white,' colored, and Indian communities on the western border of the town. I was allocated to the surgical unit of Professor Cedric Bremner. His unit, one of the three in Coronation, was structured the same as all twelve units affiliated with the university department. It had a head, another full-time consultant, two rotating registrars, a bunch of interns (3-5), and an occasional SHO. Add to it the voluntary faculty – two or three private surgeons who shared the call roster with the two full-time consultants; they also taught the students and joined the weekly grand rounds.

My first impression of Professor Bremner was this: in his early fifties, short, thin, hyperactive, clownish – a typical funny confused professor. Only later, when working under him as a registrar and even later as a consultant, would I realize what a kind and educated person he was. He was the first to prove that acid reflux is the cause of Barrett's esophagus, and he was considered a leading international authority on the esophagus. I would also hear that after his mentor – the former Chairman du Plessis – had retired, Bremner was exiled to this lowly, shabby, and messy 'colored hospital' by his new boss, Myburgh. A contemporary analogy would be a professor of surgery at Manhattan's Cornell New York Hospital on the East River, banished over the stinking Harlem River to the 'dump' called the Bronx Lebanon Hospital. But privates do not know much about their generals, and young doctors are often not aware of the actual value of their superiors.

My first encounter with Prof. Bremner was the morning after my first 'intake' – when our unit was on call. It was like this: 7.55 a.m. sharp – the male ward. Sixty patients lying on beds organized in four straight rows, like in a Victorian hospital with Florence Nightingale in charge. The sun shines through the tall windows, illuminating the flies buzzing around. A bunch of giant cockroaches hide in the corners, awaiting the night and yet another feast of human excreta and blood. The surgical team stands at the door awaiting the Prof: the residents, Jeff F. and Toni M., and five interns, all nice English-looking boys, all freshly shaven, in dark dress pants, white shirts, blue ties, highly polished old boys' black shoes, and white coats – like on parade in Oxford or ready for church.

Eight a.m. The Prof. appears, dressed exactly like his disciples. He walks and talks fast, visibly energetic, visibly keen to help all these wretches he has been forced to care for. But above all, he is eager to teach — teaching is his life. "Good morning, chaps? How's it?" He glances across the room and sees no stretchers between the beds. "You slept well, chaps, ha?"

"Good morning, Prof. Yes, the intake was light," says the tall, red-haired Jeff.

"Good morning, Prof. It wasn't too bad, thank you, Sir," adds the shy, dark-haired Toni.

The Prof. looks at the bunch of interns. "And where is our new SHO, the Israeli chap?"

"We don't know, Prof. He must be somewhere around."

8.05 a.m. I appear, dragging my feet in white, blood-stained wooden clogs; my white coat — its pockets exploding with syringes, tubes, notes, and manuals — hardly covers the white scrubs, which are stained in clotted blood and dry pus. I am sleepless but euphoric: this was my first real South African intake — I feel as if returning from a raid across the Lebanese border. I feel elated.

The Prof. opens his mouth, but no sound is emitted. He looks at me in disbelief. During his thirty years in JHB's medical environment, he has never seen such a scruffy intern, SHO, or registrar. Imagine: unshaven and no tie — for the professorial rounds!

The team observes us in silence — what will the Prof. do to him?

The Prof. stabs at my chest with his index finger and says icily: "Man, this is unacceptable. Go, shave, and change, and then come back. Hurry, man!"

"But… I was busy until now. You see, the patient there is bleeding." I point to the other corner of the ward. While the team showered, shaved, changed, and ate breakfast, I had resuscitated the guy who had arrived from the ER in the early morning, vomiting fresh blood. All eyes shift across the vast room where a junior nurse is attending to a brown body lying beneath the blankets. All eyes shift back on me when the Prof. barks: "Dr. Schein. This is South Africa. This is Johannesburg. This is the University of the Witwatersrand. We wear ties, ties, ties — man, do you understand? We wear ties to respect our patients! Move, man, now, go."

"Yes Sir." And off I went and shaved and changed and put on my tie. Then I came back and joined the professorial rounds, which stopped at each bed, where we discussed in detail everything that had been done and should be done until — two hours later — we arrived at the bed of my bleeding patient, still lying under his blankets, but now cold dead. I opened my mouth to present the case, but Jeff intercepted me: "Prof. a colored man, alcoholic, known esophageal varices, ascites. A recurrent bleed, came up to the floor on a Pitressin drip…"

This prompted the Prof. to a mini speech about which treatment modality is better: the sclerotherapy of bleeding esophageal varices mastered by Prof. Terblanche's Cape Town group or the splenorenal shunt advocated by Prof. Myburgh in Johannesburg. Then to me, now kindlier, the Prof. said: "Moshe, next week you'll give us a short talk on the emergency management of bleeding esophageal varices. And, man, your tie is horrible, go and get yourself a bunch of decent ties, man."

But the picture of that brown man slowly exsanguinating in the corner of the room with ten doctors discussing ties, and rounding a few yards away, haunted me then and still haunts me today. During the many years to come, I got used to many things but never to apathy.

During that rotation, I did my early solo surgical procedures. The first was a dorsal slit of the foreskin for phimosis, complicating a penile human bite, which was not an infrequent injury in these parts... The second was a below-elbow amputation of a gangrenous arm. I remember doing both operations while consulting the relevant pages of *Farquharson's Textbook of Operative General Surgery*, with the old anesthetist looking over my shoulder, *kibitzing*.

* * * * *

Even in hindsight, many years later, I am impressed by how technically capable a few of the junior registrars (residents) were. One of them was Carlos de Nobrega, who was younger than I was. He was a fair-looking man of Portuguese-Mozambique extraction with a bushy blond mustache, blue eyes, and a permanent naughty smile. Assisting him at night, watching him remove shattered organs, and repairing complex injuries, I was amazed at how well such a trainee operated — how smoothly his fingers danced through the tissues. He told me that during medical school, he spent his vacations in some remote bush hospital, where "they let me do whatever I wished." He used to operate on fresh cadavers, training himself to perform major operations such as esophageal and pancreatic resections. We became good friends. Later, Carlos moved to cardiac surgery. He could perform a coronary bypass faster than his boss could but repeatedly failed any written or oral examination he had to take. He was a master technician who could not qualify as a surgeon. He became a general practitioner somewhere around Johannesburg and disappeared from sight. Eventually, somebody mentioned that Carlos had emigrated to New Zealand. I cannot find a trace of him on the web. But I remember him fondly and how any operation looked like a 'piece of cake' in his young hands. Oh yes, I also recall that Carlos made me smoke the first (and last) 'joint' I ever tasted.

* * * * *

Another memory entrenched in my mind from those early Coronation days is of Mr. Stephen Eisenhammer (1906-1995). One day Professor Bremner said, "did you meet Mr. Eisenhammer? Go and see him. He sits in the outpatient clinic once a week, seeing anal cases. No one understands the anus like him." Reluctantly — *who cares about the anus* — I complied. In a tiny room in that shabby clinic, I encountered an ancient, feeble looking thin gentleman who mumbled to me a few words. I left after a few minutes. Only later I learned that this old man was the real pioneer in the anatomy, physiology, and treatment of all those common anal diseases that we see and treat each day. He was the one who accurately described the etiology and anatomy of fistula-in-ano. He was the one that understood the pathophysiology of anal fissure and described its treatment with an internal sphincterotomy. The late Sir Alan Parks, a renowned colorectal guru from St. Mark's Hospital in London, later 'stole' many of Eisenhammer's ideas and published them without citing the latter. When I returned to Coronation a year later, Eisenhammer was already dead. Message: to receive credit for your innovations, to have a novel procedure named after you — you must possess a proper pulpit.

On January 1, 1981, I commenced a year of the formal 'SHO circuit' at the New Jo'burg Hospital. It started with a most devastating post-Sylvester hangover — the worst. It was a beautiful summer morning when I crawled out of bed and collapsed on the stony kitchen floor into a pool of half-digested red wine, champagne, brandy, and other unidentifiable fluids. Heidi resuscitated me, loaded me into our 'yellow submarine,' and drove me to the hospital: "Pull yourself together. This is your first day. He wanted you to be there at 7 a.m." My head was pounding as if hit with a ten-pound hammer. All I wanted was to fall asleep. I hardly knew where I was going, only that he was Professor James Chase, the Chief of Pediatric Surgery, which was to be my first rotation. At the hospital, Heidi schlepped me into the pediatric wing and up to the surgical unit, where she dropped me off and drove home.

In the conference room, I found my new comrades: Moshe Fayman, the other Israeli on the SHO circuit, now a plastic surgeon in Jo'burg, and George Louridas, a delightful Greek South African, who later became a great vascular surgeon and a good friend (tragically, in 2007 he passed away in Winnipeg from a brain tumor). The professor looked at me coldly and hissed: "You must be Dr. Schein, eh? You are late. As of tomorrow, you will be starting at 5.30 a.m. I will round with you at 6 a.m. daily, understand? And Schein, this is not Tel Aviv; we are not orthodox Jews. We shave, OK?"

"Yes Sir!"

Thus started the most unpleasant three months of training under a difficult man. Prof. Chase, blond, tall, slender, in his mid-forties, was a talented and erudite pediatric surgeon. But he was an obsessive, boisterous, authoritative maniac who ran his consultant, registrars, and SHOs, like slaves in a concentration camp. He would often arrive at the unit at 4 a.m., round on all new patients, wake up the SHO on call, and give him hell… Next, he would round again with the entire team. In the late afternoon, the Prof. would conduct prolonged seminars criticizing everything we said. His evening rounds often continued into the night. The overall atmosphere in his unit was hostile to us, the two Israeli SHOs, and anti-Semitic. His bunch of stiffly starched lesbian nurses, who looked like matrons, discussed the "Jewish doctors" in Afrikaans as if we did not understand. Over more than forty years of practice out of Israel I never had experienced such overt anti-Semitism except in that department. Obviously, one never knows what is being said behind one's back.

One of Chase's 'hobbies' was watching newborns with Down's syndrome dying. When a newborn with Down's syndrome, and some associated anatomical abnormality, was admitted to the unit, Chase would subject the distressed parents to a solemn lecture, depicting a hopeless situation. His advice was always to do nothing and let the wretched babies die. The poor chubby and pink cute babies were then placed in a side cubicle, deprived of food and fluids, condemned to a prolonged death – often it took five to seven days to die – from dehydration and starvation as if left unattended in the desert. Twice daily, at the end of the rounds, the psychopath would take us into the room, where the babies were howling, and marvel at their human strength – polling us on how many days it would take for a specific baby to expire. Between us SHOs, we started to call him Dr. Mengele.

On the morning of our last day in his unit, Chase said to the three of us: "Well, let's have a farewell lunch at Sunnyside, OK?" Sunnyside was a fashionable colonial hotel near the hospital, a popular but expensive watering hole. The lunch on the sunny terrace, under the shade of tall trees, included seafood and two bottles of chilled Bellingham Premier Grand Cru. It seemed that Chase was relaxed and enjoying himself. No one stirred when the black waiter dropped the bill on the table; we looked at Chase, waiting for him to draw out his wallet. But the Head of Pediatric Surgery kept his red-haired hands on the table and said: "Oh, I never carry any money with me." With a heavy heart, George, Moshe, and I extracted a hundred rands each and placed it on the silver tray. When Chase left, we spat in his direction. As I am writing this, I find on Google that he, in his eighties, is still practicing pediatric surgery somewhere in the Western Hemisphere.

I still can hear the small Down syndrome babies shrieking — like starving puppies.

* * * * *

Like daily newspapers, these pages tend to focus on the negative and the sensational. For who would care to read about pleasant, everyday events, about all those who welcomed us to South Africa, treated us well, and taught us surgery?

However, I should mention another SHO rotation during that year. It occurred in thoracic surgery. Here I realized how excellent 'first world' surgery can be applied under 'third world' conditions — if somebody cares and has the initiative. That somebody was Mr. Alan Conlan, a South African-trained Irish surgeon who, in Leratong, an outlying black hospital, had established a center of excellence for thoracic and esophageal surgery. The unit was swamped with up to a hundred esophageal cancer cases per week. Because of environmental factors, this devastating cancer is endemic among South African blacks, mostly presenting in advanced stages. I remember how gently Mr. Conlan used to approach these cachectic patients. They sat apathetically in their beds, drowning in their own saliva — which they could not swallow — staring into space and puffing on homemade cigarettes. A nauseating smell of halitosis emitted from the obstructed esophagi permeated the air. Mr. Conlan would speak to them in his soft Irish accent as if they were gentlemen from Cork. I also gathered that one does not have to work at the Mayo Clinic to publish meaningful clinical papers. Later, I believe, Mr. Conlan practiced thoracic surgery in Massachusetts.

In some countries, after a notable academic surgeon retires, his colleagues often celebrate the events with a *festschrift* — a collection of articles by the surgeon dedicated to him or about him. Reading such collections, I enjoy examining the surgeon's list of publications, noting his development or decline reflected in his writing and where it was published. Typically, and almost invariably, the first publication is a clinical case report, and the last is an editorial — mostly on philosophical, non-clinical aspects of surgery. I know that no *festschrift* will ever be dedicated to me. Still, during that first year of training, I wrote and published my first paper in the *South African Medical Journal* entitled "Penile tumescence — a complication of peritoneal lavage." I remember seeing my name in print, for the first time, on the glossy paper of the journal. I was hooked, and this was the beginning of an addiction.

* * * * *

Left: Professor Cedric Bremner. Right: George Louridas (died in 2007, aged fifty-three).

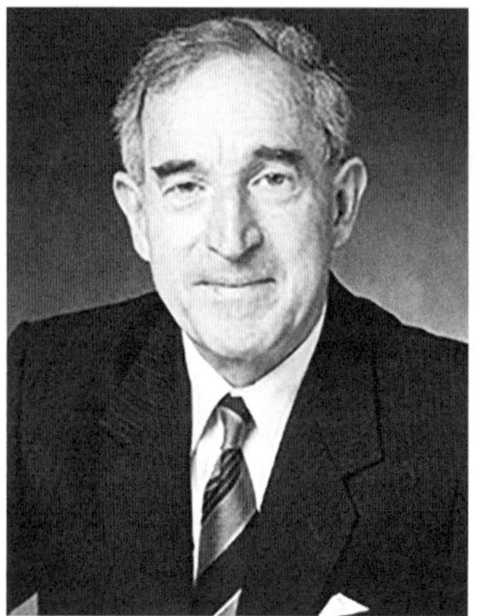
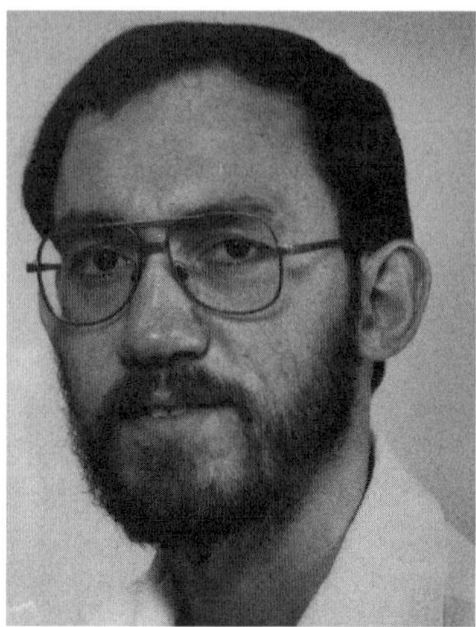

Sixteen

See one, do one, teach one

"In this Department, my dear chap, you'll learn how to cut and cut," muttered the soft-spoken Professor "Buddy" Lawson with a fixed smirk. He was the Chairman of Surgery at Baragwanath Hospital.

This was January 1982, my first day of residency in his department, which comprised five units, each treating up to a hundred patients simultaneously. The professor's was probably one of the world's largest academic general surgical departments. Prof. Lawson, who looked like a fox, was known to be the first to correlate gastric metaplasia and cancer with duodeno-gastric bile reflux.

The professor ushered me into the surgical unit led by the notorious Mr. "Bokkie" R. — whose other nickname was "the cowboy." This title was founded on his athletic frame — always clad in a white-starched safari suit — his rough military attitude and bearing, and above all, on the huge handgun bulging under his white safari jacket.

When I arrived at Bokkie's all-male ward — a hanger-like structure of 80 beds, I found Bokkie, a tall, robust man with a pink face, a prominent Jewish nose, and a bald scalp, inspecting his doctor troops. I introduced myself and straightaway received what was known as Bokkie's standard welcome speech. It included Bokkie's gospel on surgery which consisted of pearls such as: "You should always open the abdomen with a blade, and in one stroke," or "In my unit, there is no place for closed cardiac massage, I want you to crack open all chests," and "No round abdominal drains in my unit, only flat ones, is that clear?"

At the end of his tirade, Bokkie, the 'cowboy' towered over me, poked me in the chest, and concluded: "Hey Schein, just remember, I won't tolerate any Israeli cowboy in my unit, understand?"

Led by the senior registrar Dimitri, I joined the troops on morning rounds. We followed Bokkie from bed to bed. With a servile smile, Dimitri (and the rest of the team) tolerated an ongoing stream of abuse and an inane sense of humor, which was also directed at the patients. The only discussions I heard on Bokkie's rounds were comprised of "Yes Sir" or "Yes, Mr. R." At 10 o'clock sharp, Bokkie looked at his watch and commanded, "Chaps. Teatime." The entire unit would retreat for the ritual tea, with milk, served with cute little triangle-shaped sandwiches of anchovy paste or marmite.

On that first day, during tea, while Bokkie lectured the team on politics, surgery, and guns — "Yes Sir" and vigorous head nods were the universal response — I read a reprint of a surgical paper. Bokkie swallowed another anchovy sandwich, eyeing me suspiciously: "Schein, show me what you're reading!" He looked at the paper with disgust: "Pericardiocentesis in penetrating heart injury? *American Journal of Surgery*. Tell me, what on earth do Americans understand about stabbed hearts?" He contemptuously threw the paper to the floor, "I don't want you to read this crap while in my unit. No one can teach us how to treat cardiac injuries — we lead the world. Pericardiocentesis... fools." So began my short but memorable stint in Bokkie's unit. Almost immediately, I sensed that my prognosis was grim.

Surgeons don't have patience for tall ancient tales. *Who cares what this old fart did thirty or forty years ago!* For most young surgeons, anything that does not belong to the present, or the future, is useless. But even those who would not care to listen would find my Baragwanath stories hard to believe. How can they — products of today's tightly supervised training — imagine a surgical program guided by the motto of "see one, do one, teach one?"

Baragwanath Hospital (we called it "Bara") is located at the heart of Soweto — a swarming black township of several million. It was an urban battle zone then and probably still is today, albeit today, fought with better weapons — guns are replacing knives. The great 'wars' would regularly erupt on Friday (payday). With fresh cash in their pockets, the locals — propelled by cheap wine or homebrewed ale (*kaffir* beer) — became victims of violent crime or its perpetrators. The feast of fury, persisting through the weekend, would overwhelm the on-call unit with a constant tide of horrendous injuries. The surgical receiving area, locally called "the pit," would resemble a dressing station in Stalingrad (or perhaps Gaza, 2024). There were patients on stretchers, chairs, and floors with crushed skulls, stabbed chests, shot abdomens, and mangled vessels — the smell of sweat, shit, piss, pus, vomitus, and old blood permeating the air.

Still, the chaos was semi-organized. Those surviving the triage, and the resuscitation room, were wheeled to the nearby operating rooms. The latter worked non-stop, day and night. What made the scene so singular was not only the unbelievable volume of severe injuries — imagine a night with seven laparotomies, four explorations of the neck, two shot subclavian arteries, three stabbed hearts, three peripheral vascular injuries, not to mention the bread and butter of emergency general surgery — but the absolute surgical independence we, the trainees, were permitted to 'enjoy,' often at the patients' expense.

The contrast between the day and night was stark. During the day, academic professors taught us surgery; then, they would depart, leaving us as the kings of the stormy nights. The chief king of the night in Bokkie's unit was our senior registrar Dimitri — a shrewd thin Cypriot who had taught himself to become a master trauma surgeon. At night, he was there to supervise, control, teach, and assist us, while during the day, he was a humble 'yes man' to Bokkie and any other South African professor. This was the secret to his success, which would later make him the Baragwanath surgical boss, and later one of the most notable trauma surgeons in the United States.

* * * * *

Bara Hospital. I see a huge WW II era complex, one story and tin-roofed, of military barracks converted to patients' wards — barracks left behind by the British military as they did across Africa and the Middle East. The barracks are interconnected with paved passageways, roofed with galvanized tin but open to the elements.

I see patches of grass between the barracks, where under the shade of tall eucalyptuses, groups of young patients in torn pajamas, drains dangling from their chests, exercise under the watchful eyes of a blonde physiotherapist. Inside the barracks — freezing in winter and scorching in summer — smells of sweat, clotted blood, dried pus, spilled urine, lost feces, rotting flesh, cigarettes, Lysol, human breath, and food permeated the air. The food provided to Bara patients was basic: bread, jam, lumpy porridge, thin soup, an occasional piece of tough meat; tea or coffee, which tasted the same — a far cry from what white patients received, from the same hospital administration, at the 'white hospitals.'

I see a chilly dawn, the barracks immersed in smog emitted by millions of fires burning in nearby Soweto. Bloodstained and sleep-deprived, we round on the numerous patients admitted the previous night — the critically ill lie on stretchers near the nursing station. We have nowhere else to put them because the intensive care unit is always full. Others lie on beds and mattresses, between the beds, and even beneath the beds. Those with 'minor' injuries, such as a simple puncture of the lung, spill into the corridors. They sit patiently on hard, wooden benches, smoking hand-rolled cigarettes made of crude, black Zimbabwean tobacco, coughing and bubbling air into the water bottles connected to their chest drains. For hours, we stroll from patient to patient. Sometimes we find a corpse under a bed: a 'missed' injury.

But where the real action takes place is the notorious 'pit.' I see a line of stretchers along the long and shabby corridors leading to the pit's shock room doors. On the stretchers, slouching and stoic, are young males to whom suffering is no stranger. Most of them are semi-comatose from intoxication or loss of blood. At first, I ran from stretcher to stretcher to see which of the victims, wrapped in thick, stained woolen blankets, is bleeding to death from a thoracic wound — forming a red pool under his stretcher. "But Moshe," Sam B. — a middle-aged experienced ex-Russian surgeon, now one of Bokkie's lackeys — admonishes me, "you can't save 'em all. Don't waste your time. First come, first served."

Here in the pit, we pick our stabbed hearts or bleeding subclavian arteries; running, we wheel them to the nearby OR, shouting "stabbed heart" or stabbed something, compelling the OR team into a frenzy of action.

* * * * *

See one, do one, teach one. Yes, this is what we did and how we learned, but it was an abnormal learning process. A standard, conventional course of learning would start with a couple of hernias, or varicose veins, under supervision. However, here the first operation I did was to repair an acute diaphragmatic hernia, with Sam B. standing behind my back, shouting in his Russian-English mixed with some Hebrew, "*chort,* take bigger bites, *kadima.*" After assisting on numerous stabbed hearts, and doing one, helped by Dimitri, I started doing them on my own — I saved a few but lost some that, most probably, could have survived — if operated on by Dimitri himself. I found the freedom exhilarating. However, I had already realized that our independence was immature and harmful to our patients. I remember being sent to do a technically demanding arterio-venous fistula for hemodialysis after only seeing one. I noticed that those who teach one after doing one often teach it wrongly. I cannot forget watching a third-year Portuguese registrar 'teaching' a junior how to repair an inguinal hernia — the repair they performed was placed in front of the spermatic cord and not behind it, as it ought to be.

My career in Bokkie's unit did not last long. Predictably, my personality was inherently opposed to any ruthless dictator. And so, I did not comply with his commandments.

Even when I did comply — things turned out wrong.

Thou shalt use only open cardiac massage.

This crazy rule I took too seriously. I find it hard to believe I am not dreaming about what I will describe. One morning as I was strolling through the busy recovery room, a nurse pointed to a male lying on a stretcher with a bandage over his abdomen: "Doctor, he's not breathing." I noticed the guy had a tube in his trachea, obviously waking up from some abdominal operation. I felt for his femoral pulse — nothing.

Carotid? None. Monitors? No monitor. There were not enough monitors for everybody. *He has arrested*, I thought — *he needs a cardiac massage*. I looked around for help but only saw a few nurses. *Thou shalt use only open cardiac massage*, Bokkie had said. "Give me a knife, nurse... come on, keep bagging him." It took thirty seconds for my ungloved hands to grasp a heart that, my right hand felt, was full of blood and pumping beautifully.

"What the hell are you doing?" asked a young surgeon with a Greek accent whom I had never seen before.

"An open massage, he arrested, your patient, eh?" I said laconically, as if what I had just done was the most commonplace thing to do.

"Um, he has a normal pulse now; what's his BP, mama?"

"One hundred and twenty over eighty," said the fat mama.

"Strange," the Greek shrugged, "Nurse, continue to bag him, give him some morphine. He's waking up. I will organize a theatre. We have to close his chest."

I left. I realized I had done a stupid thing — I opened that poor man's chest for no real reason. I was awaiting the repercussions, which luckily never arrived.

Thou shalt not be a cowboy.

I agree with this statement, although the system forced me to be one.

One morning after tea, Dimitri ordered: "Moshe, they have asked for a tracheostomy in the ICU. You have done a few, right? So take an intern and do it." I selected a female intern. I forgot her name and how she looked. But I remember well how we both 'killed' that young girl beginning to recover from tetanus after two weeks of mechanical ventilation and muscle paralysis.

"Moshe, can I do it?" begged the intern on the way to the ICU.

Teach one! "Sure," I said, "you'll do it." We performed it at the bedside under inadequate lighting. Everything went well until I committed a classic error. The intern opened the trachea — a spray of air and blood rushed out — exposing the endotracheal tube. "Withdraw it," I commanded the nurse, not instructing her to do it slowly and leave the tip of the tube just above the hole in the trachea.

Instantly, the tube was out in the nurse's hands. The intern attempted to insert the tracheostomy tube, but it did not enter the trachea. "Come, let me do it," I hissed. After several attempts, the tube was finally in the correct position, but the monitor showed a flat line. The poor girl's heart did not tolerate even a short period of inadequate oxygenation.

I will never forget the bearded face of the director of the ICU when I came out of the cubicle and told him that the child — the girl for whose life he had fought for two weeks — was now dead. He turned white but said nothing. I could read contempt and hatred in his accusing eyes.

Then he turned his back on me, leaving me speechless and humiliated. Repercussions? None. When Dimitri informed Bokki, he mumbled something about the silly, fat black nurses.

Thou shalt not use round drains.

Late one chaotic night, two months into my residency, I took to the 'theatre,' — yet another abdominal gunshot wound. Knowing by then the holy rule that any organ has a potential entry and exit wound, I repaired the anterior and posterior injuries of the stomach, the fourth part of the duodenum, and the transverse colon. The body of the pancreas appeared bruised, so I left a large, round 'sump' drain in the lesser sac. Why did I use a *round* sump, ignoring Bokki's dictum? Because of what I had read in one of the American surgical books, which I was then devouring. It said: for the pancreas use sump drains! The operation was a great success for the patient, who eventually did well, but it brought only misery for his surgeon. The following day during rounds, I observed Bokkie's face turning red. "What's that?" he asked Dimitri. All eyes were on me.

"A sump drain Sir," I replied.

"Leave my unit immediately. Go and wait for me in front of the Prof's office."

I stood in Professor Lawson's office listening to Bokkie's ranting about my impudence and *chutzpah*. "He has to be thrown out of the residency," Bokkie demanded. When Bokkie left, the Prof. fox-smiled at me: "Moshe, as of today, you are working in my unit, on probation." At that time, Prof. Lawson was fifty-six years old. He looked ancient to me, although now, as I am writing this, I am much older than he was then, but I feel younger — perspectives of what's old and young change with aging. That 'old' man — Professor Lawson became old indeed, eventually dying in Johannesburg in 2019 at ninety-four — saved my surgical career.

Obviously, the see one, do one... practice I described must be denounced. Still, at the same time, we should not forget that forty years ago, the teaching pattern in certain American inner-city hospitals was not much different. Whatever critics may say, the surgical care provided to the masses of Soweto in those days represented one of the best available to African blacks.

On the day I left Baragwanath to continue with the second year of residency in another affiliated hospital, I felt almost like an accomplished surgeon. Was I?

Our residents today would not believe my Bara stories. Looking back, I cannot accept them myself.

* * * * *

Top: after a night in the 'pit' at Baragwanath Hospital. Bottom: the Baragwanath Hospital, Soweto, Johannesburg.

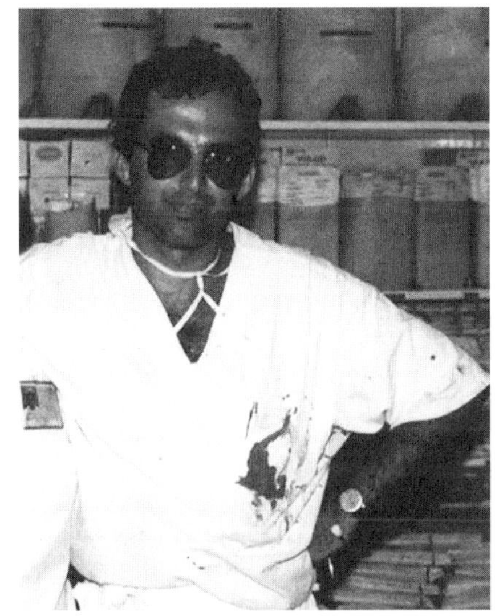

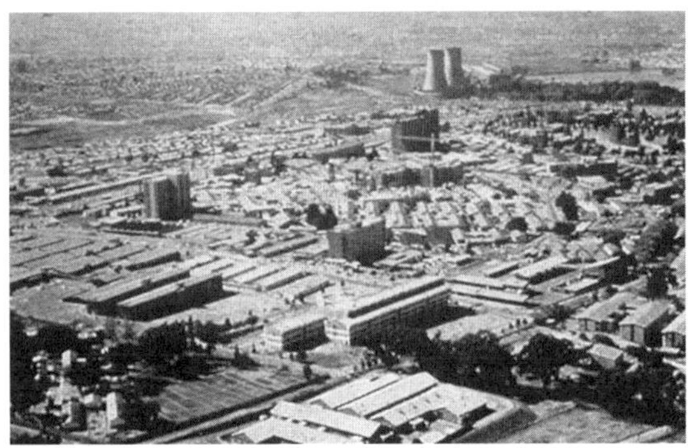

Seventeen

The 'colored' hospital

On January 1983, I was posted back to the 'colored' Coronation Hospital, now as a second-year registrar. It was a stark deviation from the original plan of training, which had been promised, in writing, by chairperson "Bert" Myburgh: "After completing a year as a rotating SHO, contingent on you passing the step I ('primary') examination of the South African College of Surgeons, you will be appointed a junior registrar in one of the affiliated hospitals. The last three years of residency will consist of rotations through the various surgical units at the Johannesburg Hospital." But a year into my residency in Johannesburg, two years after I passed the 'primary' exam, the famous chairman gathered us junior residents, solemnly announcing that he had decided that, from now on, only South African citizens would be allowed to continue training in his "all white" top-notch professorial unit. The others, namely the foreign citizens, would have to continue their training, rotating through the four affiliated hospitals — away from Myburgh's unit at the Johannesburg Hospital.

"I must train surgeons for South Africa. Those who will eventually leave are a second priority," the great professor declared solemnly, a burning cigarette in his hand. Myburgh's act affected three junior residents — two Israelis and a French Jew.

Was Myburgh an anti-Semite? Yes, it was possible. Many Afrikaners tended to be so, also xenophobic.

I resented Myburgh's decision but sympathizers, such as Hymie Green and Cedric Bremner, advised me to shut up. Another casualty of Myburgh's discrimination was a new friend I had made in Bara — Roger S. Roger, a French medical graduate, who had arrived at Bara following a few years of training in the UK, was condemned to continue with me on an "alternative residency pathway." Years later, before immigrating to Canada, Roger was to become a professor of surgery and head surgeon in Baragwanath. Roger, dark, slender, agile, sharp, brainy, philosophical, occasionally brooding and moody, sometimes euphoric, eloquent in literary, French-accented English, could be an interesting 'character' to develop. But to write or not to write about an intimate, living friend is a common memoirist's dilemma, and I choose not to.

I was 'full of myself' when I arrived at Coronation Hospital. I could open chests, fix hearts, tie arteries, explore shot abdomens, cut out the bowel, and hook up its ends. I could repair diaphragms and remove perforated appendices. *What can they teach me?* I thought.

I was allocated as the second registrar to Mr. Weisfish's unit.

Weisfish, Max was his initial name, was a short, thickly bespectacled orthodox Jew. On the eve of my first 'intake,' I asked Weisfish: "Sir, do I need to call you before taking any patient to the theater?" He looked at me as if I was out of my mind: "Of course, who do you think you are? I want to know everything, even if you take somebody with a perianal abscess. Everything. You call me for everything and anything, understand?"

But my first intake in Coronation was crazy. Coronation had no surgical 'pit' and so emergencies were triaged in a shabby casualty department by even shabbier casualty officers. Moribund patients were dispatched to the surgical floors with a tiny intravenous line, dripping a few drops of saline per hour. Alone with three interns, I would 'fish out' those who needed an operation and take them up in the dilapidated elevator to a rundown theater, where an elderly Indian female anesthetist would leisurely administer anesthesia. It was a far cry from Bara. That first intake, I operated throughout the night: a thoracotomy for a stabbed internal mammary artery, two laparotomies for stab wounds, a foot amputation for gas gangrene, an appendectomy, and as usual, an extended 'septic' list of abscesses and hand infections. I did not call Weisfish even once and never called him for any case thereafter. He did not appreciate it.

A few weeks into my stay in his unit, Weisfish summoned me to his office and declared: "Moshe, I'm trained in graphology. What I did here is to analyze your handwritten operative notes, see?" He spread copies of my notes on the table. "Unfortunately, I have to tell you that I found solid evidence, and I do not doubt my findings, that you are mentally disturbed — a *meshuggener*." He removed his glasses and polished its thick lenses with the tip of his soiled necktie, "Yes, talented, maybe — but a *meshuggener* — what should I do with you?"

However, gradually we got used to each other, and Max taught me some elective general surgery. I also assisted him in major operations but never appreciated his painful-to-watch, obsessive-compulsive techniques, including closing the duodenal stump in three layers in an interrupted fashion, using silk — it took an hour to accomplish.

Weisfish is entrenched in my memory as a weird fish. I remember sitting with him one afternoon in the 'breast clinic' he had established. I saw a young colored girl complaining of alleged breast lumps. She was simply stunning. A lovely face, incredibly statuesque — top model-like. This had rarely happened or would happen to me in clinical practice, but I felt attracted to the girl. I called Weisfish for a second opinion. He examined her breast rapidly, said, "It's nothing," and escaped. Later I asked him: "Gee, did you see her? Impressive, right?" He did not reply. Weisfish ended up in Israel practicing vascular surgery. The last time I looked him up, in 2020, he was advertising his private wound clinic on Facebook.

From Weisfish's unit, I moved on to Mr. Leni Stein's. He was an elderly, white-haired Jewish gentleman who had returned to a full-time hospital position after a distinguished career in private practice. Mr. Stein was an excellent general and vascular surgeon and a superb teacher, the old school fatherly type. He was the one who implanted in me the concept that excessive use of antibiotics and antiseptics is unnecessary and harmful, and that high fever is not a disease per se that should be treated.

A young boy was recovering from a gunshot wound of the rectum and sacrum – surgically treated with a colostomy – and running a high fever. I changed the antibiotics, but his fever continued to peak. I stopped the cheap antibiotics and prescribed a more expensive modern regimen, but each evening his temperature rose to 39.5° Celsius (103.1°F). I started irrigating his open sacral wound with betadine. The fever persisted. In desperation, I tried the archaic chloramphenicol. And then Mr. Stein stepped in: "Moshe, what are you doing? Stop poisoning him with antibiotics; stop burning his tissues with betadine. Just let him spike. Fever is a good sign that he is fighting his infection. Let him sweat it out. You know, when I was with Field Marshall Montgomery in the Western Desert, we always saw it. Luckily no such gimmicks were available to us then." I looked at him with disbelief but did as he ordered. A few days later, the temperature dropped, and the patient went home. Mr. Stein showed me the light, and I was forever converted into an antibiotic minimalist. From then on, I started using the term 'gimmick' for anything we doctors do unnecessarily. There were, and still are, so many gimmicks around.

When on call, the aging Mr. Stein cherished his sleep and would deal with all problems strictly over the phone. The following is a reconstructed dialogue on the telephone:

"Mr. Stein, sorry for waking you up, but I have just opened up this young chap who arrived earlier, shocked, acute abdomen, free air, no history available."

"Come on, Moshe, do you need to wake me up for this? You patched ulcers before, right? Just mobilize some omentum and patch the bloody hole, good night."

"But, but Mr. Stein, please don't hang up. There is nothing to patch because there is no stomach and no duodenum. His entire foregut is missing, and everything is black. I don't know what to do. Would you come, please."

Silence. "Mr. Stein, are you there?"

"Yes, I'm here, and you're talking *kak* (South African idiom for shit). What d'you mean… there is nothing? Are you dreaming? Wake up, find the ulcer, and fix it. Good night now." Click.

Depressed, I returned to the operating table where the intern was snoring, his body supported by the retractors he was still holding on to.

"Wake up, John. He won't come. He doesn't believe me." Only then did I realize that the esophagus and the surface of the pancreas were melted as well. *Probably swallowed battery acid — a suicide attempt or it was forced down his gullet by his 'friends'. Hopeless.* He was unsalvageable.

* * * * *

What else do I remember of that year in Coronation Hospital? I remember patients undergoing a three-stage esophageal resection and succumbing to complications in a poorly equipped, understaffed, pseudo-intensive care unit. I remember Estelle, who was one of my best interns — very thin, with a fresh layer of red lipstick permanently smeared on her full lips. When she came to my room to shake me out of sleep — "Hey, Moshe, hurry, wake up, his chest tube is bleeding like a hosepipe" — the scent of her French perfume was strong enough to wake up the dead.

And I remember when and where exactly I met my good old Scottish friend. It was one late evening on the second floor, in front of the operating room's elevators. I saw a tall, dark-haired young man dressed like a don at Eaton, struggling with a combative patient.

I approached and observed this: the patient attempting to jump off the stretcher, spraying blood in all directions, his hands desperately pointing to the gushing hole at the center of his neck — "I can't breathe!" The tall man tried to force the patient back, flat on the stretcher, shouting something to another registrar, but I could not understand what he was saying — *was it English*? As a Bara graduate, the solution came to me reflexively. I jumped on the stretcher and sat on the man's chest; "come, sit on his legs," I instructed the registrar; "give me a tube mama," I screamed at a nurse. Next, I shoved the endotracheal tube into the trachea through the stab wound. "Fix it," I told them. "That's all — just dress it, the operation is finished." I walked off. The following day I learned that the tall man with black hair and blue eyes was Paul Rogers, who had just arrived from Scotland, and the language he was speaking was Glaswegian. Paul had already been a Fellow of the Royal College of Surgeons and thus was addressed as a mister rather than doctor. We started a long friendship, which survives until today.

For some reason, I cannot omit from this chapter a passing recollection of the tall, middle-aged Belgian surgeon whose name I forgot before trying to remember. He immigrated to South Africa to escape Nostradamus' prediction of the "King of Terror," who would come from the sky in the seventh month of 1999. He seemed to believe that in Africa, he would be saved from this doomsday. I do not know why, but he could not obtain a license to practice surgery in South Africa. However, the good-hearted Professor Bremner let him into the department as an 'observer.' As such, he would assist us in the OR from time to time. We mostly ignored him, as it took a lot of work to decipher his rudimental French-accented English. One day I found myself repairing an inguinal hernia, and the Belgian was assisting. As I was fiddling, trying to dissect out the large hernia sac, the Belgian said, *laissez-moi le faire* — "Let me do it, OK?" "OK," I said, watching, in astonishment, his long, agile fingers pulling, pushing, and squeezing within the operative wound. In less than sixty seconds, the hernia was ready for repair. A few minutes later, the suture repair — we did not use mesh those days — was completed. *Voilà,* the Belgian said and left the OR. That episode taught me that even a non-licensed surgeon, or one who cannot speak English, could be a master surgeon.

A year later, the Belgian succumbed to an aggressive cancer. Nostradamus had followed him to South Africa…

* * * * *

With Paul Rogers (right) at the Coronation Hospital.

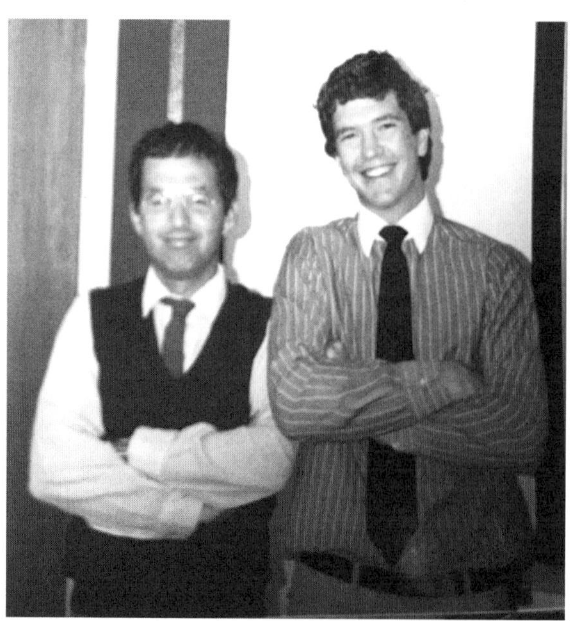

Eighteen

Gown versus town

It was in Coronation Hospital that the concept of the surgical "gown versus town" first came to my attention. In Johannesburg, in those days, the two entities were strictly separated. The 'gown' surgeons were full-time, salaried employees of the university-affiliated hospitals. Their salary was modest, and private activities to supplement it were prohibited. They drove humble cars and wore white coats; some were true academicians. However, I observed, many of them remained in 'gown' for the easy life — we cut, registrars do all the work, we sleep well. Many, particularly the young ones, after gaining some experience, absconded to 'town.'

The 'town' surgeons wore fancy dark suits, silk shirts and ties, and expensive British shoes. Their car of choice was a Mercedes-Benz or a Jaguar, and they lived in large mansions. They worked in private hospitals serving the privately insured white population. Many private chaps were affiliated with the University as "voluntary faculty." They were attached to the various units where, once a week, they taught medical students, participated in grand rounds, and took calls, on the phone mainly.

Mr. Finkelstein was such a voluntary consultant on Mr. Stein's unit. He was a second-generation South African Jew, tall and dark, wearing elegant suits and large gold rings on his fingers. "Finki," his nickname, was an entertaining addition to our grand rounds. He was witty but always positive and complimentary: "Oh how lovely! Mosh, you did such a wonderful job," or "hell boys, you saved this bloke's life…"

One day after rounds, Finkelstein approached me: "Hey, Mosh, you aren't on call on Tuesday, are you? Want to earn a buck? Why don't you come and assist me at my Hillbrow clinic? Yes, afternoon."

The clinic where Finkelstein operated was not one of the upper-class palaces but a modest building in Hillbrow. We scrubbed. The first case was the wiring of a radius bone. "Mr. Finkelstein, I didn't know you also do orthopedics?" I asked.

"I do everything." A chuckle.

Looking at the patient's X-ray, it seemed to me that the fracture was well set, and there was a callus, so why was there a need for an operation? I said nothing.

Next patient — a young male. "Oh, he has had a peptic ulcer for many years. Intractable pain." It took Mr. Finkelstein five seconds to insert a gastroscope into the patient's duodenum: "Mosh, see? An ulcer!" The scope moved so fast that I saw nothing at all. A few minutes later, the abdomen was open, and Finkelstein's long, thick fingers were tearing the esophagus away from its bed: "See the vagus nerve?" He removed another white strand of tissue — "right vagus, see?" Obviously, nothing was sent to pathology to confirm that the 'vagus' was indeed the vagus nerve. Next, he dug at a tiny hole near the pylorus, immediately closing it with a few quick bites of chromic suture. Another five minutes and the abdomen was closed — to my horror, with rapidly dissolving chromic sutures. "See, boy, vagotomy and pyloroplasty in under twenty-five minutes. Are you impressed?"

Last case. Repair of a direct inguinal hernia. With a few bites of silk, it took thirteen minutes from skin to skin. Obviously, the 'hernia' was non-existent.

"That's your share of the bounty. Enjoy!" Finkelstein popped a few hundred rands in my pocket. "We had a good time, eh? So long." Alone in the car, I counted the bills. I liked the feel of this quickly earned cash during one brief afternoon. I knew that the nailing of the radius was pointless, that there was no ulcer, that the vagotomy was not a vagotomy, and the pyloroplasty was not a pyloroplasty, and that even if there was a hernia the repair was not a repair. At home, I handed the money to Heidi, who was elated: "Now we can buy the new pram for Yariv."

I hoped that Finkelstein would invite me again, and he did, for three additional consecutive Tuesdays. Just when I was getting addicted to this steady source of extra, tax-free income, it stopped abruptly. Another registrar was invited to assist Finkelstein.

An older registrar explained: "Finki doesn't retain any assistant for longer than a month. It's his rule. How many goofy operations would you assist before blowing the whistle? Anyway, you know, he's a heavy gambler. Sun City. He's always in need of cash."

This was my first direct encounter with 'gray' surgery and the temptation of easy money to be made by unnecessary surgery. It would take me years to realize how prevalent unnecessary surgery is — wherever there is a fee for a service as a prevailing system — including in the United States of America.

* * * * *

In parallel, we slowly blended into a humble Johannesburg existence. In 1982, Yariv, our second son, was born. Heidi got a secretarial job at a German construction company. Trafina looked after the two babies, and

Moses did the garden. My involvement with the boys during the five years of residency was meager. I came home mostly to eat and sleep. With help from Heidi's parents and my mother, we gathered a small sum of money and took a mortgage on our first home. It was a small, old, red brick house in Westdene, yet another predominantly Afrikaner, blue-collar neighborhood. We lived on the steep Banbury Road, which served as a thruway from the purely Afrikaner suburb of Triomf, to the bohemian-artistic Melville to our east.

Moses helped us surround the house with a brick wall, which he painted white, and closed the tin-roofed *stoep* with bricks to become my minute study. The living room and bedrooms were tiny and suffocating, but this seemed like a palace. We had to have a swimming pool. In Johannesburg, a house is not a house without a pool in the backyard; summers are intolerable without the sounds of kids splashing in the water and the rhythmic pulsations of a Kreepy Krauly pool-cleaning machine in the background. Paying in installments, we squeezed in a small pool between the kitchen's stairs and Trafina's shed. We enjoyed it over the summer. But during winter, the walls of the pool started to cave in. By then, the pool contractor had vanished from the Yellow Pages.

We were poor but happy, as the cliché goes. After leaving South Africa, we would never socialize as much as during those years. According to Alan Furst, "For people living abroad, life is commonly a separate country — Expatriatia — populated by citizens of the world." And so was ours. The people we socialized with were rarely South Africans but ex-pats, like us, from Israel, Rhodesia, and Europe. I recall long Sundays in the garden, on the yellow grass, under the warm winter sun, or on green lawns until the evening summer rain started drumming on the tin roofs. The kids were running around or splashing in the pool, with the adults preparing a *braai* of mouth-watering, coronary clogging *Boerewors*, and sipping Cape wines from five-liter boxes. In the background, the black nannies changed the babies' diapers, washed the dishes, and conducted a parallel *braai* around their sheds — the quality of which depended on the generosity of the individual master and madam.

And from the nearby *koppies*, sects of blacks were gathering for the Sunday church service (i.e., political meeting); we could hear a muffled thud of Zulu drums. These were good years.

* * * * *

Top: Heidi with Omri and baby Yariv in the Westdene house. Bottom: a weekend on the Magaliesberg range, with Heidi, Yariv and Omri.

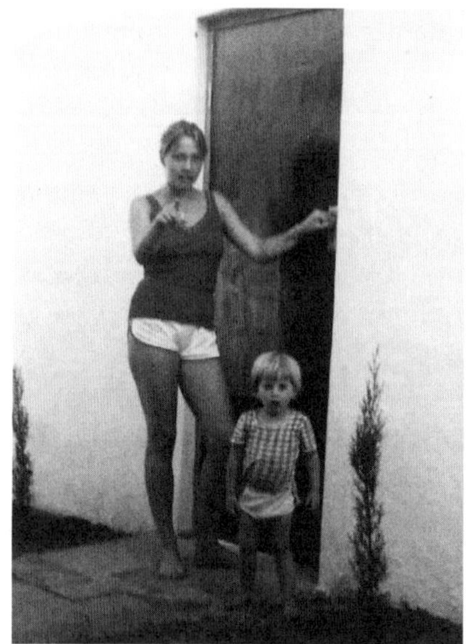

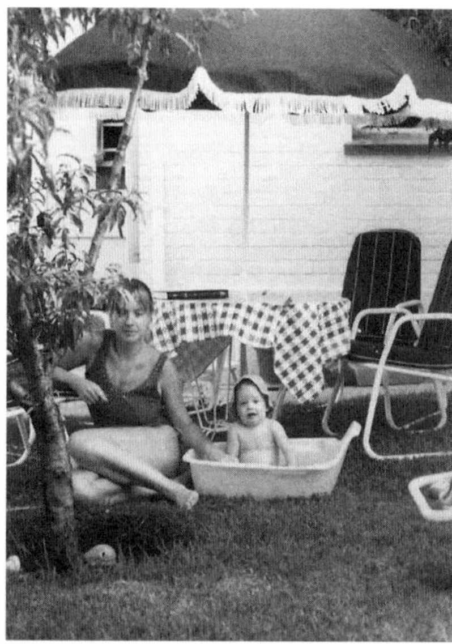

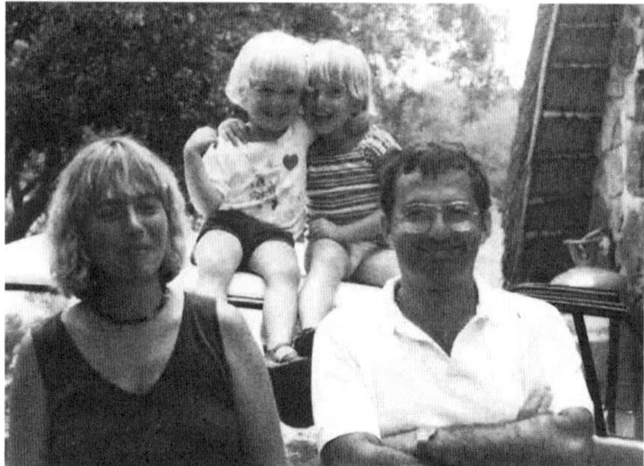

Nineteen

The man with the scar

Towards the end of my year in the Coronation Hospital, Prof. Bremner announced: "Bert Myburgh wants you to move to the J.G. Strijdom Hospital" – the "JG" in the local jargon. *Oh no,* I thought, not because I had anything against relocating to a large, public, purely 'white' hospital administered by Afrikaners for Afrikaner patients – aptly named, as almost everything else in the Transvaal, after an ex-Afrikaner Prime Minister. It was *oh no* because the head of surgery at the JG was the notorious Mr. George A.G. Decker, known commonly as GAG. Until then, I had not been formally introduced to GAG but often bumped into him at medical school activities. In his early 50s, average in height, robustly built, blue-eyed, and balding – women considered him handsome. Whenever I saw him, winter, or summer, he was dressed in a white safari suit and matching white *Veldskoens* (also known as "van de Merwe shoes") – the type of shoes favored by Afrikaners, worn with knee-long tropical trousers (long trousers in winter) combined with knee-high, heavy socks.

Years later, GAG disclosed the secret behind his ever-white, fresh safari suits: "You buy three pairs of safaris. One pair you wear, the second is in the wash, the third pair hangs drying on the line – never let the maid do it, do it yourself!"

GAG was a man of few words at academic meetings; occasionally, Myburgh would address him, "Say, George, this was your patient, right? Wouldn't it have been better to operate on him sooner?" To this GAG would nod, say a few words, and always agree with the big Prof., who, allegedly, knew everything and was always right. Registrars rotating through GAG's department at the J.G. Strijdom Hospital spread horror stories about his unpredictable and ever-changing moods, his aggression, and his ruthless dictatorial regime as if the few months they had spent with GAG equaled exile in Robben Island.

What I heard about GAG from people in the Coronation Hospital was scarcely more comforting. Albert, a Jewish anesthetist, said: "I warn you, Mosh, the man is brutal. I was a student at JG. I saw with my own eyes how he lifted an intern and threw him out of the theater, just like that, only because the bugger spoke without asking permission. He's not too tall, but man, he's strong." When Dr. Weisfish heard about my imminent departure to JG, he smiled sardonically: "Knowing your crazy personality, I predict you have no chance whatsoever. Not only does GAG hate Jews in general, but you're a foreigner too. Do you know what GAG stands for? Really, you don't know. Guess? George, Adolf, Goering. To tell you the truth, I suspect that the original George was Gerhard. He's of German stock, and his parents probably supported the Nazis like all *chates* at that time." (South African Jews called Afrikaners *chates*; a term derived from the Hebrew, *chot'im*, meaning "sinners.")

Only Mr. Stein managed to calm me a little: "Don't worry. George is tough but fair. Anyway, he's a cultivated Afrikaner. He spent a few years in England, has a British wife, it mellowed him a lot. If you work hard, everything will be all right."

Then there was GAG's mysterious scar. People told me: "He has a long, red scar on his forehead. When it turns white, be on your guard, this is when the storm erupts." There were many rumors as to the etiology of this scar, including clandestine *Broederbond* activities. Only many years later, we figured out the truth. An elderly lady recounted: "Oh, that charming scar on George's forehead? It happened after he fell off his potty."

Early morning on the first of January 1984, I parked my ancient, red Alfa Romeo Alfetta GTV in a bay marked *chirurgie,* in front of the tall, long, red brick building — the J.G. Strijdom Hospital. I was dressed in a new white safari suit and white wooden clogs — all purchased for the occasion. On the preceding *Sylvester* night, we stayed home, and I remained sober. But I did not sleep well. I was thinking about my surgical training: three years passed, and what did I know? OK, I had gained some knowledge and experience. I could cut. But will I become one of those self-made Bara surgeons? Only two years to go until the end of my training, and I had not found a *real* mentor — somebody I could look up to, try to emulate. And now, I must work with a fascist…

JG was recently built. Pretentiously grandiose and extremely ugly, like most public buildings erected by the Afrikaners, it looked like a minor replica of the Jan Smuts Airport — as if built by Albert Speer for the Führer. Everything was vast and unattractive: the building itself, the long corridors, the entry hall, the operating rooms, and even the typically massive Afrikaner nurses — well, a few were attractive. All the walls were covered, floor to ceiling, with mousy-gray linoleum.

I remember climbing up the marble stairs leading from the parking area to the deserted lobby where the statue of J.G. Strijdom greeted me. Off the main corridor on the third floor, separating the two wings of GAG's department, I found the meeting room, where the new bunch of interns, the other registrar — one of Myburgh's boys — and GAG's junior consultant were waiting. Just then, I noticed GAG approaching down the corridor: he walked fast, his head tilted down and to the side, as if counting the number of gray shades of linoleum. A heavy chain of keys dangled from the belt of his safari suit. *No gun in sight. Good.* As he walked, he repeatedly knocked on the wall with a clenched fist of his right hand. We almost collided at the door of the meeting room. I said good morning. He just nodded, looked me up and down, from my noisy clogs to my round framed glasses — still dark tinted from the sun — shrugged his shoulders and entered the room.

I sat behind the interns and held my breath to see what came next. I already knew what to expect because, looking up, I noticed that GAG's scar was pale. Thus started my true surgical training.

* * * * *

Each of us can point to a defining period in early life. The same can be said for a professional career — when one becomes what one will be.

The five years I was to spend at the J.G. Strijdom Hospital, first as a registrar, then as a consultant, produced the type of surgeon I became. Not a racing horse surgeon — no virtuoso, a surgical Paganini — but a humble violinist playing the nights away at weddings, a working horse — like GAG. As is often the case, I realized only in hindsight — years after leaving his department — that GAG was my sole surgical model. My mentor.

GAG's surgical department functioned like a Swiss watch. I had never seen, nor would I ever see, a surgical system so closely controlled by its boss. It worked like this: the two registrars, each supported by a team of two or three interns, shared the calls and the sixty-something patients. Each patient belonged to a given registrar and his team from admission to discharge. Period. There was no cross coverage, no "sign off," no "I'm off, could you do this case for me?" You started looking after a patient. You had to always be with him or her — until discharge or death. You had to know your patients, really know them. This was crucial for survival, as I learned on the first day.

GAG rounded every day, including early Saturday mornings; on operating days, he rounded in the afternoons. He led the procession from room to room, bed to bed, always serious, never smiling, and talking in quiet and measured tones, that, one could sense, masked a palpable, incandescent anger. At the bedside, an intern would present the 'case.' Not in the chaotic fashion typical of today's trainees — who often start with what "the CT showed" — but a structured presentation: name, age, main problem, past history, comorbidities, physical examination, lab results, what was already done, the plan, and so forth.

GAG would then examine the patient: expose the wound, percuss the chest — looking for anything the intern had missed. Throughout this ritual, the responsible registrar stood in the background, seemingly passive but on alert. The moment the terrified intern failed to give a required detail — which operation the patient had fifteen years ago, or what the serum amylase level was — GAG focused his piercing eyes on the registrar, blaming him for the utter ignorance of his intern (*Why didn't the two of you discuss it?*), who had to provide the correct answer at once.

GAG's motto: this is your patient, he is *your* responsibility, *you* must know everything about him, his fate depends only on *you* — no one else. To avoid embarrassment, I learned everything about my patients, memorizing their recent blood work each morning. It proved not overly tricky, and until today, my mind automatically registers each patient's level of urea, albumin, potassium, and so forth.

* * * * *

On afternoons before operating days, GAG would divide the cases between his consultant and him, each working in his own theater with one of the two registrars. GAG had received solid training in Cape Town and England; he was a careful operator. He had an outstanding knowledge of anatomy — something one seldom sees in today's surgeons — he re-edited the classic *Lee McGregor's Synopsis of Surgical Anatomy*. He was not a 'cowboy' and knew well what he could or should not do. He would summon Mr. A. Conlan for esophageal cases, and liver resections were shipped to Professor Myburgh. But unlike the latter, who was a prima donna, doing it all himself — "watch how good I am" — GAG was actively teaching and assisting us.

Unlike many South African consultants, GAG was only partly guilty of the main weakness of South African surgical education: registrars either operated independently or assisted the consultants. Of course, the North American custom is extreme in the other direction: a resident rarely operates alone, and God forbid an attending asking a resident to assist. Instead, the attending gets his coronary spasm assisting the residents, who thus seldom learn to assist.

Operating with GAG, either assisting or being assisted, was a stressful experience, not only for me but also for interns and nurses. He demanded absolute silence and that each movement in the OR be strictly controlled by him or his temper. I remember his short, stubby fingers — he liked to use them for finger dissection of tissues. His warm breath came across his mask, his perspiring forehead so near, almost touching mine. To the nursing staff, he would talk in Afrikaans, ordering a *skalpel*, *pinzette* or *schere* — the *sch* not soft like in German but harsh like in Dutch, the c like k; but to us, he spoke English.

Each of our movements was painfully scrutinized. Each knot had to slide home perfectly — any imperfection was met by a grunt or a hiss. One was exhausted after a gastrectomy with GAG, but the gastrectomy was perfect, like the ones he had done with his old British masters.

Eventually, the alternate night calls, the total responsibility, and the constant scrutiny by these seemingly unhappy pair of eyes caused me to develop severe dyspepsia that I treated with large amounts of nauseating antacids. Histamine-2 antagonists were only then being introduced. I was not the only registrar who had developed ulcers while working under GAG: I gastroscoped at least two rotating registrars whose gastric lining was sloughing off under GAG's influence. My friend Roger told me this: "I never had an ulcer while working for GAG; but even years later, every time I parked my car while visiting JG, I felt a gush of acid burning my gastric mucosa. I had, effectively, been transformed into Pavlov's dog!"

During the first weeks, I followed Mr. Stein's advice: work hard, and everything will be all right, and it seemed that GAG treated me as he treated everyone else — like a slave. But a few incidents gave me a glimpse beyond the facade.

It was my first repair of an inguinal hernia at the J.G. Hospital. The hernia was as gigantic as the postoperative hematoma that developed on the following day. I must have missed some arterial branch because, during my 6 a.m. rounds, I found the blue skin discoloration extending from the umbilicus to the knee. I was petrified. It was Wednesday, and grand rounds with GAG and the voluntary consultants were soon to start — *what should I say? Is there any excuse for such a hematoma?* After the tea break, the rounds reached my hernia patient's room.

My heart was pounding. My hands were sweating. Two weeks at the JG and now the end of me was nearing. As usual, GAG entered the room first, approached my patient's bed, and said: "*Goeiemôre meneer, hoe gaan dit met u*?" Good morning, Sir, how are you?

"*Goed dankie,*" replied the patient. Good, thank you.

Just when we — the rest of the entourage — entered the room, GAG uncovered the patient, froze a second or two, and instantly replaced the blanket as if encountering a snake under it. "*Baie goed meneer, totsiens.*" Very good, Sir, goodbye, and he moved to the next bed.

When the intern presented the next patient, I noticed GAG looking at me — was that an amused smile? The following day the hernia patient went home.

One night, a month later, I encountered a patient with a ruptured abdominal aortic aneurysm (AAA). He had been initially diagnosed with sciatica and was admitted to the orthopedic floor (remember, ultrasound and CT were not yet available). After feeling the tender, pulsating abdominal mass, I rushed the patient directly to the theater. I summoned the voluntary consultant on call, Mr. L., a 6′6″ tall, middle-aged man.

The consultant opened the abdomen, sternum to pubis, with a swift knife movement. We found ourselves looking at a giant pulsating hematoma. Now, Mr. L. inserted his huge (size 9.5 glove) right hand and dug into the deep recesses of the upper abdominal cavity. While doing so, he mumbled to himself something like, "holy shit, this one is big, a supra-renal, thoracic aneurysm."

I stood on the other side of the table, elevated on a high step to match the height of Mr. L., whose forehead dripped sweat. Finally, after five minutes of futile manipulation, he said: "Look, this fucking thing is inoperable. It starts in his chest. He's done!"

"But Mr. L., maybe it is just juxta-renal? Shouldn't we dissect a little higher and clamp above the renal arteries?" By then, I had already assisted in several AAA operations and read the relevant chapter in *Rutherford's Vascular Surgery* – I knew that genuine ruptured supra-renal AAAs are rare; commonly, what seems to start above the renal arteries, is actually a bulging infra-renal AAA.

"*Kak* man. No way. He has had it. Close him up, man, will you?" Mr. L. removed his gloves and was ready to exit the theatre.

"And what then, Mr. L? Should I take him to the ICU?"

Mr. L. wiped the sweat from his face with the lower part of his XXXL-sized scrub shirt, "ICU? What for? He's dead already. Take him to the floor, extubate, a large dose of morphine, you know, the dying man's friend."

"Yes, Sir."

Mr. L. left; it was 5 a.m.

I closed the patient's tummy rapidly – only the skin. I wheeled him to the ICU, which was run by us surgeons, and kept him oxygenated and perfused the best I could. I was awaiting GAG, who stormed into the ICU at 6:55 as he did each morning.

In a few sentences, I recounted the events of the night. I was expecting an explosion, but there was calm instead. The following minutes remained etched in my mind: GAG approached the patient, grabbed his wrist with his right hand, feeling for the pulse. With the left hand, he rubbed the scar on his forehead. He stood like this for a minute – like a 'thinking surgeon' in some old oil painting.

That minute seemed to me like an hour.

Then: "Let's take him back to the theater, now!"

We did, and he survived. Mr. L. was instructed never to operate on an AAA again.

Without noticing it, GAG gradually became my model, who I started to imitate. For example: during extended operations, when events turned hectic, GAG would suddenly pause, turn around to the water basin behind him, immerse his gloved hands in the warm water, look at them, and contemplate — for a few mute minutes. *Calm down, think, plan, take it easy man…*

In my own cases, I started doing the same.

I do not know why and when it started to happen, but GAG began to spare me. He tormented and persecuted the other team members but left me in relative peace. He would not infrequently arrive at dawn and ambush a late-arriving intern or registrar — a traumatic event to watch, but I was left out. Instead, I became his registrar. While others came and went — I remained.

* * * * *

Top: Professor George Decker (1931-2013). Bottom: J.G. Strijdom Hospital.

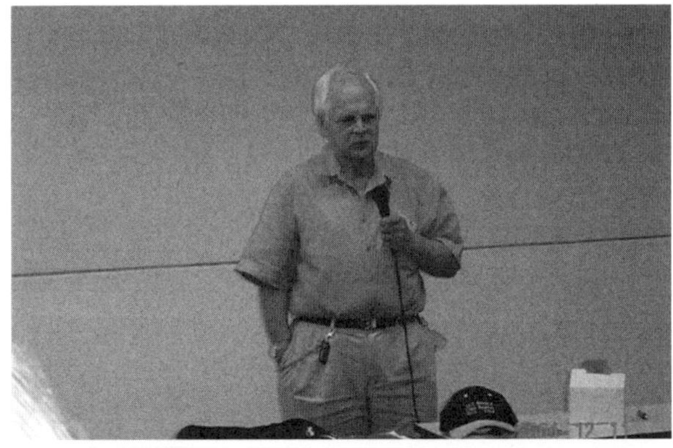

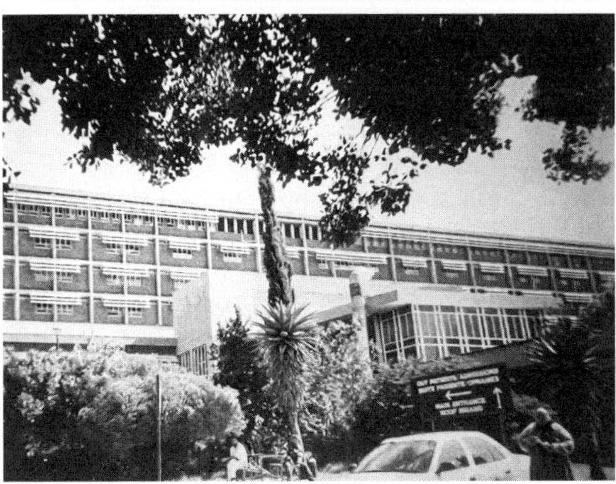

Twenty

The virus of academia

As a permanent surgical registrar at the J.G. Hospital, I had lots of pathology to learn from. The hospital treated predominantly poor Afrikaners — some of them representing the local equivalent of 'white trash' — who, like white trash everywhere, smoked like chimneys, drank heavily, used drugs to alleviate the habitual hangover, and ate crap. Thus, in addition to the rampant peripheral vascular disease and the general surgical 'bread and butter,' this stressed and neglected population suffered from terrible epidemics of peptic ulceration — supplying us with an endless stream of perforated, bleeding, 'intractable' and recurrent ulcers to operate on, and complications of such operations to deal with.

During operations for peptic ulcers, GAG repeatedly pointed to the fat, juicy lymph nodes surrounding the stomach and the poor dentation in many of these patients. "This must be an infection, Moshe," he said, "causing all these ulcers; poor hygiene of the mouth, persistent contamination. You should be culturing these nodes to look for the responsible bacteria, then an antibiotic would cure the ulcer, no need for our knives, and you will receive the Nobel Prize."

I laughed, not knowing that a year prior, Marshall and Warren had already published in *The Lancet*, a paper entitled "Unidentified curved bacilli in the stomach of patients with gastritis and peptic ulceration." The rest of the story, which took a few more years to evolve, is well known. Effective eradication of the responsible bacteria, *Campylobacter pylori*, with antibiotics, in combination with modern acid-suppressing medications, made anti-ulcer surgery obsolete. Likewise obsolete, became some ten papers I wrote at the JG about the management of peptic ulcers, including an article on "Five hundred operations for peptic ulcer disease at J.G. Strijdom Hospital, 1980-1987."

John Shaw Billings recapped it aptly: "There is a vast amount of… worthless material in the literature of medicine… nine-tenths, at least, of it becomes worthless, and of no interest within ten years after the date of its publication, and much of it so when it first appears." During my academic career, I published more than 400 papers, and edited, or wrote some sixteen books, but I never took myself too seriously — I know that some of what I have published is already obsolete, and what is not outdated may become so very soon. So is the nature of medical publishing as opposed to, say, the publishing of historical manuscripts. Yet, a brief account of how I started a prolific writing career at the JG could be of value to the young surgeons who may stumble upon this text.

I took my idea from the famous American surgeon Robert M. Zollinger who had said: "Take two squirrels, knock their heads together, and if one of them gets a headache, write a paper." In other words, if you want to write and publish, look around you: there is always something to study and write about! I found a gold mine at the JG: GAG's virgin and unexplored departmental archives.

These were still non-digitalized days when information was hard to store and retrieve. But GAG forced his interns to dictate a detailed summary of each discharged patient, which the single departmental secretary transcribed (carbon copies included). On Saturday mornings, GAG detained us to proofread the typed summaries, at the end of which he would approve and sign it himself.

When you have good data, with access to *Index Medicus* (remember those pre-MEDLINE days, when one spent hours looking for one reference?), a reasonable library, and a second-hand typewriter, you can write anything. I started with retrospective studies on perforated ulcers, bleeding ulcers, etc.

I remember showing a draft on perforated gastric ulcers to Professor du Plessis — the retired Chairman and Vice Chancellor of the University, considered the father of Johannesburg's surgery, and mentor to Myburgh, Bremner, and GAG. His job then was to supervise registrars' academic projects. It was my first and last encounter with the tall, silver-haired grand old man. He held my manuscript with his beautifully manicured fingers, and said: "Dr. Schein, a neat manuscript, um, you certainly see lots of perforated gastric ulcers at the JG, interesting, but, um, I would advise against publishing this. The mortality rate is much too high. I would suggest, um, you chaps have to question your peri-operative management and surgical technique. As to publishing — why don't you hook up with Professor Hinder. His lab's looking at the apoptosis of gastric mucosal cells." And so he went on and on, and I lost him and thought: *you're talking kak Prof. High mortality? What do you know about it — did you ever look at your department's clinical statistics? There is not even one paper about perforated gastric ulcers from South Africa, and you want me to look at gastric cells.*

I went ahead and published the paper — the first one of mine to enter an American journal. From then on, I showed my papers to no one and selected my own co-authors — this, I would learn later, did not make me too popular with Myburgh. Professor du Plessis later succumbed to dementia — was he already afflicted when we met? His life story has been elegantly outlined by GAG in *Digestive Surgery.*

GAG's department was a tertiary referral center for provincial hospitals across the Transvaal. Private surgeons would ship their postoperative complications to us once they could not provide the necessary intensive care and/or the patient's private insurance ran out. It burdened us with a continuous stream of complicated postoperative, 'septic' abdominal catastrophes. It allowed me to develop a specific interest in managing surgical infections, intestinal fistulas, pancreatic necrosis, and similar disasters. I was still a trainee, but GAG gave me almost free reign in managing these patients.

Commonly they were transferred to us with a large hole gaping in the middle of their abdomens, through which intestinal juices and feces poured out — a total mess. Together with Roger, John Jamieson (deceased), and GAG, we developed a method to control this dirty muddle using a synthetic mesh, an adhesive sheath, and suction tubes interposed between the layers. We called it the "sandwich technique" and it became our first of many publications in the *British Journal of Surgery* (1986). As commonly is the case, people started using it worldwide, 'improving' it, and publishing their 'new' technique without citing us. Finally, the industry adopted the concept of applying a vacuum to the wounds. It introduced the costly and lucrative vacuum-assisted closure (VAC) wound system that is now widely used and advocated for all sorts of 'problem wounds.' Nowadays, any innovation is registered as a patent in the quest for fame and money. But we were too naïve to think about such things during the 1980s. To the best of my knowledge, our *BJS* paper was the first ever published description of negative pressure management of wounds. Sometimes, when a commercial representative is trying to sell me one of those negative pressure management wound apparatuses, I say: "You know, I invented the VAC system." The rep's response is invariable: a nod of the head and smile — he must be kidding or dreaming…

A complete discussion about surgical publishing would deserve a book; years later, I produced such a book, *A Surgeon's Guide to Writing and Publishing* (2001, tfm publishing, UK), together with the late John Farndon and the living Abe Fingerhut. Before ending this tiresome academic account, I must mention that the J.G. Hospital provided the experience and many of the concepts which subsequently would mature into our book *Schein's Common Sense Emergency Abdominal Surgery*, presently in its fifth edition.

* * * * *

Twenty-one

Senior registrar

Thus, two years passed – permanently on call, rounding on weekends, studying, writing in between, and falling asleep as soon as I reached home. What I mainly remember from that time is GAG, his temper, and our coexistence. I never asked him about this, but if one could question him, he would probably tell you how difficult I had become to manage. Not only did I argue with him – questioning and ignoring his policies – such as routine drainage after cholecystectomy or mandatory vagotomy and hemi-gastrectomy for pre-pyloric ulcers – but also my general attitude had become brash and smug. Over the phone, I insulted referring doctors from small Afrikaner towns: "What?! What do you mean you don't know what his blood pressure is? Do you want to transfer a corpse?" I would be cocky and arrogant to the pretty senior superintendent of the JG who tried to reprimand me: "Ag, Dr. Schein, you can't use the F word on the phone." I kicked an internal medicine consultant out of my office who had been complaining that I had abused his junior registrar. I emptied a wash basin on the head of an irritating circulating OR nurse and then maltreated Mrs. Malan, the head nurse, who came rushing in to investigate why her nurse was dripping wet and hysterical.

Since I do not know why I behaved this way, I must blame it, perhaps, on the specific type of psychopathology that draws certain people to become surgeons, a pathology that tends to mellow with the passing years, a pathology that would not be tolerated these days. I also do not know how he did it and why, but after each such incident, GAG, with some effort, managed to save my butt. Luckily, this was before the era of strictly enforced political correctness.

One incident remains clear in my mind. Towards the end of my second year at the JG, the team of physicians and anesthetists, led by Jeff L. (now a leading intensivist in Australia), who had controlled the general intensive care unit (ICU), managed to also take over the surgical ICU, that hitherto had been under GAG and his surgical team. The first week of the takeover, during which Jeff – a short, ambitious, arrogant Jew – was trying to establish his authority over the care of our critically ill patients, was traumatic to us. Then, I admitted a ninety-year-old man with a perforated colon and diffuse peritonitis to the surgical ICU. When I entered the unit, I found Jeff with his band of doctors around my patient's bed. "What do you want to do with him, Schein?"

"Oh, I'm preparing him for a laparotomy."

"Never! The man is ninety; did you see his chest X-ray — the emphysema? Look how blue he is. You don't want to operate on cadavers, eh?"

What? Now they're telling us on whom to operate and on whom not to. I exploded.

Next, I removed that patient's perforated colon; Jeff discharged him from the ICU a day later — to die on the floor. I instructed my interns: "This guy must survive. Understand! If he survives, I will buy you the best meal in town." The old man survived. Before he went home, I brought my camera, told him to raise his right hand in a Churchillian V sign and smile, and I took his picture, which I enlarged and sent by internal mail to Jeff L. The enclosed text said: "Goodbye Dr. L., I am going home — [signed] Johan van Klerck."

Jeff never talked to me again, but a while ago, I received a friendly e-mail from him. Some of us calm down and mature as we grow older.

* * * * *

Professor Myburgh's surgical department provided numerous learning opportunities. An academic program took place each afternoon at the department's medical school site: registrars' seminars, journal clubs, gastrointestinal and vascular forums, and guest lectures — attracting registrars from all affiliated hospitals and units, and consultants from both the 'town' and 'gown,' but nothing could beat the Saturday morning meeting in the grand auditorium of the medical school. Here the entire Johannesburg's surgical community would gather in white coats or dark suits for case presentations, invited lectures, and lively discussions — followed by the omnipresent tea with milk.

Myburgh presided over those activities: coughing between frequent pulls on his filtered cigarettes, emitting a constant stream of pearls from his eloquent lips. Not only did he read 'everything' late into the night, but he also traveled extensively around the surgical world. He used the department's travel budget almost exclusively for himself — thus when he was standing up to conclude, he sounded like an updated textbook in the making: what is known, what has been written, who said what, and what does he, Myburgh think about it. Perfect! Never again did I listen to such a tremendous surgical mind that knew to part with knowledge but, unfortunately, not to mentor copies of itself, thus, eventually, leaving a vacuum behind.

In 1985, towards the end of my residency, I took my final (South African) College of Surgeons examinations — the local boards. The examination had two steps: written and oral. The written part was not one of those American multiple choice examinations but consisted of eight broad questions, each covering an entire field, such as "Discuss the surgical management of acute pancreatitis" or "What is your approach to bleeding esophageal varices?"

A whole day was provided for the writing of these eight essays. A week or two later, the oral part took place. All South African chairmen of surgery would gather in Johannesburg for this grand event. At night, they would be stuffed with food and soaked in alcohol; during the day, they would examine. Each candidate had to assess four pre-operative patients and then present and discuss each case before four examining committees, each of three members. It lasted the entire day. I had studied hard throughout the years of training, supplementing textbook knowledge with journals, reviews, and monographs, and when one writes papers, one covers the entire relevant field. Thus, towards the end, just before the examination, I could feel how the whole body of knowledge fits into what I had seen and experienced. Then I realized how much I had not known before and how many errors I had committed out of ignorance.

I remember GAG calling me at home after the oral examinations. "I'm informed that the examiners elected you as the best candidate of this year," he said dryly.

"Thanks, Mr. Decker," I replied. I sensed that he was proud: his boy, the one he had trained, is the number one candidate in South Africa, first among a large bunch of locally bred boys. I was proud too: Myburgh had shunned me from his ivory tower, but now I showed them, like I, the foreigner in Italy, showed them, and later the 'Italian' in Jerusalem showed them. Thus deepened my self-image of the habitual outsider who functions on the system's edge but shows them. In the years to come, I would cherish and enjoy this image of a successful non-conformist — the stranger. But eventually it would hamper my progress. For to climb to the top and stay there, one has to belong and be part of the system.

* * * * *

What else do I remember from those years? My memory flickers on and off and recaptures Sister Heggy, who was perhaps the best surgical head nurse I had ever met: she knew the patients better than us; with gentleness and humor, she advised us and held our hands. I see the chubby Australian surgeon John C. He was a talented surgeon but an awkward chap who avoided small talk and any direct social contact. Most of all, he liked to perform major vascular procedures and to do it alone — never to teach or assist. Now, in my last year of training, I complained to GAG that I had to start doing more aortic cases. After talking with John, GAG returned to me: "Tomorrow, John will assist you with an aortic aneurysm." The following morning, John, as usual, placed himself on the patient's right side, sliced the abdominal wall from the sternum to the pubis, and exposed the nine-centimeter aneurysm. I was pale with anger — over the last year, I had assisted John in numerous such cases — *why won't he let me do one?* John continued operating, and I assisted and sulked; eventually, after he controlled the neck of the aneurysm and clamped it, clamped the iliac arteries, opened the sac, and sutured the lumbar back-bleeders, I had had enough. "I don't feel well," I said and stepped out.

"I won't be scrubbing in with him anymore," I declared to GAG and left the OR. The second registrar was sent in to replace me. The following day I saw John taking the patient back to the OR because of bleeding from the renal vein, and then again back to the OR, and then the patient died. Did I somehow contribute to this poor patient's outcome?

One image most engraved in my brain — I wonder whether GAG had ever been aware of this case? — is the middle-aged businessman I admitted to our ICU late at night with bleeding esophageal varices. I injected a sclerosing agent into his varices through the endoscope, but he continued pouring blood as if from a faucet.

"Bring me a Sengstaken-Blakemore balloon tube," I asked the nurses — one of which was Woody, an emaciated chain smoker; she was a lesbian, as many of the ICU nurses were.

I tried to insert the tube into the stomach, but the balloon — designed to tamponade the bleeding varices — simply would not slide down; it curled repeatedly in the patient's esophagus while fresh blood was bucketing from his mouth as from a soda fountain. I tried again and again and again in a frenzied madness; my mind obsessively petrified. At the same time, the patient, despite the blood transfusions rushing into his veins, became grayer as life exited his body. Why didn't I call for help? Was I paralyzed? I knew — I 'killed' him — as I had previously 'killed' that poor tetanus girl at Bara.

And I cannot forget the many interns who passed through my hands — each staying with us for six months. The young medical graduates produced at that time in Johannesburg were a great brand of doctors: knowledgeable, practical, keen, enthusiastic, and disciplined — significantly better than their counterparts I would later encounter in Israel and the United States. The best example would be Graeme Pitcher, now a pediatric surgeon in Iowa. The interns, most of them living in the hospital's dormitory, occasionally invited me to their wild parties. I recall how the huge ICU nurse Ella — a six-footer, 250-pounder, a large hairy mole above her hairy upper lip — popped cans of Castle beer into her mouth. She did it like this: shake the can, pop it open, open the mouth and let the pressurized fluid gush directly into the stomach — no swallowing necessary; one can per two seconds. Then Ella would try to 'have her way' with the interns.

And how can one forget Dr. Lebo — our Chief of Anesthesia. Crippled with severe hip distortion, he could not effectively tie his scrub trousers, which at the end of extended operations tended to be situated at his ankle level. And what about the old Australian anesthetist who, after putting the patient to sleep at night, would collapse on the floor, his head supported on the wall — the patient cruising as if placed on an anesthetic autopilot. "Please wake up and wake the patient up. Operation finished," we would shout. Both Lebo and the Australian died many years ago.

* * * * *

In parallel, our small life continued in our tiny house in Westdene. I remember, however, little of it: ever on call, ever tired, specific events are blurred and difficult to reconstruct. On her way to work in the morning, Heidi would deliver our two little boys to their kindergartens. At some point, however, the three-year-old Yariv would stubbornly refuse to step into her car (only years later, he told us that the rough Afrikaner kids in his public kindergarten tortured him); so he would stay home with our maid Trafina.

One cold winter day, I returned home early; the house was empty — no Trafina or Yariv. I rushed through the garden to Trafina's shed, where I found her lying comatose on her bed, stone drunk. The little boy was sitting, astounded, huddling the open paraffin fire. I picked him up and carried him away; he was a cheerful and stoic little boy who never cried or complained. We knew that Trafina had a long flirt with alcohol; often, on Sundays, her days off, when she came to the house for food, her speech would slur, and a wave of cheap wine reeked from her. We ignored it — let her have fun in her free time — but now she was endangering our son's life. The following day I gave her a motivational speech and a warning, "Next time, we find you drunk…" However, there was no next time because two weeks later, Trafina collapsed while hanging the washing on the line. We lifted her into Heidi's Volkswagen station wagon, our two boys with her in the back, and drove her to Hillbrow Hospital, where a day later, she died of a massive stroke — a common fate of the unknowingly hypertensive blacks. A bunch of unknown distant relatives came to bury her and share her meager possessions. A few weeks later, her son, Moses, disappeared.

In December 1985, our third son, Dan, was born on a beautiful summer day.

* * * * *

Admission to the South African College of Surgeons. Professor John Terblanche of Cape Town (standing); Professor Myburgh, second on the left.

The
College of Medicine
of South Africa

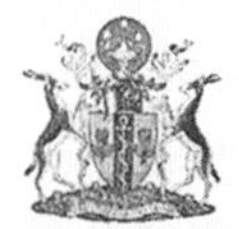

Die
Kollege vir Geneeskunde
van Suid-Afrika

Admission Ceremony 26 October / Oktober 1984 Toelatingsplegtigheid

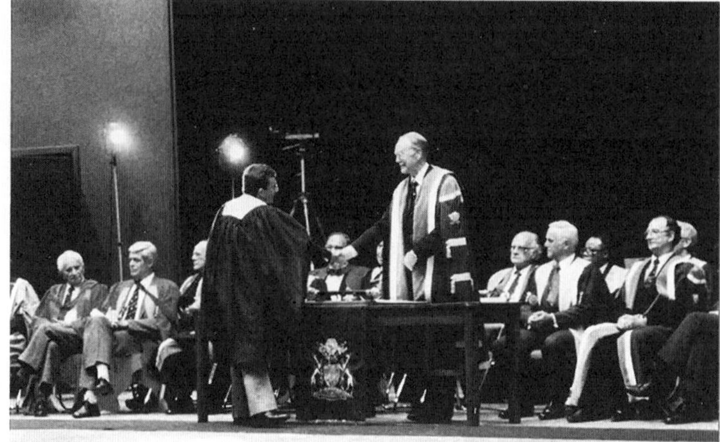

Twenty-two

Consultant

Hard work and luck alone are insufficient to expand and maintain a successful and notable professional career. So, with my residency nearing its end, we asked ourselves, "What's next?" Back home to Israel? Too early. Cavafy's *Ithaca* ringing in my ears: "Always keep Ithaca in your mind. To arrive there is your ultimate goal. But do not hurry the voyage at all…" One does not wish to return home as a junior surgeon. Go into private practice? I already knew that private practice — the fee-for-service system — did not fit my attitude and personality. I sensed that my place was in academia; I knew that I had to develop a subspecialty niche for myself — why not in vascular surgery — didn't I enjoy the drama of major arterial surgery? There were no formal postgraduate subspecialty fellowships in South Africa, but the renowned Groote Schuur Hospital in Cape Town had a unit dedicated to vascular surgery. I approached Prof. John Terblanche, the Cape Town Chairman, who contacted GAG, and (surprisingly) I was given a junior consultant position in Cape Town's vascular service. This was surprising, considering that historically, Groote Schuur Hospital had previously not admitted surgical faculty from outside of Cape Town. We put our house up for sale. The plan was to move to Cape Town in December, immediately after Heidi delivered our third son. However, in early November, GAG informed me excitingly that John, his Australian consultant, had resigned: "You are going to Cape Town, but if you wish to change your mind, you can have John's consultant job as of January the first."

It took Heidi and me only a minute to make up our minds, so on the first of January 1986, I became Mr. Schein — no more Dr. — a consultant and second in command to the notorious GAG at the J.G. Hospital. I do not regret that decision. The following years were enjoyable and fruitful, but in terms of career planning, it had been the first error in a series of mistakes.

Prof. Terblanche (1935-2023), the famous, tall, and loud boss in Cape Town, was furious.

* * * * *

Melville, Johannesburg, 1986. "Certain memories are what you long to take with you…" wrote James Salter. Here is one such memory on a late summer Sunday morning. Sunrays glimmer on the grass, still wet from the previous night's rain. Two small boys jump, dive, splash, and laugh in the clear, blue, oval pool, surrounded by high walls, completely covered with dense shrubs of red and violet and yellow bougainvillea, intermingled with blossoming and fragrant jasmine. We, and Dan, the baby, sit around a small metal table under an apricot tree laden with ripe fruit, drinking coffee, eating fresh croissants from the neighborhood bakery, and reading the Sunday papers. Paul Simon spills out through the French doors leading from the garden to the living room. It was an old, white, one-story, Victorian house, half-encircled with an enclosed porch, surrounded by bougainvillea and jasmine bushes. Two old avocado trees produced fleshy fruits left to rot on the ground — we were not yet acquainted with that delicacy. Ancient lemon trees carried lemons the size of grapefruits and shaded the ten stone steps leading to the wooden front door, with its stained-glass windows. The rooms were large, walls freshly painted, but a few cracks peaked through. The ceilings were tall, of decorated pressed steel; the single bathroom could not mask its Victorian origins. The wooden floors were polished and squeaked loudly underfoot. The kitchen was old-fashioned and opened to the back garden, which led to the guests' cottage, and the servant outbuilding — the domain of Shirley — who had replaced Trafina — and her husband, Johannes.

When one changes houses and addresses every few years, each remains engraved in memory to the smallest detail, marking a certain point in the long journey. But this house, which we bought in 1986, in the hilly and sleepy Melville, on a side street shaded by tall Jacaranda trees, with its purple blossoms in October, has a special place in our memories. Melville, just a few blocks east of the blue-collar Westdene, was adopted and transformed by Johannesburg's artistic and gay communities into a pseudo-Greenwich Village. Here one lived in secluded houses behind white or purple, or blue walls, surrounded by lush vegetation, with the main street only a block away with its galleries and art shops, cafés, and a few of the best restaurants in town. The lovely Emmarentia Dam, with its vast Botanical Gardens, was a jog away. The J.G. Hospital was four minutes by car to the west, and the medical school with its library was ten minutes to the east. My salary was modest — not more than the equivalent of $2000 per month, but we lived in a small paradise — or so we thought.

Johannes, our maid's husband, worked as a truck driver. A big and muscular man, always smiling and mild of character, he was also an excellent handyman who, in his free time, was willing to earn extra money by doing small jobs for us. One day I told him: "Johannes, why don't you paint your shack, put some tiles on the concrete floor, add a roof on your porch, and replace the old shower. We will pay for everything."

"Yes, master," he smiled but typically never did anything to improve his and Shirley's dwelling, where on weekends and nights, many of their guests celebrated and often slept — illegally. Blacks had to possess a permit to work and live in the white-only sections of town.

On a sunny Sunday morning, I was washing my car in the driveway when a short black man, his head shaven, dressed in rags like a hobo, appeared, stopped, smiled, and said nothing. I recognized him immediately: "Moses, where have you been?" We had not seen him for many months since the death of his mother, Trafina.

"Yes, master," he smiled, pointed his finger to his mouth, and continued smiling. *Hungry*. After devouring a large pot of *mealie pap* (corn meal), topped with meat gravy, with a Lion beer in one hand and a cigarette in the other, smiling happily, Moses, in his broken English, recounted his experience: about how the police had arrested him on the street — he had not been carrying his permit — about the prisons, beatings, and hard labor that followed. That was nothing extraordinary — a regular occurrence for many black men in South Africa.

We rehired him as our gardener; Roger, who had just moved to Westdene, had a vacant servants' shed in his back garden — it became Moses' palace and harem.

* * * * *

My first year as a consultant in GAG's departments was mainly agreeable.

I was starting to enjoy the pleasures of mentoring surgical trainees. Naturally, you can mentor, and share whatever you know, only with those who want to be mentored by you and are teachable. From then on, wherever I would go, I was always lucky to find a few of those young surgeons who were thirsty to learn and chose me as their teacher. I would treat them as equals, like friends, and in return, would expect only one thing: loyalty. Over the years, some of these young men would overtake me, becoming better surgeons, more successful, or more prosperous. Some would disappear, others would contact me for letters of reference, but a few would remain good friends for life.

I talk about loyalty but what about myself? Was I always so loyal to those above me — in Johannesburg, Haifa, New York? Yes, I was, to some extent, but it did not prevent me from speaking my mind. Loyalty stops whenever those to whom you are loyal misbehave or double-cross you. And it is open to different interpretation — I wonder what my superiors would think.

Three registrars of the many who had passed through the JG deserve to be mentioned. Each was different but served as a model of the ideal surgical apprentice. One was Gary G., a short and lean Jewish boy — a classical 'bagel': a local nickname for a wealthy Jewish boy, driving a brand-new BMW, bought by daddy, sporting a heavy Swiss timepiece and vacations in Mauritius — then the dream holiday target for affluent Johannesburgers. Gary had all the qualities to bring him to what he would eventually become — an immensely successful surgeon in Long Island. He worked like a horse, was dedicated to his patients, extraordinarily educated and knowledgeable, demanding of his interns, and supportive and loyal to his superiors — he would do anything to make you happy. The second was Wolfi; he was the opposite of Gary: tall, heavy, phlegmatic, not a millionaire's son but the son of a blue-collar Jewish family.

I will always remember Wolfi's first day at the JG. It was a Friday. Around lunchtime, I took him through a cholecystectomy that had turned out to be rather tricky. "Let me show you," I said, completing the procedure in twenty-five minutes, and then went home. It was my weekend off — now I was a consultant — and Wolfi was on call. I went to a dinner party. I enjoyed myself very much and continued enjoying myself after dinner, sipping one KWV brandy after another.

Around 11 o'clock, Wolfi paged me. "Hey, you know, the gallbladder we did earlier is not doing too well. He's very distended and tender all over, and I am having difficulties in maintaining his blood pressure."

Shit. Now forced to think, I realized how much booze was soaking my brain.

"Wolfi, let's take him back to theater. I'll be there in ten minutes." I returned to the dining room, swallowed a cup of black coffee, parted from the hosts, guests, and Heidi, and started the Alfa Romeo that seemed to drive by itself. It was the first time I scrubbed on a case while drunk — and the last one — never again.

As predicted, the ligature had come off the cystic duct, and the belly was full of bile. Under my slurred supervision Wolfi resutured the duct. After the operation, we took the patient to the ICU.

I remember the events of the night. 2 a.m.: the patient is unstable, and his blood pressure is in the fifties. I grab a chair, placing myself by his bed — determined to save his life. Wolfi takes another chair at my side. 3 a.m.: blood pressure still very low. Wolfi starts infusing dopamine. 4 a.m. "Go to sleep," I tell Wolfi — "I'll stay here. It was my ligature which came off. I fucked up."

But Wolfi does not move from my side until 7 a.m. when the patient's blood pressure is above ninety and urine appears in his catheter.

Many years have passed since I met Wolfi, who became a successful private surgeon in Johannesburg. But the image of his extreme loyalty to the drunken consultant, whom he had first met a few hours ago, will remain in my mind forever as a shining example of surgical comradeship and steadfastness.

The third registrar was Herman Gerding. Poor old Herman. Herman did not come to us as the other registrars — on rotation from Myburgh's program — but had applied for the job after years of general and surgical practice in mission hospitals in Africa and Asia. In other words, when he came to us, he was already an experienced surgeon but without formal training. We saw a tall, fair, handsome, athletic Afrikaner. We were a little worried about such a name and his missionary past. But rapidly, Herman proved the best of registrars — keen, able, responsible — and an excellent friend and companion: calm, modest, and always in good spirits.

A few months after he arrived, we started a study on whether sutures placed deep into the first part of the duodenum could reach the common bile duct. Books and articles warned us that under-running bleeding duodenal ulcers may damage the nearby bile duct. Still, we could not find any documentation that such disasters had occurred — that this danger was real. We decided to study the question on cadavers and contacted the Johannesburg municipal mortuary. "Come early Monday morning," we were told.

The gray and low sprawling morgue was situated on Joubert Street in Braamfontein, just behind the Old Fort that served as a prison. A black security guard let us through the gates. A surreal, medieval, nauseating sight unfolded in front of our eyes: corpses everywhere, in the open yard and the vast roofed sheds; corpses on tables and on the concrete floors; white corpses and black corpses, but mostly black; corpses of young men predominated, but here and there, a shriveled old body or a minute corpse of a baby was to be seen.

A large group of black technicians in soiled white gowns carried or worked on the bodies. One could hear the chainsaws digging into the crania. The stench of old blood, fresh feces, putrefying guts, and decaying flesh was unbearable. I looked at Herman — he was pale and sweaty — and took a few deep breaths to suppress my gagging.

A tall, elderly white-haired man in a neat gray safari suit approached us. He drew deeply on his cigarette — I noticed how his hand shook — and said, "I'm the Chief Pathologist. What do you want?" Strong Afrikaans accent. *Rude.*

"We are the surgeons from the J.G. Hospital. I called you yesterday," said Herman.

"OK, but what do you want?"

I started to explain, but he did not seem interested and interrupted: "OK, Nelson will show you the cadavers. How many do you need? You must rush; by lunchtime all this," he pointed with his cigarette to the killing fields around us, "has to be disposed of. It's Monday, you know, lots of work after the weekend." Now I noted his red nose and bloated face, which explained the shaking hands and how he could bear this place.

Nelson, a giant black technician, showed us a pile of cadavers in one corner of the shed. "They are fresh, last night. Help yourself." A white grin appeared on his face when he saw the fancy surgical instrument extracted by Herman from his bag. "Planning a heart transplant?"

What did we do next? To refresh my memory, I retrieve a yellowing reprint from a crumpled cardboard box that contains reprints of my old publications. "Twenty block specimens of the liver, biliary system, pancreas stomach, and duodenum were obtained from fresh human cadavers... there were fifteen men and five women, age range 20-78. The common bile duct was cannulated supraduodenally with a size 8F feeding tube, which was then passed into the duodenum. The duodenum was opened via a longitudinal duodenotomy. The distance, mucosa to mucosa, between the duodenum and the common bile duct was measured at three places using a needle and Vernier caliper. Next, several stitches and 3mm Ligaclips were inserted into the posterior-medial part of the duodenum adjacent to the common bile duct, which was then opened longitudinally to see if any of the stitches or clips had entered its lumen." They didn't.

Yes, we worked like crazy. At the end of each 'case,' we placed the 'block' back into the empty abdomen, which was then closed by Nelson, who used silk mounted on a reusable needle. By lunchtime, we had only worked on six cadavers, so we had to return on two successive days — finding the place as terrible as the first day.

Two weeks later, Herman, a reserve medical officer in the South African Army, went on a duty tour to Angola. On a dark bush night, the side of the ambulance he was riding in was torn to pieces by an incoming truck. When I heard about his death, all I could see were the rows of the cadavers in Johannesburg's mortuary; *now, I thought, he is one of them.* He was buried. We published an obituary about him — I cannot find it and forgot what we wrote. All that is left of Herman is that one modest paper published sometime later by H. Gerding, MB BCh (deceased), and M. Schein in the *South African Journal of Surgery.*

* * * * *

My first year as a consultant passed rapidly. One memorable aspect was the difficulties I encountered while trying to master major abdominal vascular procedures — with little preliminary experience. Remember, my predecessor John C. had never agreed to help me on these cases. Eventually, I learned, but the learning curve was painful.

I remember one ruptured abdominal aortic aneurysm (AAA) at night. A straight tube graft to replace the ballooned main abdominal artery proves unpractical, as both iliac arteries are severely diseased. So, I insert a bifurcated Y graft down into the groin's two femoral arteries. It clots. *Junk — clots, in the graft?* I clean the graft and irrigate it with heparin. It clots again. *Distal thrombus? Distal emboli?* A Fogarty balloon catheter is inserted into each limb and irrigated. The graft clots again. The resident falls asleep, and the nurses are desperate — the anesthetist curses under his mask. The room is cold and the patient colder, but I am hot; I sweat like a pig. No one to call — now I'm the consultant. *Is the runoff, the outflow vessels, adequate?* On the right, the superficial femoral artery is occluded, but *is the profunda femoris artery adequate?* I expose the poplitea and insert a 'jump' femoropopliteal graft. Let's unclamp — it clots again. *Fuck.* The night is almost over, and this stupid graft refuses to remain patent. *It must be the fucking upper anastomosis — did I 'include' the posterior wall with my anterior line of sutures, thus occluding the aorta?* Meanwhile, the clock is ticking, the patient is asleep, and his limbs are without a blood supply. *Not good.*

"Dave, please, please expose," I tell the registrar. I re-apply the proximal aortic clamp and re-expose the lumen of the aorta — perfect. *What now?*

I turn around and do the 'GAG maneuver' — hands in the hot water: *think, relax, think, you idiot. Shit, I know… the stem of the Y is too long, the limbs of the Y emerge in too wide an angle, turbulence, thus the repeated clotting.* I clamp the aorta yet again, excise the excessive inch and a half of the graft, and join the graft to graft. "Push fluids, I'm unclamping." It works — finally, after nine hours. The patient survives, but this is the wrong way to learn major abdominal vascular surgery. The next case and, the many that followed were smoother. I enjoyed being a plumber of arteries and veins, saving limbs and lives. Later, I would officially qualify in Israel as a vascular surgeon. Unfortunately, my vascular career would end in the USA, which I do not regret, as that noble specialty has now become chiefly endovascular — non-invasive, high-tech, and involving much less 'drama.' Some thirty years after I operated on my last ruptured abdominal aortic aneurysm, I can still 'do it' in my mind and in my dreams. I believe that I could still do it in real life… call it my 'vascular nostalgia.'

* * * * *

Another 'career' I started then was to *not* mind my own business. Many of the complicated cases transferred to our care at the J.G. Hospital came from the private sector after being badly butchered by sleazy or incompetent surgeons. One of them was Dr. Potgieter, an Afrikaner from an outlying hospital in the Transvaal. His hobby was to perform a Nissen fundoplication (a procedure treating gastro-esophageal acid reflux) on any patient he could lay his hands on and to perform it poorly, destroying the lower esophagus. Then he would mismanage the complications and transfer the dying patients to us.

I complained about him to the Health Professions Council of South Africa. An inquiry was conducted, and I was called to testify. Surprisingly, one of the committee members was none other than Mr. Bokkie R. — the Baragwanath surgeon who wanted to kick me out of the training program only a few years prior. At the end of my testimony, Bokkie approached me in the corridor. He offered me his hand, which I was hesitant to accept — still hating him for what he wanted to do to me. "Schein," he said, "I was wrong about you. I hear you are doing very well…" Reluctantly, I shook his hand. Bokkie would pass away twenty-eight years later. The outcome of the inquiry was the Afrikaner surgeon would lose his license. I was proud — I knew that I did the right thing. But obviously, others looked at this from another angle.

This incident foreshadowed a pattern in my future role as a 'surgical vigilante' — a whistleblower. I always found it challenging to mind my own business. A personality defect?

* * * * *

At home in Melville.

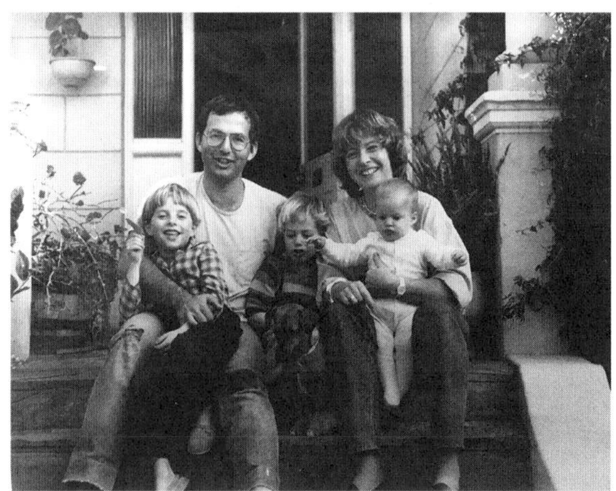

Twenty-three

A try in Bern

1987. Life was good, but I remained unsettled. We knew that, eventually, we would have to leave South Africa — it could never become a permanent home for us, not under the white minority regime, even less under black leadership. The winds of political instability were gathering, and changes seemed imminent. One day, after attending a funeral in Johannesburg's Jewish cemetery, I came home and told Heidi: "I don't feel like being buried in this African soil. I hate lying under these foreign skies. We should leave while the boys are young."

The USA? I was not keen to repeat residency, which was, and still is, required for foreign surgeons relocating to the US. I tried another route: I wrote to Dr. Hiram Polk, then the Chairperson of Surgery in Louisville, a leader in surgical infections, asking for a position in his laboratory. It was a known tactic, namely, if you cannot enter a system through the front door, try the back door — get into the lab of a surgical leader, prove yourself, and hope that he will provide you with a ticket to clinical surgery. Three months later, I received a polite reply from Dr. Polk: sorry, all positions are occupied. I was surprised. By then, I had a significant number of independent publications on surgical infections. Wouldn't he prefer a qualified and published surgeon in his lab rather than one of those young postgraduate students from Japan or China who typically occupied such positions? A few years later, when I broke into my file in Myburgh's office, I found the correspondence between Dr. Polk and Myburgh. The former had shown a keen interest in my application. The latter discouraged him. "His research is immature," and so forth, wrote Myburgh.

"But why don't you try in Switzerland," Heidi kept nagging. "After all, you are married to a Swiss; a working permit and citizenship won't be a problem." Why not? By then, I had worked as a student and visited surgical departments in the German-speaking world. I was familiar with the ruthless, Teutonic surgical system, where the *Chefarzt* is also the *Herr Gott* — I sensed that a non-conformist would not last long within such an environment.

But then someone brought to my attention that Professor Leslie Blumgart of London had been selected as the next Director of Surgery at the famed Inselspital in Bern, the Swiss capital city. Every academic surgeon had heard about Blumgart, the young dentist from Durban, South Africa, who, over the years, rose meteorically to become a guru of liver surgery in the United Kingdom. I wrote to Blumgart, we spoke on the phone, and a month later, I was on my way for an interview in Bern.

* * * * *

It was late February 1987. The ancient city at the foot of the Alps was still immersed in snow. I stomped in dirty slush from the railway station, wetting my thin shoe soles, into the nearby Inselspital. *Allgemeine Chirurgie, Sekretariat*, the sign directed me to Professor Blumgart's offices where his secretary, a spinster-looking Frau Hauptli, received me enthusiastically: "Ach, Herr Doktor Schein, *Willkommen*, the professor is awaiting you in the operating *saal*."

Hastily changing into scrubs, I was led into the room where the professor was operating. "He's fixing a recurrent biliary stricture," someone whispered in my ears. I stood there, watching Blumgart rapidly inserting clamp after clamp into the depth of the right upper abdomen — "Kelly, another Kelly, another Kelly," he kept asking.

Then, at one point, he commanded his first assistant: "Hans, tie them all, will you? And do close him up, please, will you? Thank you, everybody." He turned around, removed his mask, and, still discarding his soiled gloves, smiled at me: "Oh, very well, so this is our Moshe? Welcome to Bern." He appeared in his mid or late fifties, about my height, i.e., on the short side, with a slightly hooked (Jewish style) nose under a pair of shrewd small dark eyes. And he moved fast.

With his arm around my shoulders, he guided me to a small lounge. I saw nurses and doctors smearing thick layers of butter on thickly cut slices of fresh dark bread. After five minutes of small talk, a younger surgeon joined us. Blumgart introduced him: "Please meet my *Stellvertreter* (my deputy). He'll show you around while I do a few more cases. In the few months since I arrived here, we have already become the referral center for complex hepatobiliary surgery for the whole continent. Only the continent? Nay, patients are coming from everywhere." He spoke enthusiastically in an acquired British accent; my ear could, however, detect the South African Jew of Lithuanian origin. So Blumgart continued to hop from one operating room to another — the assistants opening the abdomen and exposing what needed exposure. Then he would come in to perform the crucial step, leave the abdomen full of Kelly clamps — like a porcupine — to be ligated by the assistants. They would close up; he would have a coffee and scrub again, and all would begin again. *Like the two late great Theodors — Kocher of Bern or Billroth of Vienna — in the good old days.*

Now I was left in the company of the deputy, himself recently imported by Blumgart from the French part of Switzerland. The deputy, good-looking, athletic, exhibiting typical French body language, immediately started to examine me in correct but 'Frankonic' English: "How do you treat acute diverticulitis? How do you approach gastric bleeding?"

How do you — and on and on. Then: "I want you to assist one of our senior residents with a cholecystectomy, OK?" I scrubbed in but typically, like most immature surgeons, and many mature ones, I did not appreciate how he 'did' it, how the surgeon operated, because he didn't 'do' it like us. I kept silent until the end when the Swiss guy — or was he German? — inserted a drain into the gallbladder bed. *Why?* And yet another drain into the fat under the skin — *is he crazy?* I could not restrain myself and said: "Why? You don't need these drains."

Two big blue Aryan eyes were looking at me above the masks: "*Ach ya Herr Kollege*... but we believe in drains."

"Well, believe it or not, they are useless," I stupidly replied.

Back to the deputy who showed me around the hospital and departments: patients' rooms, medical ICU, surgical ICU, cardiac ICU, ER, library. "So how did Heinz perform the cholecystectomy?" asked the handsome, blond deputy, "he's our top senior resident."

"Not too well, I believe. I didn't like the two silly drains he left." The *Stellvertreter* did not reply. *Mistake.*

Late afternoon and it was time for the evening report. Under the old European system, morning and evening 'reports' were conducted daily to update the boss about recent developments in his sprawling surgical kingdom. A large meeting room with all surgeons present, everybody in white shirts, trousers, gowns, and clogs or shoes — almost a hundred doctors were gathered. Blumgart, the only one clad in a three-piece dark suit — a British surgeon forever — presides, but the deputy conducts the event purely in English. Everybody is now required to force his or her tongue into his foreign language. That is until the boss acquires some German. On his turn, each of the section heads stands up and reports: "Herr Professor, today my section performed two cholecystectomies, three resections of the sigma, five hernias... everything went well... all patients on the floor are in good shape, no new complications. For tomorrow we have..." — a long list followed. "I'd like to bring for discussion the case of Herr X with the question of what to do..." *Like in the Wehrmacht,* I thought.

Next, we moved to Blumgart's private office. "Come, Moshe. You can't walk around this hospital in your funny corduroy jacket. Take it off, let's hang it up… here, take my white coat, yes, put it on, now you look better. Join me, please. I'll round on my private patients." Together we rounded on patients from Iran, India, the Netherlands — they all came to be operated on by the maestro. After leaving a room where a French patient was recovering following a hepatectomy, Blumgart commented proudly: "You see, with all of their big French hepatic surgeons, she came to me." In the last room lay a bloated young girl. "She's from Tel Aviv, a recurrent hepatoma, caudate lobe — no one would touch her. I did. You speak Hebrew, eh? So talk to her Mom, tell her this…" As he was walking around, he touched everybody — the patients and their families — holding their hands, hugging their shoulders. A trait I recognized from home — definitely not British.

Back in the professor's office, on his black leather couch, Blumgart unlocked a wooden cabinet and presented a bottle. "Glenmorangie, eighteen years old," he proudly declared, "you like single malt, don't you?" He uncorked the bottle and poured two generous portions. *"L'chaim!"* Blumgart retrieved a large brown pipe from his pocket and fed it gently with tobacco from a small square tin. I took out my own pipe, "May I?"

"Please help yourself," he pushed the tin towards me. We lit up, filling the room with blue smoke and the marvelously distinctive aroma of Latakia-based English tobacco. Now, in the warm room, snowflakes falling outside the dark windows, Scotch in our veins, came the time for a soul-searching discourse — or a monologue. The overall message was simple: he is the best and had had enough of Britain. Here in Bern, he would develop the best surgical center in Europe. He needed to inject some fresh blood into this stagnant Swiss environment — a wink. Well, they want him to learn German — a chuckle. He needs somebody trustworthy to look after the department when he or the deputy is away. "Yes, you seem the guy I need, but I must sell you to *them*. You see, for many locals, it is hard to swallow the idea of me running this Inselspital department. You can only guess what they'll say." *A foreign Jew brings in another foreign Jew* — he did not say so, but I completed his sentence in my mind. "But leave politics to me… tomorrow I want you to operate and walk around. I would've loved to have you for dinner, but my wife is still in London, and tonight I must continue with the private German lessons." A wink. "Another small drop of the Glen? Like it? The best, huh? Don't forget your jacket. Cheerio, take your bag now; my deputy will drive you to the hotel. All is paid. Eat as much as you wish and wherever you want, bring all receipts to Frau Hauptli. Please don't order expensive single malt. Stick to local wine." Wink.

The hotel was a block away from the hospital. The deputy dropped me off: "Sorry, Moshe, we'd love to have you for dinner, but my wife is in Geneva, and I have to lecture the local physicians. We need their business, you know," — a deep sigh. "Just walk into the reception. Your room is booked." I dropped off my bag in the room — 12 feet by 9 feet, a narrow single bed, washbasin, mirror, shelves; the toilets and shower were outside at the end of the corridor. Spartan. I started wandering the frozen, deserted streets of the medieval city, looking for a place to eat. A lonely pizzeria, a rude Yugoslavian waiter, some pasta, half a bottle of Chianti — toasting myself. 9 p.m. Back in the hotel — did you ever see a hotel without a lobby? There was no TV in my prison room, but there was a phone, and I dialed Johannesburg and spoke with Heidi for forty-five minutes.

"Blumgart's impressive. I like him. It's a great opportunity. I think the job is mine." I slept badly. Trains were vibrating on the nearby railway trucks. There were constant noises — doors slamming, laughter, beds squeaking above my ceiling.

Next morning, 7 a.m. The morning report, on an empty stomach — the hotel does not serve breakfast, and the department does not provide free coffee. The almost hundred white-coated foot soldiers are gathered before their British professor, who alleviates the military atmosphere with sporadic comments. The surgeon in charge from the recent night reports that there was yet another suicide attempt from the tall Bern railway bridge — a number so and so this year. Blumgart comments about suicide attempts in general and appoints a surgeon to conduct a retrospective study on "Suicides from the Bern railway bridge."

On the way to the OR, I manage to stop at the gleaming cafeteria. It looks like a typical coffee house. I purchased a coffee and a croissant — five Swiss francs. At the OR, I am told to do the lower end of an abdominal perineal resection (APR) for a low-lying rectal cancer. It goes well, but I have a small argument with the senior guy doing the top side. He refuses to understand that by folding back the divided rectum and letting me grasp the proximal edge from below, he can rapidly finish peeling the rectum off the prostate in front.

Lunchtime but no lunch — are they all gobbling sandwiches in their private rooms? We gather at the spacious radiology amphitheater. White-haired professors of radiology present the radiological images. There is a professor of ultrasound, another for CT, and yet another showing the angiographies. Again, English is spoken, and we see the most bizarre liver cases. I sit near Blumgart, who whispers in my ear: "See the pathology?" Afternoon, semi-starved, I am led yet again to see the various ICUs. Finally, I am deposited in the departmental library to busy myself.

Six o'clock. I wonder into Blumgart's *Sekretariat*. "The Herr Professor is busy with the *Spitaldirektor.* He'll see you at 8 o'clock."

Blumgart looks tired. "Lots of politics with the Swiss, lots. You did well today with the APR — so I was told. I'm trying to sell you to them, some resistance." A wink — the magician can solve everything. "Be patient and enjoy yourself. There are good restaurants in this town. Don't forget the receipts."

Another lonely dinner. Tonight, I drink more to help me sleep. But at 2 o'clock, I wake up to a loud concert of lovemaking behind the wall. *Is this a whorehouse?* I can't sleep.

Day 3. Morning report. I'm bored. No one pays any attention to me. I try to converse with a few young surgeons, asking many questions — no one asks me anything. I join them on rounds, but they seem impatient, albeit polite — *what does he want here?* So I leave the hospital and wander around the streets, under the metallic sky and chilly wind; snow is falling. I visit a museum, a palace, and an art gallery. A coffee. A beer. Suddenly I have had enough. I walk back to the hospital and storm into Blumgart's office. He looks up, surprised: "Having a good time in Bern, Moshe?"

I still remember exactly what I told him because it was one of the most significant errors in my professional life. "Professor, look, you brought me here, you asked me all the questions, your deputy asked me all the questions, you saw me operating, I've seen your department, and I like it. So instead of roaming the empty cold streets of Bern, please permit me to catch the train back to Schaffhausen where I have a family and some friends, and you'll let me know about the final decision, whatever it is."

Blumgart produces a cold smile. "I see. I see. Well, let's do it this way. Go and have the best dinner money can buy and come and see me tomorrow at 6.45 a.m. — just before the report. OK? Don't forget to bring the receipts. Good night then."

6.45 a.m, in front of Blumgart's desk. "Moshe. Last night I spoke to my wife in London. I always consult her before making any major decision. I told her about you. She said that I should recruit you. But I have this angst." He repeated the word *angst* a few times. "Here, I'm trying to arrange things, and you walk like this into my office with an ultimatum. I must think about it. I'll let you know. Before you leave, please hand all receipts to my secretary. Cheerio." A brief handshake. I passed by his secretary's desk and said, "*Auf Wiedersehen* Frau Hauptli."

"Herr Doktor, please let me have your receipts. We'll have to reimburse you."

"Thank you very much, but I pay for my own food." And I stormed out. I knew that I had lost this opportunity. I returned to the hotel, took my bag, and walked across the reception towards the revolving doors. "Herr Doktor, are you leaving today? The elderly receptionist asked. *Is she the part-time madame from the night?*

"*Ya, Auf Wiedersehen...*"

"But Herr Doktor, you have to pay first!"

"My bill is paid by the hospital, *Chirurgie*, OK!"

"Ach ja, ja, but the phone bill. You must pay for the phone. Three hundred francs." *Shit.*

Why do I go into such detail, recounting what appears to be a banal event: a young surgeon botching up an interview? Because as the years went by, I understood that this had been the most significant *opportunity* I had ever had to reach the surgical summit.

During his career, most of Blumgart's protégés continued to become eminent hepatobiliary surgeons. He could have been the mentoring surgical *giant* I needed. A few years under his tutelage, learning all the hepato-pancreatic-biliary tricks would have opened large doors.

So why did I fail? Young and provincial, lacking any previous exposure to the European surgical world, my innate impatience? I should have researched the war zone in advance. I should have dressed appropriately and instructed myself to limit my comments to the agreeable and pleasing — but this applies to interviews anywhere. When I returned to South Africa, Heidi said, "I should've come with you." She was right.

* * * * *

About eleven years later, I visited Blumgart in New York City where — after almost a decade in Bern — he became the director of hepatobiliary surgery at a renowned Manhattan cancer institute. I entered his small and crowded office at the end of the corridor. Blumgart emerged from behind his desk — aged and stooped somehow but with the same vitality and shrewd dark eyes. He puffed continuously on his pipe, filling the room with dense smoke, illuminated by the gray light of Manhattan peering through the windows.

Smoking in a New York Hospital! Only Blumgart would dare to do it.

We had a few minutes before going to the OR. I asked a few surgical questions and decided to avoid the past. Suddenly he said: "Moshe, I did you a favor by not letting you come to Bern. Those Swiss would have made your life as hard as they did mine. In my experience they are not exactly Jew lovers."

His fellow entered the room: "Professor, the patient is on the table." In the USA, of course, no doctor is called "professor" by his colleagues, but later that day, the fellow told me: "For all of us here, he is *The Professor*." Then I saw him operating; now in his late sixties, he was still unbelievable — the magician. So they used to call him.

Professor Leslie Harold Blumgart, a giant of modern hepatobiliary surgery, died in New York in September 2022. He was ninety years old.

* * * * *

Professor Leslie Harold Blumgart (1931-2022).*

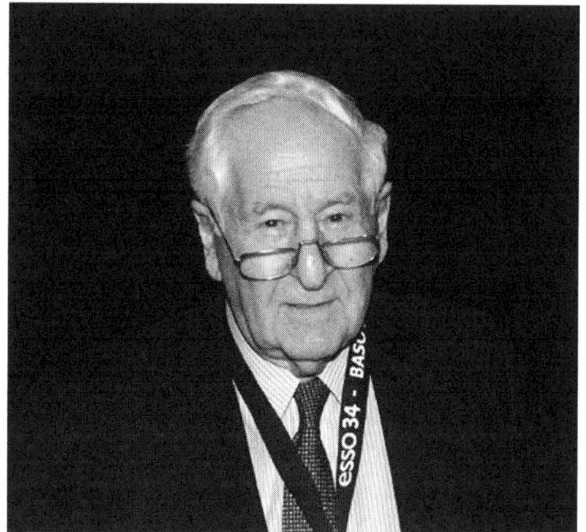

* Reproduced with the kind permission of Professor Graeme Poston.

Twenty-four

A fellowship in Leeds

Each year, the Department of Surgery in Johannesburg selected a young surgeon for a traveling fellowship. A few months after returning from Bern to Johannesburg, I was nominated as the traveling fellow for 1987. I could choose to visit any 'surgical' destination in the world – multiple destinations were acceptable – for six months, all expenses paid, including the salary at home. Where should I go? Japan? The Mayo Clinic? Australia? All the above?

"I won't go with you," Heidi declared, "not with three little boys, aged one to seven, surviving on a ridiculous allowance, in a little rented hole, in some inner city, near a hospital where you'll be buried day and night. You go alone."

Should I try in the USA? I thought. It might be helpful in the long run.

"I've arranged for a colorectal spot in Minneapolis," I proudly told Myburgh.

But the Prof. was not impressed: "Why America? In this department, we follow the British tradition. Why don't you spend some time with David Johnston in Leeds? He's doing a superb job in peptic ulcer and colorectal surgery. Their work on ileal pouches is splendid. I'll write to him immediately." My fate had been decided – goodbye to the American dream.

In those days, the name Professor Johnston of Leeds had become widely known – I mean surgically – for his 'invention' of the 'highly selective vagotomy,' an operation for peptic ulcer disease. Whether he was the one who had invented the procedure was controversial since Professor E. Amdrup of Aarhus had described it in parallel. Later, in Leeds, I would hear that the idea germinated in John Goligher's (the great colorectal surgeon and Johnston's predecessor) brain and that the failure of Johnston to acknowledge Goligher's contribution had led to a rift between the now-retired professor and his follower.

I prepared myself thoroughly for the Leeds affair. I read widely on anorectal physiology and its clinical application. My goal was to return from Leeds as an expert on anorectal physiology and all common and rare anorectal diseases. In my naïve mind, I saw myself as an established South African consultant surgeon going for a study sabbatical with his equals in the United Kingdom. Little did I know.

No one welcomed me at the Leeds railway station on that rainy summer Sunday evening when I stepped out of the Manchester train. I schlepped my heavy suitcase — winter clothes and books included — to the 'grand' Victorian era hotel. The hotel was a hundred quid per night, but the drowsy night porter eyed me briefly, allowing me to continue schlepping my load.

The following day I took a cab to the nearby Leeds General Infirmary on Great George Street — an impressive Victorian structure opened in May 1869 by the Prince of Wales. Since then, it had been expanded and patched up, but its proud walls were darkly stained by many decades of Yorkshire pollution. I walked through an imposing entry hall, with statues, and pictures of past illustrious physicians and surgeons who had walked these corridors, including that of the great Lord Berkeley Moynihan, who in 1920 had founded the Association of Surgeons of Great Britain and Ireland.

I located the professorial surgical unit. Lynn, the professor's personal secretary — tall, blonde, heavily made up — welcomed me: "Oh, Prof. Johnston's touring Australia. I managed to arrange a room for you at the International Student Hostel in Headingley." Another cab took me to the hostel at the northern edge of town — a cheaply built structure surrounded by lawns and shrubs. The superintendent — a retired army sergeant? — handed me a key: "Sir, gates close at 11 p.m., no cooking in the rooms, payment upfront."

I climbed up to my room: tiny, with a narrow hard bed, a wash basin, and a balcony. Loud African music was blasting from downstairs. I explored the communal bathroom. The sink and floor were covered with a carpet of tiny curly black hairs and discarded condoms in the corner. I investigated the kitchen on my floor. Five black kids and girls sat eating, singing, and laughing hysterically to a Caribbean Afro mix. Two fat Pakistani girls were busy cooking something in the corner — completely ignoring the blacks.

The same day I bought myself a second-hand three-speed bicycle. Until late autumn, I would spend my time in the hospital or on the bike, touring the countryside — avoiding the international hostel as much as possible. Two months later, when a misty winter grasped the town, I managed to transfer to the hospital nurses' dormitories.

* * * * *

Finally, Professor Johnston returned from his ever so frequent international trips. He was in his mid-fifties, of medium height, and trim — a marathon runner — a Scot who had lost his original accent. The professor met me in his secretary's office — his own was non-useable as the desk, floor, and chairs were stacked with journals and charts to the ceiling. "Would you join us for dinner tonight?" he asked almost immediately.

A few hours later, I was sitting in the prof's little Polo VW, driving towards his modest bungalow in the suburbs, where I was introduced to his modest-looking and much younger second wife. Following a tasty dinner, the prof. fell asleep in his easy chair, spilling cognac on his trousers.

Riding a cab back to my third-world hostel, I was rather elated. I could envision a fruitful period of clinical and academic cooperation between the professor and his important South African guest. I also looked forward to many similar cozy, tasty, and boozy social encounters with my most genteel British hosts. I could not guess that this was the last and only English family house that I was to see from the inside. The following day, as I cycled to the hospital on my new bike — like any English consultant, I was clad in my new dark suit, trousers suspended with wooden pegs, like Dr. Watson in a Sherlock Holmes movie — I had to face the new reality.

"Moshe, you wouldn't mind using our research registrar's room, would you?" proposed the charming Lynn and ushered me into a tiny cubicle — a converted storage room.

"Good morning, gentlemen. May I introduce you to Dr. Schein of South Africa? Please do make some space for him." *Dr. — not Mr.*

Three young faces above white collars and ties peered at me. They were sweating in this stuffy room, a warm sun spilling in through windows glued to their frames by many layers of old thick, white paint. They introduced themselves. Mark T. and Mark R. were doing a year of research before becoming surgical registrars. The third young man said in a distinct Arabic accent: "My name is Hafez. I'm a qualified Lebanese surgeon from Beirut, here as a clinical observer." I arranged a square foot of desk space opposite the window and squeezed a chair between the two Marks. "Chaps, are there any computers around? Typewriters?"

"Wrong address, old boy. This is the University of Leeds, not Harvard or Princeton," said the smaller and thinner of the Marks. He had a public-school accent, his hair pitch black and eyes slightly narrow — later I found out that he was half Scot, one-quarter Japanese, and another quarter Indian.

"Welcome to Yorkshire, Dr. Schein," said the taller and stouter Mark. He looked at his watch. "Well, chaps, enough jacking off. Let's go to the pub." He did not try to conceal his Yorkshire pronunciation where any "u" comes out as "oo" — *poob*. "Hafez, you wanker, coming with us?" The Arab sulked and said nothing. "Bloody Muslims, teetotalers, sick," the big Mark said goodheartedly. Then to me: "Do join us, tossers like us need a pint of Tetley's bitter before lunch." And so, the three of them, fifteen years younger than me, became my only friends in Leeds.

From the start, I tried to act as a regular clinical team member — but in vain. The more I tried to be one of the boys, the more I was rejected. I discovered that some English people knew how to snub you passively by letting you feel that you were a nobody — like thin air.

My first day in the operating theatre was for a scheduled esophageal resection by Mr. M. — Johnston's second in command. I introduced myself to the senior registrar on the case, a totally Anglo-Saxonised Indian: "Could I scrub in, please?"

"Ewoooo, um, why don't you scrub in as the second assistant?"

The English Indian started the operation, and M. joined in mid-case. At some point, he hooked his finger around the vagus nerve, which was adherent to the lower esophagus, saying, "This is the vagus, see? This is the nerve which is being divided during a truncal vagotomy." It took me a few seconds to realize that he, the great consultant, was uttering this exciting piece of information to enlighten me — the humble second assistant, on a pilgrimage to this center of excellence, from some unknown third-world country.

After the operation, M. vanished into the consultants' OR lounge — off limits to mortals — where lunch was being served on porcelain and white tablecloths. He was a tall, dark-haired Celt with a square jaw — mountain climbing was his passion.

Like many competent and brilliant operators, M. seemed addicted to technical gimmicks, always trying a new one, for example, using a liver ultrasonic surgical aspirator to resect the distal pancreas — painful! This fondness for gimmicks would probably make him a pioneer of the emerging field of laparoscopy a few years later. I had scrubbed with M. on numerous cases, but he never acknowledged my assistance or existence with even one personal question or comment. Initially, I had diagnosed him as a sociopath, but gradually I grasped that what in other places may reflect psychopathy, in the UK is no more than everyday eccentricity. Here oddballs were respected, cherished, and successful.

The attitude of others was no better. If I wanted to scrub in on a specific case, I had to arrive an hour earlier and plainly 'fight' for my place at the table. Otherwise, one of the senior registrars would say: "So sorry, but Helga will scrub in on this case," Helga being an attractive German exchange medical student.

In addition, my ambition to learn practical anorectal physiology was short-lasting. The anorectal laboratory was run by a registrar who, from morning to night, shoved balloons in patients' anorectums. I pestered him for a few days: "Teach me, let me do these tests," but all he wanted was to get rid of me and to continue writing his thesis. Frustrated and bored, I went to the professor and asked for a few research projects.

A month later, I started handing him completed manuscripts of studies. He would take each home and return it a day later with his comments in red ink. I would spend the nights revising the manuscripts and handing them back again to the professor, who would never return any of them to me. I kept the copies with me.

During my sojourn in Leeds, numerous international visitors passed through the department to visit the distinguished professor and see what was new in foregut or rectal surgery. A few stayed a day or two and gave a lecture; others, French and German, arrived for a month, rented a flat, hired a car, and explored the Yorkshire countryside. I noted these were the favorable guests: "Show your face in the OR for a case or two and do not bother us."

I also observed that the Britons, in addition to their rigid class system, used a non-official method to classify foreign doctors based on their origin, race, and language. The ex-colonials, such as Australians or South Africans, topped the list; I mean authentic ex-colonials with the correct accent, not recent immigrants from elsewhere. Americans, preferably whites, were also welcomed – after all, one could always, one day, benefit by visiting them in the USA. Then came the Western Europeans – the French more respected than the Germans and the Italians even less. Eastern Europeans? The Poles would do – didn't they fight with us during the war? *Ruski*? No, no, no. Indians had a soft spot in the English psyche – reserved for humble, dedicated servants. Middle Easterners were at the bottom – just above the blacks from Africa.

What about Jews? The topic seemed taboo, but I was surprised at the extent of the latent British anti-Semitism. Leeds had a large and thriving Jewish community since the 16th century, but I did not see any Jews around. Once in the cafeteria, somebody pointed out a doctor to me and whispered, "He's a Jew, you know?" *Really, is it a secret?* And a secret it seemed to be. Somebody mentioned Professor Norman Williams, M.'s predecessor who had moved to London, "He knows how to write papers but not to operate. He's a Jew." *A Jew called Norman Williams?* Then one day, a senior registrar in vascular surgery approached me while I was sitting in our converted storeroom. He looked around to confirm we were alone and murmured, "Are you Schein? I've heard about you. I'm John Stevenson." He brought his mouth to my ear, "I was born in Tiberias, you know, on the Sea of Galilee. I speak Hebrew." We chatted in Hebrew, and he left hurriedly. A week later, I came across him in some lecture hall. "*Shalom* John," I said loudly and continued in Hebrew. He looked away as if I was addressing the wall behind him, turned around, and left. *What's wrong with them?* I asked myself. The great massacre of Jews in York occurred in 1190, so why are they still hiding?

I was lonely. All my life, wherever I went, I had been surrounded by family and friends. This was my first experience of almost total isolation — an absolutely alien feeling. Weekends were the worst. I remember walking the streets, scenes of cozy family lives playing across large Venetian windows of massive Victorian houses. I felt like those Turkish or Albanian laborers one commonly sees, in their shabby Sunday suits, shuffling, hands behind their backs, in the deserted streets of Western European cities. I learned how foreignness, loneliness, and non-belonging breed resentment — a resentment that may produce dangerous energy.

As long as the weather permitted, I had my bike. I explored the magnificent Yorkshire countryside: the Dales, the Moors — the Bronte sisters' green and quaint country. But the winter found me imprisoned in the dormitory between a bunch of spotted, cottage cheese-faced nursing students. A permanent fog and drizzle engulfed the town — John le Carré's English weather. Each night, as I jogged away my solitude in the park, I expected secret agent George Smiley to emerge from the milky mist.

And there was the equally lonely Hafez, who prepared hummus for me in his moldy Dickensian rented room. And there were the two young Marks who saw to it that I regularly joined them in the pub, always followed by a dinner at the neighborhood's Indian joint where, allegedly, the food was extra spiced to hide the flavor of cat meat in the 'mutton' curry.

* * * * *

It was from Leeds that I traveled to visit Karen in Denmark (see Chapter 7). Another unconventional trip I took was to Spain. In Leeds, I met Carlos, a young surgical resident from Seville. His father, the local head of surgery, had arranged a short 'fellowship' for his son — watching the British surgical giants at work. The two Marks and I would treat Carlos for beers at the pub. "Come to visit Seville," he encouraged us before returning home.

Mark T. and I were on an Air Iberia evening flight from London to Seville a month later. Mark had arranged tickets, but I had no idea about the details. After about ninety minutes, the airplane started descending. The captain announced something in Spanish. "What's up?" I asked Mark, who had some Spanish from school. "I thought the flight to Seville takes more than three hours." "Well, it seems we are to land in Santiago de Compostela for passport control," replied Mark. Where is Santiago? Looking at the map in the back seat, it appeared that Santiago was not far from the northern coast of Spain, while Seville was much more to the south.

It was pitch dark when we landed. We were told to leave our things on board — "take only your passports and other documents."

All passengers were lined up on the edge of an empty tarmac area in front of a small, white-washed building. Uniformed sentries, armed with submachine guns, patrolled the perimeter. I saw two uniformed men inspecting the passports in a lighted window in the building — a scene from World War II or taken from the movie *Casablanca*. The line moved fast. Each passport was stamped and returned to the passenger, who turned around and returned to the nearby airplane — my turn. Mark was behind me. I handed over the blue passport. The Spanish border police official, with a funny-looking hat on his head, took my passport, turning it around. He was paging through carefully as if looking for something. A few minutes passed. Finally, he looked at me, pointed at the passport, and said: "*donde esta la visa?*" I understood the term "visa" and the question mark in his tone. "Visa?" I replied, "Why do I need a visa? I am Israeli, a doctor, a surgeon, you know. Going to a surgical meeting in Seville." After ten minutes of futile protests, no one on the other side of the window understanding a word in English, I was removed from the line. They led me into a closed room behind the front office. "Mark, they are taking me away," I managed to tell my British friend — his burgundy passport now being rapidly stamped. Half an hour later, I could hear the screech of a jet engine — my flight leaving for Seville. Just then, two police officers entered the room, my luggage in their hand — I knew that they had had to search for it in the plane's baggage compartment. "*Ven con nosotros por favor*," one of them said.

"Where are you taking me?" I asked.

"*No Ingles*," they responded, "*venir*."

We climbed into an old, rattling, military-type Land Rover. The road was dark and empty. It was nearing midnight. *Where are we going?* I do not remember being overly anxious. Yes, the situation was a little surrealistic, but I knew that Franco had died more than ten years ago, and Spain was now a democracy. I perceived that passengers, who enter the country without visas, would be deported — not executed with a bullet to the nape of the neck on some desolate hill of Galicia. About fifteen minutes later, we drove into a graveled courtyard and parked in front of an old-looking white, well-lighted castle.

The two officers carrying my luggage led me up some marble stairs. We entered an elegant lobby. *A five-star hotel?* They received a key from the concierge napping at the front desk, guided me up soft, red carpets to a spacious room, dropped off my luggage at the entrance hall, and said, "*buenas noches*." With a head nod, no smile, they left.

I tested the doors. It was not locked. Good, I am not a prisoner. On the other hand, I am not entirely free, for I don't have a passport. I collapsed in the four-poster king bed and slept like a king.

A pale autumn sun was shining through the windows when I woke up. Half a mile below, I could see a small walled town — ancient palazzi and many church towers. In the haze of the morning, the vista of Santiago was magnificent.

I was hungry. I went down and found the large dining room. It was empty. The waiter led me to the table, served me coffee, and pointed to the breakfast buffet. Who is paying for all of this, I asked myself. This place must be expensive. I had the phone number of Carlos' home in Seville. I called, but there was no answer — time to explore Santiago. I found a map in my room and left the hotel. The concierge smiled and waved at me. The door attendant opened the door. A free man without a passport. From my long stroll around Santiago, I remember the intoxicating smell of fresh coffee permeating the air, the fabulous cathedral, and the fried calamari in an outdoor café. I returned to the hotel in the late afternoon. I had a snooze and returned to the dining room. Here the portion of calamari was huge. I will never forget how good they tasted. They were tenderly fried, served with wedges of lemon along delicate potato fries. A bottle of chilled white wine was easily consumed. Back in the room, I tried Carlos' number again. It rang and rang. *How long will they keep me here?*

I fell asleep.

I woke up to banging on the door. It was still night. "Wait," I shouted. I dressed rapidly and opened the door. Two police officers, I recognized one of them from before. "*Venir por favor,*" he said, pointing to my things and luggage, "*Todo, todo…*" take everything. The Land Rover was waiting. Back to the airport, through the gates, directly onto the tarmac, and in front of the ramp stairs leading to an Air Iberia airliner. The plane's engines were roaring. It was ready for take off. I am being deported back to London, I thought. A short dark man with a mustache, tie, and jacket was waiting at the bottom of the stairs.

He smiled and shook my hand and introduced himself in English. I heard the word "inspector." "Sir, you will now be flying to Seville." He led me up the stairs and to a first-class seat. A policeman followed with my luggage. "Have a nice stay and see you soon," he said. I think that I was a little bewildered — *what's happening here? — where is my passport?* "I need my passport," I said. The inspector smiled: "Your passport stays here. See you next week." Fifty minutes later, we landed in Seville.

Fast forward a week. The flight from Seville to London stopped over in Santiago de Compostela. A few passengers join the flight. A slight, mustachioed man in a dark suit walks towards me down the aisle. I recognize the inspector. He smiles, shakes my hand, and hands me back my passport. "I hope you enjoyed Seville. Next time you come to Spain, please do it with a valid visa. Goodbye." A happy ending.

In Seville, I found out how it was all arranged. When Mark arrived with the news of my 'disappearance,' Carlos' influential father immediately activated his contacts in the police and the Ministry of the Interior. A day on the phone and apparently, it worked. And Seville? What is left in my memory from that hot Andalusian town is the elegant old house of Carlos' family, rooms permanently shuttered against the sun, dinners eaten into midnight, the streets waking up at noon, a few strong coffees in the bars to kill the hangovers, long siestas, eating lamb chops in an outside restaurant — throwing the bones on the pavement. But the best memories are the flamenco bars. Late at night, standing at the smooth zinc bar, sipping another glass of red wine, munching green olives, those guitars, the rhythmic clapping of hands, the women's flamenco heels tapping on the wooden floor, the guttural laments of the male vocalist, everybody dancing, including little children — all so intoxicating and sensual. Hemingway described it better. I lost touch with Carlos soon after.

* * * * *

February 1988. The two Marks and Hafez drove me to the airport in Manchester. I returned to Johannesburg twenty pounds lighter and without a new surgical hobby. Anything surgical I learned in Leeds became obsolete a few years later or was never of any value to me. But I learned that a surgeon out of his town, or his hospital, is a nobody, and, above all, I learned how not to treat foreigners and outsiders — and this would become of great practical value to me in the future. It would take the two Marks fifteen years to become surgical consultants in England. I am still in touch with Hafez — the poor Lebanese, ignored and shunned in Leeds, is now a successful surgeon in Paris.

Back in Johannesburg, I wrote to Professor Johnston and inquired about the fate of the manuscripts I had written for him in Leeds — did he intend to publish them? He did not reply. I waited a few months and then published one of my Leeds studies alone. In a footnote, I thanked "Professor David Johnston for the permission to study and report on his patients." When the paper appeared in the *World Journal of Surgery*, I mailed him a reprint. He faxed me frantically a week later: "Dear Moshe, congratulations on the paper. Please do not submit the others. We are busy finalizing them." I never heard from him again; the other studies on which I had worked for long days and nights in Leeds ended up in my garbage bin.

Yet, I found the Brits excellent surgeons, educators, and researchers. That some Brits are as they are is not their own fault but an inborn error of national development, or in John le Carré's words, the British social structure is "one of the crying pities of the modern world."

* * * * *

Left: roaming around the Yorkshire countryside. Right: Leeds 1987, with buddies Mark R., Hafez S. (top) and Mark T. (bottom).

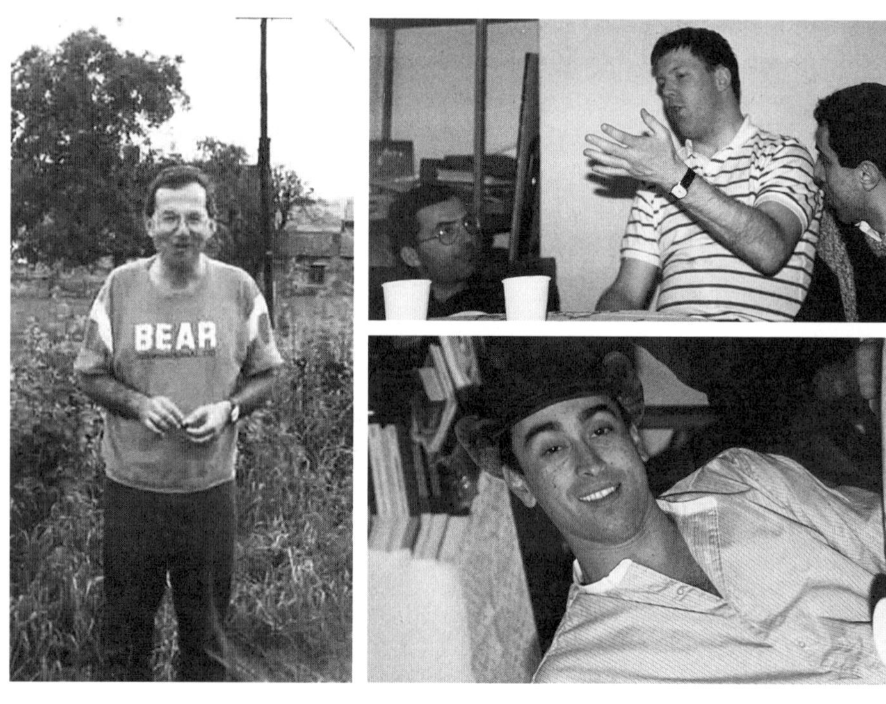

Twenty-five

My own unit and goodbye South Africa

My little son Dan did not recognize me when I returned from Leeds to Johannesburg. "This is your *Aba*!" he was told.

Back to the J.G. Hospital. It seemed to me that GAG, after savoring a six-month interval without Schein, was finding it hard to readjust to my reappearance.

The tensions so common between teachers and their up-and-coming protégés, were mounting. Not only was he constantly criticizing my alleged deviations from certain surgical routines — considered 'holy' in his eyes — but he also expressed unhappiness with the type of papers I was writing. "Physiological scores? APACHE II scores? Who needs such BS? You want to assess a patient? Just look at him." In retrospect, GAG may have been right.

What I suffered most, however, was GAG's 'weekend syndrome.' For unknown reasons, GAG would often develop foul moods on weekends; it seemed that his remedy for such moods was to operate on something or anything. It was probably the act of surgery, which produced a surge of soothing endorphins — for the surgeon, not the patient — which calmed his mind. On my weekends off, GAG would round on Sundays. On the following Monday, I would find my patients, whom I was preparing for semi-elective procedures, had already had the operation. I clearly remember a patient with a controlled leak from his duodenal stump after a partial gastrectomy; I managed him non-operatively and hoped for a spontaneous recovery. However, on one of his black Sundays, GAG took him for a re-gastrectomy. Only a surgeon knows how it feels to have your patient undergoing a reoperation by another surgeon without your consent.

The situation exploded one Saturday morning before the weekly grand departmental meeting at the medical school. Atypically, GAG was five minutes late for the rounds. When he appeared — a button missing in the top piece of his white safari suit, remnants of shaving cream drying in his right ear — I could sense the gathering storm. He rushed from room to room, irritably criticizing the interns and registrars, and sarcastically rejecting my comments. It was an elderly lady, admitted just an hour before the rounds — abdominal pain, low blood pressure, borderline peritonitis, the 'nonspecific belly' declaring "I have dead bowel" — which triggered

GAG's terminal explosion, now directed towards the house staff. I left the room without uttering a word and marched towards my car. My pager beeped ten minutes later: "GAG wants to see you." I turned around. He closed the door behind us in the doctors' room and hissed — GAG never shouted: "Why did you leave the round without saying anything? What's the source of your resentment towards me?"

"No resentment, I simply can't tolerate your attitude… how you acted today towards the residents, the interns, it wasn't fair. They didn't have time to assess that lady properly."

"You don't understand," GAG stopped me mid-sentence, his pale eyes desperately burning through mine, "You don't sense how stressed I am in front of a sick patient." I can't help it — that's how I am, his eyes added.

I am unsure whether I understood him then — later, I would, but I perceived that I must move on. GAG had made me a surgeon and gave me whatever he could, but now there wasn't enough space for us in his little kingdom. Luckily, at that time, a head of a unit at the Hillbrow Hospital announced that he was leaving for private practice. I expressed an interest in this position. A month later, Myburgh announced my nomination.

* * * * *

Early 1989, 8 a.m. I was in the elevator, together with a bunch of medical students. It was my first day at the Hillbrow Hospital.

"To which unit are you allocated?" asked one of the male students,

"We are in Prof. Bremner's," replied one of the other students. Prof. Bremner, my previous boss at the Coronation 'colored' hospital, had meanwhile been 'upgraded' to lead the Hillbrow department.

"We are in Mr. Schein's unit," the two female students replied. I smiled to myself. *Mr. Schein's unit*. It sounded good. I could hardly believe my ears — eight and a half years in Johannesburg, nine and a half years after medical school, and now, at thirty-eight, I was the boss. At last free. Fate decided that my 'freedom' would not last long. However, the almost two years spent in the Hillbrow Hospital are engraved in my mind as the most exciting period in my surgical life.

The Hillbrow Hospital was previously the Old Johannesburg Hospital — the main university hospital before it had moved to the monstrous building on Parktown Ridge. It later became the urbane hospital for 'nonwhites' — serving the blacks who worked in the city. It was considered an upgraded, more civilized, albeit smaller, version of the Baragwanath Hospital. Its colonial stone buildings were situated in the middle of Hillbrow, then, a sort of declining mini-Manhattan: apartment buildings, restaurants, shops, cafés, bordellos, and nightclubs. In 1989, Hillbrow was still formally a 'white zone,' but the illegal invasion of colored and black people from the townships had already started. Today, I am told, Hillbrow is strictly a 'nonwhite' area controlled by armed hordes of the Nigerian mafia — a war zone.

My unit treated an average of sixty inpatients at all times and was on 'intake' every third night. The other consultant — my 'deputy' — was the charming Jim Howell. He was a tall, white-haired, red-faced, aging surgeon, twenty-five years my senior, who had come to Johannesburg after a long surgical career in the gold mines in Zambia. Jim would have been an ideal actor for a movie about an old colonial British surgeon. He was immensely experienced — he had seen and done everything — abdomens, bones, endocrine, vascular, trauma, head and neck, just everything. He was also well-read and knowledgeable. Jim was tired of operating, but his enormous hands were still steady — despite a steady consumption of Scotch — and there was no better assistant than him: calm, patient, active, supportive, humorous — at times hilariously funny. An example: during a ward round, we got to a 'colored' female patient sitting on a wooden chair next to her bed. From her looks, her make-up, and her cheap jewelry, she was unmistakably a Hillbrow prostitute. She also had had her incisor teeth removed — a common practice in the profession supposedly meant to enhance fellatio skills. Jim wanted to examine her abdomen; he said dryly, "Could you hop on the bed, dear, and lie down, a position that you are, no doubt, most accustomed to." No procedure, however major, new, or threatening, was scary, with Jim's hands exposing the operative field and his calming voice suggesting, for example: "OK Moshe, we did enough, let's just leave here a few swabs, let's go for tea." One of his mottos was, "Never finish an operation during which more than half of the patient is sent for pathology." Many years have passed since I had last heard from Jim or about him. He must be gone by now. To me, this modest, kind, and funny man was a surgical giant — even though you cannot find him on Google…

My unit had three registrars: two rotating and one, the most senior, was permanent. The latter was Angelo, who had emigrated from Italy. (I mentioned Angelo in "*Life Means Nothing Behind the Green Wall*" in the (real) stabbed heart scene, which I 'moved' from Hillbrow to Brooklyn.) He proved hard working and loyal, a dexterous surgeon with a solid mind. His ideas concerning pancreatic pseudocysts were original and translated into a few well-cited papers. Angelo, a classical espresso-plus-a-cigarette-per-minute Italian, was, however, not too fond of the English language, and while completing the equivalent of two residencies, he did not care to take any examinations. Consequently, and unfortunately, this talented surgeon finally ended up as a general practitioner in Johannesburg.

These were great surgical years. We did it all: massive thyroid goiters, esophagectomies, giant abdominal tumors, mesoatrial shunts, vascular procedures, and of course, lots of trauma and other emergencies. It was my last opportunity to savor the pleasure of traditional 'big' general surgery before moving to other countries where general surgery had become fragmented into multiple sub-specialties. So, whereas most surgeons reach the top and continue climbing at 50 (see the Epilogue), in hindsight, I was at my surgical summit when I was 40. From then on, it would be a gradual decline as I migrated from place to place, finally becoming a 'bread and butter' surgeon.

* * * * *

Meanwhile, Moses, our gardener, did very well for himself. He was now fully scheduled – tending the gardens of many of Roger's friends and ours. Moses accommodated a continuous stream of black maidens in his modest shed behind Roger's house. Like many young and older blacks, he did not know what this might inevitably bring. Then, one day, while crossing the main street of Melville, a fast car hit Moses. He flew a few meters into the air and landed, on his head, on the opposite pavement. On the following day's rounds, I was surprised to find Moses connected to a ventilator – a tube sticking out of his mouth – lying on the first bed in my unit's male ward. Severe head injuries – there were so many of them – were treated by us general surgeons, on the floor, by supportive means only. We managed Moses very carefully, and four weeks later, he emerged from his deep coma, recognized me, and smiled. A fortnight later, I drove him home. Anyone who had known Moses before now claimed that the severe blow to his head did something to improve the synapses in his brain – thus his intelligence. However, Roger and I managed to classify him as "permanently brain damaged," which earned him a lifelong government pension to supplement what he earned gardening, an occupation to which he returned with great vigor.

On a sunny, late winter Saturday morning, as I was leaving the medical school, I saw a tall white-haired black man, surrounded by a group of younger blacks, walking in my direction on the plaza. Even from a distance, I immediately recognized him, as I had seen his image repeatedly on the TV and in newspapers. As I passed him, I nodded politely and said, "Good morning." I continued walking, but he stopped me: "Doctor, Sir, would you be so kind as to show us the way to the hospital? We are lost." The soft but strong, confident voice, the warm smile. "Sure," I said, "just follow me, please." I turned around, leading him to a shortcut, across the medical school, to the hospital. I pretended not to recognize him – as if I would make such a long detour for anyone. The tall man chatted to me, asking questions: my name, what I was doing, where I lived, and my long-term plans. The others were following us at a respectful distance. We arrived at the hospital's main corridor. "Here you are, Sir. From now on, you can't get lost."

The tall man smiled down at me, grasped my hand with his large and warm one, and gave me a firm handshake and sincere thanks. Then he left, but I could still feel his immense charisma. As you must have already guessed, the tall man was Nelson Mandela, who had just been released (February 11, 1990) after twenty-seven years of imprisonment.

Although 'protected' from the true picture by the State-controlled and censored South African media, we understood that huge political changes were knocking at the gates. After President P.W. Botha had been forced to resign, Frederik Willem de Klerk became the 'Gorbachev of South Africa,' calling for the end of apartheid laws and freeing Mandela. South Africa was changing rapidly. What about us?

The exodus of whites — a constant trickle during the latter part of the 1980s — now reached significant proportions. Anybody who had somewhere to emigrate, and the means to do so, seemed to be leaving — people knew what happened to Rhodesia after it had become Zimbabwe. Hence, the value of property plummeted. So, we asked ourselves: should we go now? Where to?

The answer was provided to us unexpectedly: my mother in Haifa was diagnosed with metastatic breast cancer and needed close support. Moreover, my friends called from Haifa about an opened promising position.

We sold our Melville dream house at a significant loss, divided our furniture among friends, and shipped a few boxes of books and paintings to Haifa. It was early summer, perfect for a farewell party in our garden for the good friends (e.g., Hatchuels, Meisters, Frohlichs, Saadias, and others) we had made in that lovely country. In some respect, it was beautiful indeed. How can one forget the beaches of Natal, the deserts of the Cape, hiking in the Drakensberg mountains; the weekends on a lonely Highveld farm; the cozy Victorian hotels and 6 a.m. tea with milk served in your room; the country inns — a black waiter taking your order and rushing to the kitchen with his finger on the relevant entry on the menu.

A lovely country that, however, never captured my heart. Perhaps because I could not bond emotionally with, or lacked empathy for, the cause of any of its communities and factions. Thus, over eleven years, South Africa had never become to me — what America eventually would be — a second home.

Do I feel guilty for benefiting from the apartheid system — enjoying the good life while the blacks suffered? Should I feel bad for having learned to 'cut' on blacks? This is a surgical memoir. Hence, I avoid contemporary politics as much as possible. Often, however, I reflect on how we tend to be callous and impervious to the suffering of those around us. We bury our heads in the sand like ostriches and continue with our daily lives. I admit — this is what we did. But what could we have done? Didn't we save many black lives — significantly more than we 'killed.'

Traditionally, when consultants left the university department in Johannesburg, a farewell event would be organized in their honor — but not for me. I never found out why. However, a year later, Professor Myburgh's secretary wrote to ask for my picture to be added to those decorating the department's corridors. I am told that it is still hanging there.

We sold our cars to our handyman Johannes and German friends — both were stolen within a month — this was the emerging face of the new South Africa. And I cannot forget Moses' face when I opened before him my cupboard and told him, "Take anything you wish" — I did not have any use for suits and dress shirts in Israel. Now Moses became the best-dressed gardener in Johannesburg, but for how long? The AIDS epidemic has since destroyed his generation of urban, promiscuous — a way of life for them — South African young blacks. Moses' fate is unknown to me.

Professor Myburgh retired in 1994. He, a chain smoker, passed away in 2010 at eighty-two from respiratory complications. My mentor George Decker eventually left the J.G. Hospital to become a professor and chairman elsewhere. After his formal retirement, he continued teaching and operating in a remote, rural 'black' hospital for a few years. Surgery was his life. He could not stop. Over the years, GAG regularly communicated with me through emails. In 2013, he wrote about having a malignant melanoma removed from his shoulder. "I hope it didn't spread," he wrote. A few months later, his wife Margaret informed me about his brain metastases.

The decline was rapid. GAG died at the age of eighty-one. He was a complex man — hard, tough, demanding, ferocious, explosive, and occasionally sarcastic. However, under the envelope, under the capsule in which he wrapped himself, there was a soft core of compassion, justice, and warmth. He was a *mensch*.

My surgical father… after my father.

* * * * *

A tremendous summer storm flooded the streets of Johannesburg when Roger and David drove us to the airport, Pimpush, the Dachshund, and Goofy, the kitten, included.

We booked an El Al flight to Tel Aviv for 4 January 1991. However, in December 1990, the Americans and their allies had already deployed over half a million troops on the Kuwaiti border, facing the Iraqis — the Middle

East was set for war. A few months previously, the newspapers had reported Saddam Hussein's threats to destroy "half of Israel," if it, or the USA, attacked his country. We knew that gas masks were being distributed to the entire Israeli population.

"Shouldn't we postpone our departure? Do we need to fly into the war zone voluntarily?" asked my sensible Swiss wife.

"Come on, what war? There is always some war in this region. You cannot avoid all of them," replied the nihilistic, fatalistic Israeli in me. "Do you want us to cancel everything because of this fucking idiot Saddam?!"

The midnight flight to Tel Aviv was almost empty. The pale winter sun was high over the stumpy hills of Judea as the Boeing arriving from the south flew low over Jerusalem and then turned, westbound, towards Ben Gurion Airport.

Back to the great Greek poet Cavafy of Alexandria: "Always keep Ithaca in your mind. To arrive there is your ultimate goal. But do not hurry the voyage at all. It is better to let it last for many years…"

Were we arriving in Ithaca too early?

* * * * *

Twenty-six

Going back to Haifa

January 5, 1991. Up from the Boeing, on the right side, I saw the sun rising over the mountains of the Saudi peninsula. We flew over the Red Sea, the Egyptian desert on the left. Next, we were above the tip of the Sinai; the jet turned right to follow the course of the Gulf of Aqaba. Soon we would reach Eilat, the Negev Desert — home. Heidi and the boys were asleep, stretched over three seats each. The airplane was almost empty — who would want to fly to Israel on the eve of war? It was too late in the night and early in the morning for a Scotch, so I drank a coffee and pondered: yes, my mother is probably dying, and my sister cannot cope — they need me back home, I know. But what about the job I had been offered?

A few months prior, I had flown to Israel to be interviewed at Haifa's Rambam Hospital. Professor Meir Maccabi, the head of the department, received me in his miniature office. Under the pseudo-social Israeli system, only administrators provided themselves with adequate office space, not the clinicians — like in the Soviet Union. Maccabi welcomed me with Turkish coffee in tiny Arabic cups and delicious pastries served on white porcelain. I saw this: a short, slender man, not more than 5′4″, in his fifties; a pleasant, intensely suntanned, and deeply furrowed face, an abundance of black hair. He was dressed in a very tight, bell-shaped pair of trousers, a short-sleeved white shirt — almost bursting over his narrow chest — and an ancient blue blazer, a few sizes too small. He looked like a caricature from an Italian fashion magazine of the 1960s. It was summer — in Israel, it means no necktie — and indeed, Maccabi's shirt was wide open, proudly exposing his furry chest and a heavy silver medallion. When he stood up, I noticed that his torso was bent forward, and the belt line reached the lower chest.

"Sit down, Moshe, sit down. I'm so happy to see you. Heard a lot about you." A prolonged handshake — his small, warm, soft hand holding mine for many seconds — as if refusing to let go. "We are not buying a 'cat in a sack'" — a Hebrew expression describing an unknown entity — "you are one of us, and people in this town know you well — and of course, your academic record is impressive. So, all we have to do is to see whether you can operate. This is crucial to me," he raised his small brown hairy hands, "as you may have heard that I'm a *superlative* surgeon." He spoke a classic, correct Hebrew, using no slang whatsoever — almost biblical.

Early the following day, Maccabi led me into the operating room. I was to perform a total gastrectomy for cancer with one of the senior residents. Maccabi had not scrubbed in. He just hovered on a footstool behind my back, forcing himself to shut up — like a frustrated basketball coach watching his team without being able to tell them what to do. As we completed the last anastomosis, Maccabi said: "OK, that's enough. Doron will close, go and change. Professor Kodkod will see you in five minutes."

When I had emerged from the tiny, grimy, flooded changing room, Maccabi hugged me warmly. "Moshe, you will be my deputy — welcome home to Haifa!" Obviously, he had been satisfied that I could hack out the whole stomach. "Now I will take you down to Kodkod's chancellery, but be careful, we can't consider him among our supporters."

Professor Menachem Kodkod was the general director of the hospital. Like many senior Israeli administrators in other sectors, the professor was a retired army brigadier general. He was nominated the director of this largest northern Israeli hospital after serving as the Chief of the Israeli Medical Corps.

No one I asked could tell me how and why Kodkod had been nominated a professor at Haifa's Medical School, affiliated with the prestigious *Technion* (the 'MIT of the Middle East'). Before that time, Kodkod had been the first author of only four publications — three of which were published in low-key Israeli periodicals. "Well, it's a secret," his supporters would say, "the research he did in the army is classified." Others would roll their eyes, let their jaws hang down, mouth open, arms flexed, palms facing up, which for Jews means: "*nu, vot du you vont*," adding, "another Napoleon."

Kodkod's vast chancellery was on the first floor, just to the left of the main lobby. Interestingly, while CEOs of American hospitals tend to build their vast offices on the top floors — the higher, the better — in Israel, it was the opposite.

When his secretary ushered me into his room, the ex-brigadier general stood behind his desk. I saw yet another very short and thin man in his 50s: gray trousers, a white short-sleeved shirt, gray hair, and glasses. His handshake was flimsy, languid, and his voice was listless yet arrogant. *Altogether a gray man.*

"*Shalom* Dr. Schein." He'd pointed me to a hard chair by the door and walked back behind his desk at the other remote corner of the room. "So, you want to be Maccabi's deputy, hah? Let's see, let's see." He picked up a folder, opened it, and glanced at it above his bifocals. "South Africa? *Yohannesburg*? Eh? Why? Training in Israel was not good enough for you? We have here the *best* surgeons in the world, we train them here, and then, usually, we send them to America for advanced training, a year or two...

or, eh, perhaps you were not good enough to be accepted into one of *our* training programs?"

"Not at all. I didn't even try..." But Kodkod continued: "So Maccabi wants you as his deputy, hah? Do you know anything about his department, the political situation? Do you know with whom exactly you will work... eh... if you get the job?"

"I'm not a politician. All I want is to come back home. Haifa is my town, and I need a job."

"I assume you did serve in our army. Yes, I see it here — the Golani Brigade, a medic, hah?"

"No, I was a platoon sergeant, Company C, Battalion 13."

In his face, I read: *not even an officer*. "Perhaps you don't know, but your chairman in *Yohannseburg*, Professor Mi-bu-rg — what kind of name is that? It doesn't sound Jewish — wrote me this, I quote, 'he never had any experience in administering a large department, not as its chairman, nor as a deputy,' ha? You really want to be Maccabi's deputy?"

"Professor, it seems that my chairman in Johannesburg believes that the Israeli surgical department is equivalent to what in South Africa is, or the USA, a vast administrative complex, a system controlling multiple sections and units and numerous surgeons and trainees. How could he know that an Israeli department of surgery comprises 30 beds and a few surgeons — half the size of my current unit in Johannesburg?"

I was not surprised by what Kodkod had said, for I was carrying a copy of Myburgh's classified letter to him in my pocket. After hearing from Maccabi previously that "the letter from Myburgh to Kodkod is not favorable," I had decided to look at what Myburgh had written exactly. The departmental master key had been in my possession, so on one Sunday afternoon, I left Roger in the corridor to ambush any stray visitor and unlocked Myburgh's suite. I located a giant filing cabinet in a small backroom — it was not locked. With my heart pounding, I retrieved the cramped file that had my name on it and carefully examined its contents. Most items had been duplicated by carbon copies that I stuffed in my pockets.

Back at home, I had read Myburgh's recommendation letter to Kodkod. It was laconic, focusing on what Dr. Schein is not ("no administrative experience, no basic research experience") rather than what he is ("a well-trained surgeon," "a loner"). I was bewildered. I had been working for Myburgh for ten years. Now I wanted to go home — not to the Mayo Clinic in Minnesota but to an unknown hospital in the Middle East. So why not give me a glorious recommendation? If I was good enough to lead a unit in Myburgh's department, why shouldn't I be OK for the Haifa job?

"I don't know Schein," — like many Israelis Kodkod had the irritating military, or East European habit of using your second name — not Mr.

Schein or Dr. Schein but just Schein — "we'll have to discuss further your candidacy. We train here a large cadre of promising young surgeons who may be better suitable for such a senior position."

He dismissed me. I was pale when Maccabi walked me out to the hospital gate. "I don't know why he's against me. What's his problem?"

"It is not you but me… *yihye beseder*, it'll be OK, don't worry, leave the General to me, trust me. Now go to the Ministry of Health and organize your certificate of surgical specialty." Maccabi's hug had been warm and tight.

Later that day, Jacob, my old friend from medical school, a plastic surgeon in Rambam, had explained: "Maccabi is desperate, he's alone, and Kodkod is slowly destroying him. He needs you."

"How come?"

"Well, a couple of years ago, Maccabi had inherited the department from Schrammek. It was an empire — vascular, general, everything. Then Maccabi fell off a stepladder. He was painting a wall or something and broke his hip. They put him in a spica cast, you know, the cast which goes up to your neck and you can't move, and while he was lying like this for a few months, you know what old Schrammek did? He helped organize a revolution against Maccabi: his attending surgeons went to Kodkod and convinced him to nominate one of them as head of a new independent vascular section, with the old *schmock* Schrammek reinstated as deputy. They took the rest of the department's attendings with them, and now poor Maccabi was rotting in bed without even one attending surgeon — only with his spica." Jacob was enjoying his own story — political intrigues are considered a national and most entertaining hobby in the Holy Land.

"And then?"

"And then nothing. While Maccabi was in bed, his department was attached to Surgery A — Professor Barzilai's monarchy, but then after his spica was removed, Maccabi surprised everybody with a rapid physical recovery. The man is a small lion. He returned to his department, which existed only on paper, but, as you know, in Israel, chiefs of departments are nominated for life. Only God can fire them."

"So, what's Kodkod's problem, and where do I come into the equation?"

"You still don't understand, do you? Kodkod hates Maccabi. He considers him just a small 'homo.'"

"What?"

"Yes, a 'homo' allegedly. I bet he's hugged you today for half an hour. A long story, everybody knows, but he's an excellent surgeon — the best — and thus they hate him."

"So?"

"So Kodkod hopes to render Maccabi's department dysfunctional: no attendings, no teaching, no night cover. He wants to open a third department, bringing in his own protégé — now doing liver transplants in the US — and then place Maccabi in formalin: a professor with a room and no junior doctors, like the dwarfish cardiology professor in Jerusalem, Rogel was his name, remember? But now Maccabi is importing you, and according to the bylaws, two attending surgeons can run a department and a teaching program. And in one or two years from now, Maccabi's own senior residents will graduate; by then Maccabi will be fully recovered. Your candidacy is killing Kodkod's plan, you see?"

"And you want me to insert my head into this awful mess?"

"You told me that you want a job in Haifa near your mother. I will tell you only this, and remember what I'm saying, Kodkod will be your sworn enemy, and Maccabi is an alleged 'homo.' Think carefully about your future."

I had no problems with the 'homo' whom I found very likable; as to the little brigadier general — *we will see; first, let's return home.*

Back in Johannesburg, after the interview, I met the orthopedic surgeon Jack Yakim, who had previously spent a few years in Rambam Hospital. Jack spat out his cigarette, and spat again on the ground, saying in his typically bombastic style, as if he were the Prophet Ezekiel: "Beware Schein, beware Schein. Rambam is a snake pit, you understand? Listen to me: they are all snakes, beware Schein, and take care."

* * * * *

The airplane started descending towards Tel Aviv. Heidi and the boys woke up and put their shoes on. *Snake pit, beware.* Yakim's harsh words were replaying in my head and made me smile.

Snakes, 'homo,' Kodkod — here I come!

* * * * *

Twenty-seven

The return to the Holy Land

Early morning. Ben Gurion Airport. A representative of the Jewish Agency guided us to a side building dedicated to the reception of *olim* — 'newcomers.' Heidi and the boys were not Israeli citizens yet. Thus, we were arriving as *olim*, entitled to all the benefits the Jewish State would bestow upon any diaspora Jew who decided to return to Zion. This meant no sales tax on a new car, no income tax for a year, housing rental assistance, basic furniture, a free flight to Israel (one way), a free ride from the airport to any destination, and more. The huge reception hall was packed with at least a thousand people: old, young, and babies — standing, walking, and lying on the floor — sweating under layers of heavy winter clothes and fur caps. On side tables, old women volunteers handed out tea, yogurt, and egg and tomato sandwiches. *Is this Ben Gurion Airport or a Moscow train station?* Actually, these people did not look like Muscovites but refugees from one of the obscure 'stan' regions. Our arrival to Israel coincided with the peak of the great immigration of Russian Jews — at least a third of them *claiming* to be Jews — in the early 1990s. Each morning, one El Al jumbo jet after another would land, unloading people from all parts of what had once been the Soviet Union.

Two hours later. Our turn to confront the man across the desk: "*a vy otkuda*; where are you from?" asked a small, bald man who looked like Anatoly Sharansky.

"*Ya ne govoryu po russki*; I don't speak Russian"; this was the only thing I could say in his language — except, of course, *spasiba* and *nazdrovie*. The guy, two front gold teeth in his mouth, who probably had arrived from Russia only a year ago, looked at me in disbelief: *how come this man talks no Russian — is he retarded?* So, he tried Heidi, but by then, I was addressing him in Hebrew, which he hardly understood. This comical situation would repeat itself on many occasions in Haifa that absorbed a hundred thousand Russian immigrants — particularly for Heidi, who, with her Aryan looks, would be repeatedly mistaken to be a *Russiya* — in Hebrew, a 'Russian woman.' For many Israeli men, the *Russiyot*, Russian women, were considered beautiful and for some an 'easy target.'

We settled in a spacious flat rented from our friends Bubi and Memi, who were then living in Long Island, New York. The apartment was in Bat

Galim, a little run-down, peaceful seaside working-class neighborhood. Bat Galim was built during the 1930s by German Jews fleeing from Hitler. Now many of the two- or three-family *neubau* houses — so elegant years ago — were dilapidated by the erosive forces of the sea. Our flat was on the ground level, surrounded by a small patch of grass and a few trees, stunted by the salty winds. Above us lived an older man who lost both eyes in the War of Independence; his wife, a Hungarian Auschwitz survivor, a tattooed number on her arm, used to walk him along the beach at each sunset. "Shh, shh, be quiet," she used to admonish our boys, "my husband has a bad heart. He needs his *schlafstunde*." Years later, I was told that the woman had died, and the blind, ill man was living there with a young *Russiya*, until he died too.

Our house was less than a hundred meters from a sandy beach. A few houses to our north were the headquarters of the Israeli Navy. Further, at a five-minute walk, the Rambam Hospital and the 'white elephant' — the modern skyscraper accommodating the medical school — stood spoiling the coastline with its phallic presence. Summer and winter winds constantly blew sand into our rooms through the open windows. It was a shabby living space, unlike Melville, Johannesburg, but the Mediterranean Sea — the beloved sea of my youth — compensated for everything. You return home in the evening, put on your bathing suit, and in bare feet, run straight into the sea; you crawl three hundred meters offshore, turn on your back and watch the Carmel Mountain towering over you, the panorama of lights coming to life. That beloved sea was kind to us — much more than the actual events which were to take place.

* * * * *

January 15 1991. First day at work. Maccabi embraced me like a father meeting his lost son. "Let me introduce you to everybody," he said, dragging me for a tour that lasted into the afternoon. We walked into each of the numerous departments and labs, climbing up the floors of the ugly 'new' building, crossing the vast garden with its old palm trees into the cozy building erected during the British Mandate. We saw the deserted winter beach and ships entering Haifa's harbor from each window. These were my childhood views; on that beach, I often swam with my father — it was all so familiar yet different. Wherever we entered, Maccabi approached the section head, declaring proudly: "This is *my* new deputy." Meaning: *I'm back in the picture; my department is now in business... screw Kodkod*. Each introduction was followed with the usual casual Israeli barter — everybody expressing his love and support for Maccabi and a warm welcome for his new acquisition.

After each such series of prolonged handshakes and heavy shoulder pounding, Maccabi would schlep me on, providing me with his take on the last person we had just met: "An enemy, beware," or "a poisonous snake," or "blown-up balloon," with an occasional "*yadid*" — a dear friend. I had grown up in this town, I had studied in this country, I had done my internship and left. I had no idea how sweltering, wet, and thick the medical-political swamp was that I was entering now.

A swamp? A snake den?

* * * * *

The Rambam Hospital would provide an ideal background to a Machiavellian saga. There were so many bizarre characters, locally born or gathered from all corners of the world: Europe, South America, Morocco; Ashkenazi and Sephardim Jews, even Jews from India; and Arabs. Many doctors had been trained everywhere: Houston, the Sorbonne, Zurich, Minsk, Buenos Aires, and even Sophia, Bulgaria.

And here they were, all now speaking Hebrew in many different accents; each belonging to a different department; each loyal to another boss, each highly competitive and jealous of the other and wanting to get rid of his boss and take over; each craving the private patients of his colleagues; each continuously bad-mouthing his friends – while eating hummus together at the Arab restaurants on the beach. And each was tied to the other in invisible but gossiped about bonds of previous friendships, arguments, coup attempts, academic competition, and of course – this was considered highly entertaining – extramarital love affairs. Why? Simple: take too many potentially talented and well-educated ambitious doctors; dump them into a flailing, semi-feudal medical system, and pay them peanuts with additional income to be made 'on the side.' Now place the system in a tiny country with a population the size of New York City, where the saturated environment limits mobility from job to job, and you will get a swamp. The snakes will multiply themselves. Worst of all: these snakes were inbred – little fresh blood flowed in.

But all this knowledge was still to be accumulated. First, a traumatic period had to roll onto the stage as in our past and future moves.

* * * * *

Bat Galim, Haifa. The tall white building is the medical school. On its right is the Rambam Medical Center.

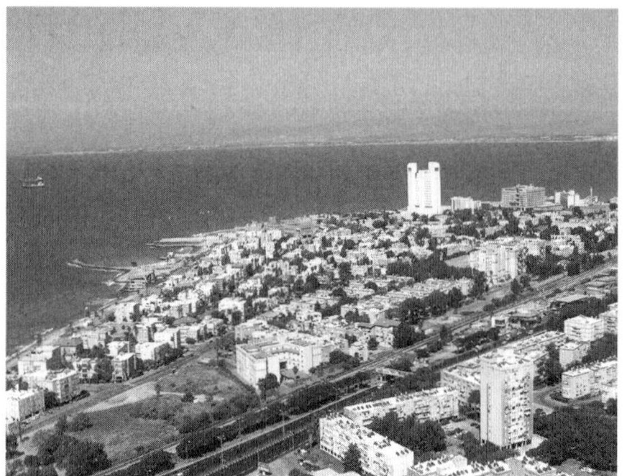

Twenty-eight

The Gulf War

January 17, 1991. A violet Eastern Mediterranean winter evening. Earlier that day, the Americans had initiated their "Desert Storm operation" with massive bombardment on the Iraqis. I walked to the hospital in pitch darkness — a total blackout had been implemented in the country in anticipation of an Iraqi attack. I heard ululating sirens wailing as I was nearing the hospital gates. Here we go again. I experienced a weary sense of déjà vu: blackouts, sirens, like in 1967 and 1973.

I rushed through the gates, where one of the Uzi-carrying security guards said in a muffled voice through the gas mask he was wearing: "Doctor, where is your gas mask?"

"I don't have one," I replied, passing him in the darkness into the hospital. Gas masks had been distributed to the entire population already some time ago. On arrival to Israel at the airport, we received our masks, except for Heidi, because of some administrative confusion. A few days later, Heidi developed viral hepatitis — incubated in South Africa — and became bedridden. She insisted: "You have to go and get another gas mask."

I reluctantly complied, joining a mile-long queue before the distribution center at the main synagogue on Hertzel Street. The people ahead and behind me were recent Jewish Russian immigrants or tourists, all evidently desperate to procure a mask that they believed would save them from Saddam's poisonous gases. I looked at the old Jews waiting for their gas masks — like, I thought, their parents, some fifty years ago, queued to receive their terminal dose of gas. Never in my life did I have to wait in a queue for that long — *with all these Russians, me, an army veteran, what nonsense!* Half a mile before the synagogue, I resigned and returned home. "You can have mine. I'll find another mask at the hospital."

I reached my department. What I saw was outlandish if not pathetic: nurses in gas masks, patients wearing gas masks, and those too weak to breathe through the masks were provided with 'active' masks — powered by batteries and wrapped around the neck and head — old patients looked like astronauts. Patients on ventilators were placed inside transparent anti-gas tents. *Ridiculous.* I descended to the ER, which was fully set to receive gas casualties; there were decontaminating showers at the entrance.

I finished what I was called to do and rushed back home on foot. The otherwise noisy town was now silent as if it was Yom Kippur. The sirens howled yet again, activated by information received from US satellites that Iraqi missiles had been launched — where the rockets would fall was unpredictable.

I remember that short walk on the first evening of that silly little war: the darkness, the tall black shadow of the Carmel Mountain behind me, the dark waters of the sea in front, the scent of the Eucalyptuses, the sirens. I remember being calm and elated: this was my mountain, my sea, my town. It was not my war, but not being in your town at such an hour of danger would have been devastating.

But as I went through our house's front door, my euphoria faded. I found the entire family — yellow Heidi, cancer-laden mother, the three boys, and Pimpush, the little dachshund dog — all packed into the tiny bathroom, which now served as our 'sealed' room. The Israeli population had been instructed to prepare sealed rooms to serve as a refuge during gas attacks. Such rooms had been sealed by applying duct tape around the windows and doors. "When the siren sounds, put your gas masks on and go to your sealed rooms" — this had been the standing order.

"Just come in fast, close the door, fast," Heidi said. She had her mask on, breathing elaborately. In his 'active' hood, little Dan was squatting in the empty bathtub with his two brothers. My mother lay on the floor — she was maskless.

"Mama, where's your mask?"

"I can't breathe through it."

"And where is yours?" asked Heidi.

"He can have mine," said my mom.

"Where is Goofy?" asked Yariv, referring to our South African cat, "can I go and look for her?"

"Poor Goofy, she'll die," added Dan.

"Nobody moves. Just shut up," Heidi snapped (this being her first war).

"Let the stupid cat be gassed," I offered my sense of humor — not well appreciated — to relieve the tense atmosphere. "Where's the radio?"

"The batteries were sold out at the local shops, like the duct tape," said Omri.

"Listen, you can stay here, but I'm going out for a smoke," said my mother, lifting herself up on her walking cane.

A loud bang, another, and more — it seemed only a few meters away. The glass window of our sealed room shattered into small pieces, falling on the boys in the bathtub — the room becoming unsealed. Heidi's yellow face turned white. "Is the roof going to fall over us?" asked Yariv.

"Stupid, if it were a direct hit, we would be dead by now. They're probably aiming at the Navy base," replied Omri.

"This is nothing," said my mom, puffing on her cigarette, "nothing like a thousand American bombers dropping bombs. They covered the sun, the darkness, the noise…" She was referring to her WW II experience.

When the siren announced the attack was over, we left the room to learn on the TV that a few Soviet-made Scud missiles had exploded above Bat Galim, our little neighborhood, falling into the sea. The Scuds continued to fly above Haifa in the following days. A US battery of anti-missile Patriot missiles stationed on the hill just above us failed to intercept them. After the first night, we became blasé about the gas masks and the sealed room. We perceived that the real danger was the conventional explosives of the Scuds, and even if gas attacks were launched, these primitive measures would be useless.

* * * * *

A month after the war, I was invited to Cyprus to operate on a sick nun in one of the convents that decorates the hills of that Mediterranean Island. On a rainy day, as we were driving the rental car at the foothills of the Troodos Mountains, we saw an older man emerging from an olive grove with his flock of sheep behind him. I stopped and asked for directions to the convent. He spoke broken English: "Where do you come from, London?"

"No, Israel, Haifa," I pointed to the east.

He smiled widely, exposing rotten teeth. "Ahh, Israel, Saddam." He then moved his index finger across his neck, from left to right, and smiled again. Ahh, Saddam is going to slaughter you all.

Funny.

* * * * *

Twenty-nine

Rambam Medical Center

Life was returning to normal after the war, and I engrossed myself in being Maccabi's right-hand man. The deputy's office, a tiny cubicle adjacent to Maccabi's, was occupied by a senior vascular surgeon — one of the 'deserters' or 'traitors' who had absconded when Maccabi was down and out. The guy (later the Chief of Vascular Surgery), a *yarmulka* on his head, used to smile at me sardonically: "Schein, how can you work with that jerk?"— pointing to the thin wall separating his room from Maccabi's. Maccabi had arranged a private office for me by converting it from a storeroom. Its door opened onto a sea-facing balcony; to enter it, I had to push away visitors and climb over patients, who used to crowd here for a smoke, fresh air, or an impromptu picnic.

I shared the attending call schedule with Maccabi; he took ten monthly calls, and I did twenty. This almost tripled my meager salary, for under the Israeli system, the basic wage was negligible; any additional income, without which one could not survive, had to be generated by diverse methods. Ours was a busy department in a major tertiary center, and we were continuously flooded with oncological, vascular, 'bread and butter' (hernias, gallbladders, colons, rectums, anuses), and emergency cases. Maccabi proved an easygoing boss: trusting, dedicated, and sharing responsibilities — while on vacation or traveling, he would leave me in charge. He seemed warm, easy to talk to, and with a peculiar sense of humor. But, above all, Maccabi was a 'surgeons' surgeon' — a virtuoso. He cherished this image for himself, as this was the essence of his life. He often said: "Moshe, I'm not a great theoretical surgeon, you are better read, but there are still a few tricks you can learn from me, and I want to teach you." And he did. He was considered *the* liver surgeon of northern Israel, so he set out to teach me how to perform major liver resections.

"You do ten with me, and then you will be ready to do it alone." But one of those ten left a scar in my mind.

The patient was a middle-aged, obese man with a large, solitary metastasis from colon cancer in the center of the right lobe of the liver. I stood on a stool on the patient's right; Maccabi was on the left, and the patient tilted my way. The right lobe of the liver was huge, as was the tumor. I mobilized the liver from its attachments, controlled, clamped, divided, and sutured the portal structures feeding the affected lobe, which now, without its blood supply, was turning pale. Maccabi grasped the mobile right lobe and twisted it to the left, partially exposing for me the long, soft blue pipe – the inferior vena cava.

"Moshe, now carefully, I emphasize, very carefully… get the hepatic veins, careful." He was sweating – it is easier to do it alone than to assist.

"But Meir," – unlike with GAG, I was on a first-name basis with him – "it is deep. Shouldn't we first divide the parenchyma and get the hepatic veins from within the divided liver?"

"Moshe, Moshe, don't argue, just get this vein… let me expose it better." He pulled gently on the liver, moving it further to the left for, perhaps, four or five millimeters, and *pop* – the abdominal cavity was suddenly turning into a deep pool of fresh blood, gurgling out rapidly – like a main water pipe exploding in Manhattan – flooding everything and draining the system. "Oops, we tore the vein," said Maccabi. "Give me a straight aortic clamp, one more, another," he commanded dramatically. Within thirty seconds, applying numerous vascular clamps, he hacked out the lobe and controlled the bleeding. "Come on Moshe, now suture everything." But it was too late. The patient had stopped bleeding because there was no blood left to bleed.

Postoperative soul searching? From Maccabi? No. After the operation, I tried to discuss what happened – to learn lessons: "Perhaps we pulled too hard," – I said *we*, not *you* – "this was a huge lobe. Exposure was hard. Perhaps we should have gone through the liver to get the hepatic veins?" I did not add, "as I'd advised." But Maccabi was not interested in dwelling on sad events which had taken place in the past, with the past being only a few hours earlier. Like great maestros, he preferred to remember only the glorious past, hoping for more promising excitement in the future. Contemplating recent tragedies was terrible for morale – why cry over spilled milk?

And like some surgical maestros, Maccabi loved seeing the blood hit the ceilings. Sometimes, he would enter challenging situations only to demonstrate to everybody how easily he could solve the emerging disaster he had just created. This was one of his standing jokes: during abdominal aortic procedures, when the time arrived to test the proximal anastomosis, he would release the clamp suddenly, spraying, with blood, the novice intern or student. He always thought this was funny and impressive, particularly when the intern or student was a handsome boy. Females did not count or matter too much to him.

That he was the best technical surgeon in the world was an indisputable fact to Maccabi. At least twice a year, he would travel to some center of excellence in Europe or North America to learn 'what's new.' Over the years, he visited the *who's who* list of international surgeons. He was not impressed with anybody – "they're OK," he would say after visiting the

Mayo Clinic, "but not *superlative*." He repeatedly used that word (in English), emphasizing that it only applied to him.

However, he was truly a brilliant technician — daring, hazardous, extremely obstinate, and persistent — a combination that makes the best surgeons but kills a few patients. For example, one day I assisted a resident with a low anterior resection for rectal cancer. The circular stapler we used to fashion the colorectal anastomosis had misfired, resulting in a large anastomotic defect deep down in the narrow pelvis of the fat male patient. I could not figure out another option but to take down the anastomosis and 'pull through' the colon through the rectum, joining it to the anus — coloanal anastomosis. I called the boss: "What do you think Meir?"

"Wait," he said, "I will scrub in." He placed a headlight on his head and sat himself on a stool between the patient's legs and very slowly — it took him more than an hour — sutured and repaired the defect in the anastomosis which was up there in the narrow dark hole — a task which to me appeared impossible and futile. Unable to tie the sutures in the deep keyhole, he fashioned sliding ligatures, gliding them upwards. His stubbornness paid off.

* * * * *

Rambam Hospital also served as the main northern military hospital. It received a steady supply of combat casualties from the ongoing, low-grade warfare between Israeli and Hezbollah forces in the South of Lebanon. Day by day, choppers, carrying Israeli and often enemy casualties, landed at the small helipad by the sea. I expected that a hospital priding itself on having the best trauma services in Israel, directed by an ex-general ('Napoleon' Kodkod), and posing an image of "we save the lives of our young soldiers," would provide organized and well-oiled care for the wounded. However, after a few weeks within the system, I realized how chaotic it was — a total *bardak*.

In theory, everything had been organized according to conventional guidelines. The wounded were to be met in the trauma room by the senior general surgeon on call and his team for triage and decision-making — who goes to the operating room, who needs further investigations, who needs sub-specialists. But in practice, it was a circus.

My first trauma call. I was told: "Dr. Schein, a chopper carrying three wounded soldiers will land in fifteen minutes. One is critical." I summoned three residents and ran down the stairs to the receiving area. It was already packed with numerous white coats and the white heads of professors: professors of medicine and hematology and even professors of microbiology — all adamant about being present to help our 'wounded boys' and, in general, enjoying the action; being captured by a TV camera would be an extra perk. I should emphasize that in Israeli society, being part of the *chevre* — difficult to translate, but it means a close group of *your* people — being seen taking part in exciting events is a way of life. Even if you cannot help, you stay to see, to *kibitz* — to give your invaluable but superfluous advice. I must admit that Professor Kodkod rarely showed his face in the receiving area. Still, one of his deputies, especially Dr. Zvi Ben-Yishai (soon to become a professor) — a non-M.D. but a virologist, a self-appointed HIV specialist — was always present, performing in front of the ever-present TV cameras.

I found it challenging to provide adequate care amidst such commotion and mayhem — swarms of plastic surgeons, urologists, orthopedic surgeons, and non-surgeons gathered around each wounded soldier, all trying to save his life.

I remember a case of a young paratrooper flown in from Lebanon after sustaining a high-velocity bullet injury to his abdomen. The Army policy—it must have been revised since — was to pick up the wounded in the field and fly them rapidly to a first aid station in Rosh Pinna, south of the Lebanese border, where a military doctor would insert additional intravenous lines and start or continue, flooding the patients with many liters of fluids. After such 'stabilization,' the wounded would be repacked into the chopper and continue their trip to our famous trauma center, receiving, on the way, more salt and water, and thus gradually swelling up. And so did our paratrooper. On arrival, his face was puffy, and his abdomen was swollen as a waterlogged balloon. He had already been intubated, and with a chest tube *in situ*; there was a large entry wound in his lower chest and a larger exit wound in his left loin. I managed to penetrate the human herd surrounding his stretcher. His heart rate was 160, blood pressure 70/?. "Move away," I said, "I'm taking him straight up to the OR."

"Not so fast Schein, first I need to change his central line. It's too small," said Dr. Mishmesh, an ex-orthopedic surgeon who was the ER and Trauma Services Director.

"But his tummy is full of blood. Let's not waste time."

Speak to the wall. I went up to the OR and waited. Almost an hour later, we explored the moribund paratrooper: his tummy was full of liters of fresh blood; his intestine, and every other cell in his body was engorged with all the excessive salt and water he had been receiving. I removed his spleen, distal pancreas, and half of his kidney (I did the partial nephrectomy by firing a linear stapler across the kidney — a method we had developed in Johannesburg. This, of course, was not included in the repertoire of the Chief of Urology, who drifted into the OR at that moment. Afterward, he would claim, "Schein is experimenting on our soldiers…"). I repaired the stomach and resected some small intestine, but only then the troubles started — the shocked and edematous organs failed. The patient was managed in the general intensive care unit, which in Rambam meant a total lack of continuity of care: you did the lifesaving operation, but all subsequent care was under the ICU doctors. So, a day later, they may call another surgeon and ask him to re-explore the abdomen because it is 'tense.' And then, yet another surgeon would be summoned to deal with the complications of the previous unnecessary exploration. The chaos would continue. Four months later, I read in a national newspaper about that paratrooper having been just discharged after surviving almost fatal injuries thanks to the superb care in Rambam: "According to Dr. Ben-Yishai, his survival was miraculous." I thought to myself: with a direct, thirty-minute flight to the hospital and an *immediate* move to the OR, he would have been home a week later.

Unfortunately, the lack of continuity of care was not unique to the trauma system but a prevalent trait in all departments, including ours. Having trained in a surgical system where responsibility for a patient is *individual — your patient is yours forever* — I was appalled by the system of *collective* responsibility: *it is my patient only when I am on call.* I was frustrated by my inability to change it. So, I would assist the senior resident Zigi Dayag in a case of advanced intra-abdominal infection; forty-eight hours later, I would want to take the patient back for a planned reoperation. Where is Dayag? I would ask. Oh, he's fishing, would be the answer. Dr. Gross would scrub instead, in a lousy mood and bored, for he hated pus. Or Gross would do an open cholecystectomy — residents were allowed to operate without supervision — and three days later, when I had to reconstruct the damaged common hepatic duct (Gross had confused it as the cystic duct), Gross would be unavailable as he had to take his daughter to the puppet theater. I could not accommodate such attitudes, which increased tension with the senior residents, collectively considered "Maccabi's boys." Maccabi had recruited and trained and spoiled them, and they were hoping to grow up and take senior positions in his department. Behind my back, they considered me a 'paratrooper' — parachuted above them from outside. Gradually I sensed that I was becoming, in their eyes, an irritating obstacle.

* * * * *

Thirty

Life in Haifa

I noticed a trend forming: whenever I needed to speak with one of my senior residents, I would find one standing, chewing the fat, at the central nursing station by the main entry to our department. It took me some time to understand why they were standing there.

During the daytime, the nursing station always looked and felt like Tel Aviv's old central bus terminal — that of Haifa's was less chaotic. Doctors would be writing orders, nurses deciphering and copying the orders, clerks screaming down the phone, patients' wives complaining that "his urine bag is exploding," or husbands lamenting that "the chicken soup is too cold." Consultants — psychiatrists, microbiologists, rheumatologists, and dieticians — would be standing, fighting for desk space to write a note in the chart. Medical students would loiter amongst the legs of all the above. Let us not forget the ancient volunteer ladies, who arrived each day to improve the mood of our 'wounded boys;' they would stand at the station, drinking lemon tea in plastic cups tattooed by burning cigarettes. Small groups of infantry soldiers in oil-stained field uniforms, carrying assault rifles — who arrived directly from Lebanon — would loaf around, awaiting the return of their comrades from the OR. Contributing to the sub-acute cacophony were the habitual *kibitzers* — porters and custodians, who, after unloading or loading a patient, or a corpse, would halt at the nursing station for a small glass of 'mud' coffee or sweet mint tea and share a racy joke with the nurses. I have visited, before and since, surgical departments in Africa, Canada, the US, Chile, Germany, Italy, Belgium, England, Switzerland, Cyprus, Moscow, and the West Bank. Still, I had never experienced anything as noisy and chaotic as a nursing station at the Rambam Hospital.

But where were all our senior residents? Where were Drs. Gross, Dayag, and Modyin — the 'three Musketeers' as I called them — what were they doing? In their early 30s, the three of them were well built and tall — that is how Maccabi liked them — but each was entirely different. Gross was thin and bespectacled; Dayag blond and handsome, an avid angler, and a ladies' man; Modyin was dark and corpulent — previously an army intelligence officer, he was cunning and manipulative. Whenever not in the OR or the ER, they would position themselves, leaning at the counter of the nursing station. Invariably they were clad in scrubs or white coats hanging slackly over faded jeans, crumpled T-shirts, and open sandals exposing furry toes. It took me a year to decode this strange behavior: why are they wasting their hours? Couldn't they read or write something or swim in the inviting blue sea just a few steps away?

Then I understood. Even as residents, they were already pre-marketing themselves to the public by being available to the patients' families amidst this pandemonium. "Yes, Mrs. Goldstein," fair-haired Dayag would say to the little lady carrying a heavy bag of oranges, "I fixed Mr. Goldstein's stomach" — in reality, it had been fixed by Prof. Maccabi — "Let me know if there are any problems… I'm always at your disposal." It was impossible to ascertain how many *shekels* or dollars — the American green banknotes were always welcomed — were dropped into Dayag's pocket the following day.

This 'terminal' served not only as a marketplace for residents trying to build up current and future private practices but for established senior (attending) surgeons who would divert patients from here into their private offices or clinics. (The complex intricacies of the 'black' and 'gray' Israeli medical system are ever-changing and beyond the scope of this narrative.)

I noticed that after 3 p.m., the hospital was emptied of all its senior doctors, myself being one of the few taking residents on afternoon rounds. I realized that most attendings spent the afternoons and evenings striving for an extra buck and that doing one major operation at a private clinic on Carmel Mountain could earn more than I was getting for being on call for a whole month. But to gain entry into private practice, one had to be accepted into one of the private HMOs. A leading HMO was Maccabi (nothing to do with our Professor Maccabi). I applied to be added to their surgeons' roster. No reply. I reapplied — nothing. I talked to their head administrator: "Your application, doctor, is being processed." Three months of silence. I asked for an interview with the deputy medical director, a middle-aged English-born lady who said, "We have too many surgeons on our list, but I will see what I can do; would you agree to travel to the suburbs?" I never heard from her again. "Oh, you want to join Maccabi," exclaimed one of my mother's girlfriends, "why didn't you tell me? The CEO of Maccabi plays bridge with us on Tuesdays." In Israel, it does not matter much who you are, but who you know and how well they are connected — and so I reached out to the CEO in Tel Aviv. "Did you ever apply?" he asked, "our Haifa branch has no file under your name."

Later, before I left Israel, I accidentally encountered another administrator of that HMO. "Didn't you guess," he said, "that your boss, Professor Maccabi, had blocked you? He befriended that English woman. I know you were his deputy, but nobody needs competition…"

Eventually, I managed to penetrate another, smaller HMO — its medical director was a remote member of my family. However, my contract excluded operative privileges — this was stipulated by the late Dr. Toledano, the chief surgeon of that HMO — a surgeon from the competing department in Rambam. When you are 'parachuted' in from the outside, it takes cunning and patience to penetrate the system — two qualities I lacked.

The endemic Israeli *balagan* or *bardak* ("chaos" in slang derived from Arabic and Russian, respectively) did not spare the weekly 'professorial' rounds led by Professor Maccabi. After passing the first or second patients' room, the large procession of doctors, students, and nurses gradually fragmented into multiple groups of individuals chatting among themselves. Eventually, hardly hearing our own voices, Maccabi and I would be left alone to discuss the patients. The others stood by, telling jokes or flirting with attractive students. The lack of discipline irritated and frustrated me, but Maccabi, to my great surprise, seemed not to be bothered at all. To survive in that environment, one had to be immune!

Formal resident education existed only on paper; teaching sessions were scheduled and announced, but it was impossible to have more than one or two residents attend. The Israeli Medical Association Scientific Council had established a curriculum, and every year or two, a few external reviewers would arrive from Tel Aviv or Jerusalem to assess whether we adhered to it, finding, of course, a solid paper trail to suggest excellent academic standards. Yet, the overall standard of the residents produced by that system was not much inferior to that which I would later observe in the United States. Just to show that surgical training is like an apprenticeship in any profession — what you need is a good mentor and practical experience — and in Maccabi's department, they had plenty of the latter and some of the former.

The competing department, Surgery A (ours was B), was led by the late Professor Ami Barzilai, nicknamed *mukhtar* — meaning "leader" in Arabic. Aptly, he behaved like a *mukhtar*: well-connected, cunning — kind and protective to his disciples, ruthless to the opposition. He was the director of the hospital's section of surgery, which existed only on paper. As Prof. Maccabi had not introduced me to him, I wondered whether I should walk into his office and say hello. This, however, proved unnecessary because Barzilai introduced himself to me the Rambam way — in the men's room. As I shook my member dry, ready to leave, the professor joined me at the adjacent urinal and undid his fly. I zippered my fly and said a dry *shalom*. Extracting his penis, the head surgeon looked straight ahead at the white porcelain wall and said solemnly without any preliminary small talk: "Schein, I warn you — never badmouth Surgery A."

"What? Who is badmouthing? What are you talking about?"

"You did already, people talk. Stop or else."

"But I only arrived a month ago; I don't even know your doctors."

"You've been warned." He was in a feeble midstream, but his monologue was over.

I recounted this to Maccabi. He shrugged: "Don't worry — it's a prophylactic measure for him."

Surgeons, in general, and everywhere, tend to be highly competitive egomaniacs. It is said, "If a surgeon were asked to name the three greatest surgeons, he would be hard-pressed to name the other two." But what impressed me in Rambam was the profound disrespect of surgeons, if not doctors in general, to each other. A Hebrew word exists — *lefargen* — it does not possess an equivalent in English. It was adopted from the Yiddish *fargenen*, which had been corrupted from the German *goennen*, meaning begrudge or resentment. But in Hebrew, the use of the word has a positive connotation — *lefargen* means the total opposite of begrudge — a combination of "to praise, to support, to appreciate, to admire, to encourage," and so forth. This was, however, almost totally absent in Rambam.

When asking a doctor the opinion of another surgeon, the response inevitably would consist of the eyebrows going up, shoulders shrugging, palms of hands being raised, sardonic smiles — all the above accompanied with long "eeehhhs." Or — if a rare occasion occurred where one would bestow a compliment on somebody, it would always be followed by a certain "but..."

It was the prevailing attitude among Rambam surgeons — the residents adopted it rapidly. Such a nonchalant macho-like attitude was probably imported from Eastern Europe, where according to Professor Plotnikov of St. Petersburg, "For a surgeon, modesty is the shortest way to obscurity," and "It is not the surgeon who does not drink pure spirit, does not sleep with the scrub nurse and does not urinate in a washstand." The 'spirits' did not apply to the average Rambam surgeon who preferred orange juice. Still, the constant and vigorous pursuit of casual sexual encounters with anybody — nurses, students, secretaries, visitors, and even patients — was emblematic. Not for everyone of course!

Yet, the early few years in Rambam were altogether not too bad. Maccabi and I worked well together and seemed to appreciate and even like each other. Clinical work was abundant and stimulating. We wrote and published quite a lot during that period. I received my senior lectureship and knew that the next step — not too far away — would be a professorship. A professorship in Israel as in central Europe (*Herr Professor*) is crucial to establishing a private practice — unlike the USA, where academic titles mean nothing to the patients. The average Jew, if forced to dish out money from his pocket, would only dish it out for a professor — not to a lowly doctor.

As in most places, Rambam included a few positive characters — highly qualified professionals who avoided the corrupting political intrigues, stayed away from the gold rush, and did good for the public — people who were termed locally as *tzadikim* (the 'righteous ones'). Like the late Dr. Isserlish, a portly bearded anesthetist, who in summer and winter wore tight shorts, a torn T-shirt and brown biblical sandals, always smiling and witty, riding on his old Vespa; and ever helpful. Later when I was kicked out of Rambam, he immediately helped me to find another job.

Or the late Dr. Teitelman — an astute senior intensivist, straight like a ruler, modest like a monk — ever engaged in combative opposition to the forces of darkness represented by General Kodkod and his band. He was the only one who stood up openly and actively by my side when I came under attack by Kodkod. The *tzadikim* in Rambam were obviously tenured; only tenured doctors would dare to speak out about their opinions without endangering their positions. Under the Israeli public service system, after three years of employment, all employees became tenured or 'permanent' — only criminal activities could result in their termination. Thus, if one wanted to get rid of somebody, one would have to do it within the first three years of employment.

But it was Ahmad, a young Israeli Arab, who made my Rambam period tolerable and even enjoyable. I saw him grow from a junior resident to an outstanding and charismatic surgeon. With his sharp intellect, curious and independent mind, overwhelming personal charm and charisma, and high qualifications of a *bon vivant*, Ahmad had become my chum from the first day I stepped into the department. Our intimate friendship earned me the title of "the Arab lover," which was added to the "South African racist" (see the following chapter). After I left Rambam, Ahmad was victimized as "Schein's friend" — an enemy. But he survived to become a professor, a leading Israeli surgeon, and finally, the Chairman of Surgery in Rambam. Ahmad is a remarkable character — easily reproducible in multiple entertaining and sad subplots. Still, as stated before, I will not be developing the characters of my close friends, especially not those with whom the friendship has survived and continues.

I should remember to mention Boris. He was among the lucky ones among the numerous doctors who had arrived from Russia. He managed to pass the Israeli licensing examinations and find a clinical job — others, doctors and professors, continued to sweep floors. He was a typical Russian intellectual — literary, fond of music, delicate, subtle, and with a warm sense of humor. It did not take me long to realize that Boris was one of the best anesthetists in Rambam. Whatever the case was — hernia or liver resection — the patients sailed smoothly through anesthesia with

Boris. Boris, his wife, and their child rented a flat in Bat Galim near ours. One Saturday, I met him walking his dog on the beach. His face was down.

"What's the problem, Boris?" I asked.

"They stopped my night calls, the budget, you know."

"So?"

"So? No calls, no money — how am I supposed to feed my wife and son?"

It turned out that Boris, who provided the best anesthesia in the hospital, was working as a slave. To be paid for a few night calls, he had to work during the day as a volunteer — for nothing. I do not remember what I replied. What could I have said — we all had our problems. But later, soon after I left Rambam, one morning, Boris was found locked in the toilet of that scruffy OR doctors' changing room (as an overgeneralization, the quality of surgical care correlates directly with the quality of the surgeons' changing room), a plastic tubing in his brachial vein, connected to an infusion of pentothal. Boris, the top anesthetist, decided to anesthetize himself forever. I was deeply saddened: is this how we, a nation of chronic sufferers and immigrants, treat newcomers? I remember with distaste the patronizing, jocular contempt with which Israeli doctors treated their new colleagues from Russia — having a Russian accent was interpreted as practicing an inferior brand of medicine. But xenophobia is endemic everywhere — later on, in the USA, I would feel it (rarely) on my skin.

* * * * *

When you return to an old hometown, it always seems different. Not only has it changed during the years of your absence, but you discover its previously unknown faces. And so it was with Haifa: an underrated jewel on the shores of the Eastern Mediterranean, where the steep green Carmel Mountain meets the sea, with miles of sandy beaches and pine forests — a pseudo-Mediterranean San Francisco or perhaps Cape Town. Haifa is a fusion of the East and West; the lower port town looks like a little Alexandria, the upper town like a mid-European spa resort — lush, elegant, and peaceful. As a 'good' Jewish Ashkenazi boy, I had grown up on the slopes of the Carmel in the 'European' Haifa, where ladies like my mother had huddled in cafés, *kvetching* in German, amidst cigarettes and strudel, reminiscent of Krakow or Vienna. I had little knowledge of Haifa's 'exotic' Arabic enclave, but now, with Ahmad's help, Haifa's Levantine delights were revealed to me. Often, after a prolonged late-night laparotomy, we would venture out to the Arab market at the *vadi* for hummus at the Allenbi restaurant. We would share a large portion of freshly ground hummus, covered with a thick warm paté of fava beans and garlic, swimming in a lake of extra virgin olive oil from Lower Galilee.

One would scoop this with two freshly baked pitas and side dishes of sliced onions, tomatoes, pickled eggplants, and broken olives, washing it down with a bottle of Goldstar beer. According to Ahmad, such a breakfast would build a solid layer of concrete in the stomach, keeping hunger away until the night. Then, heavy but satisfied, belching out garlic fumes, we would return to the hospital for yet another day.

And there was the 'Gold Fish' restaurant, wedged between the commercial Jaffa Road and the railway trucks. It consisted of one cubicle, five or six small wooden tables, broken chairs, a ceiling fan, and a noisy air conditioner. Behind the counter, in the tiny kitchen, there was a huge metal bathtub filled with ever-boiling oil, where all sorts of fresh seafood — the catch of the day — was turning yellow, brown, and crisp. The chef, who was also the manager, a diminutive, hyperactive young Arab, was assisted by one or two ever-changing blond *Russiot*. It was our favorite place. There was no need to order — a bunch of pitas, pickles, a jar of *charif* (hot sauce), and a tall mountain of fish, shrimps, calamari, whatever was caught in the net, appeared instantly on the table. This was always followed with a bottle of *Arak* served by the chef himself: "*Tfadal, tfadal* — please, welcome — it's on the house," his right hand on his heart — the Arab way.

And just on the other north side of Haifa's bay was Akko (also known as Acre), the ancient harbor town built by the Crusaders, the fort town Napoleon had attempted to conquer from the Ottomans but failed. Akko, with its old and crumbling majestic walls, Crusaders' halls, and authentic Arab market, is yet another underappreciated Levantine jewel. Here we would sit in the azure evening night, watching the fishing boats leave the harbor, which had been built by the Greeks, enlarged by the Romans, and rebuilt by the Crusaders. At Abu Christo's they would serve whole grilled fish on large silver plates, covered with parsley, dried thyme, and lemon. Slowly, across the bay, the sun would disappear behind Carmel Mountain; Haifa's lights would glitter through the white mist emerging from the dark water.

I came across a poem called "Akko" by the late Chaim Guri, my favorite Israeli poet — the man with the ever-present, legendary pipe in his mouth. It seems we both experienced the same view and emotions, albeit he conveyed it more eloquently. Here is my translation of the poem from Hebrew:

> To have lost your way in Akko, by the quay, the evening sinking on the darkening lilac sea,
> To see the weary boats returning from the open sea,
> And the faraway houses beyond Haifa's bay, fading bit by bit, turning into lights.
> As wrote Guillaume Apollinaire, who preceded me, he that loved like me this hour,

Because again, I saw local beauty refusing to part from the familiar images.
To get lost, to sense the salty breeze, steering the long waves lightly,
That end silently at the weeded rocks at the foot of the wall.
Like in soundless hypnosis that beseeches me — stay a bit longer,
For you feel good here with us and what do you care.
Even the national situation that traces me usually does not know that I am in Akko,
By the pier and the fish restaurant, with the lights trembling in the water,
With my soul, that was to me a booty, by the last seashore.

* * * * *

Top: with Heidi in Akko. Bottom: Ahmad Assalia.

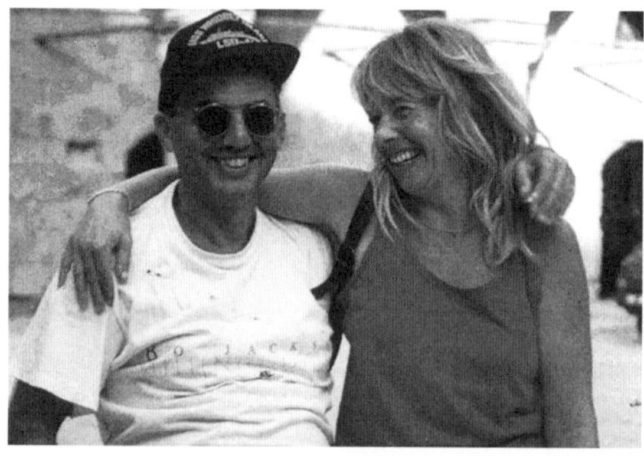

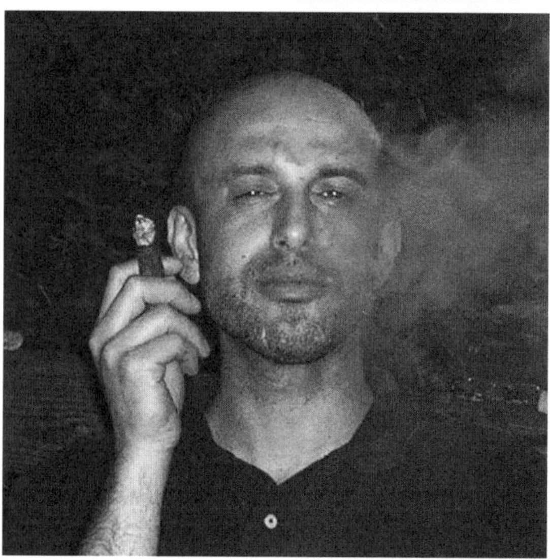

Thirty-one

Schein the 'racist'

1992. My mother was dying of metastatic breast cancer. My sister — unable to cope with the situation — was emotionally labile, and hard to get along with.

At the time, we were always short of money. Maccabi's residents were graduating, transitioning to seniority. Now they demanded to share the emergency calls with me, which translated to a significant drop in my income. My private practice provided a few additional *shekels*, as did Heidi's aerobic classes at the country club on the Carmel. But these means were not enough.

Meanwhile, as most immigrant children do, our boys were talking Hebrew and assimilating into their new environment. We had Haifa to enjoy, a few old friends were around us, and we made new friends, such as the delightful couple Shuli and Dudu, who had 'adopted' us. Dudu was the greatest optimist I had ever met. Whenever I would lament my Rambam problems, he would say, *"me'az yatzah matok"* — from the harsh came sweetness. The source of this expression is in Judges 14:14: Samson, who had killed a lion cub and discovered a beehive in the lion's carcass. From the harsh lion came sweetness — the honey of the bees. Even later, when I lost my job in Rambam, Dudu would say *"me'az yatzah matok,"* which he repeated when we were leaving for the USA. However, a while ago, when we revisited Haifa, he failed to comfort me with his beloved slogan; he said instead, "*Nu,* isn't it time to come back home?"

Well into my third year at Rambam Hospital, I felt I should escape the 'snake pit' sooner rather than later. I planned to survive a few additional years with Prof. Maccabi, attain my professorship, and, following a common pathway, get my own department in a smaller hospital in one of the Northern outlying towns. That we would stay in Israel was not a question at all.

Alas, brigadier-general Kodkod's plans were different: he was waiting for an opportunity to undo me and was running out of time. He had to get rid of me before I entered my fourth year — which meant automatic tenure — the status of 'untouchable.' In brief, he had to find an excuse for not prolonging my contract beyond the first three years.

I never understood what exactly Kodkod, the almighty CEO, had against me — one of the few hundred clinicians employed by him. Was it because he had failed to block my entry to Rambam after the Ministry of Health overruled his obstinate veto against me through my own *protektzia*? (In Israel, the term *protektzia,* the synonym being *vitamin P*, translates to "influence with people able to grant favors.") Or was he smart enough — I guess he was — to gauge me, mainly through feedback from his disciples, as a non-conformist and argumentative? A potential, if not already, troublemaker. To succeed within that system as an outsider, you must shut up, deflate your ego, and be useful to the powerful. You had to wait — wait for the tenure and your own power base. You had to stop behaving as an outsider and play the insider, a role I, as before, found hard to play.

* * * * *

Kodkod tried to harass me occasionally, like the letter he sent me a day after I passed my vascular boards, obtaining a license to practice vascular surgery in Israel. He wrote, "I wish to congratulate you for passing the vascular examination, but have to inform you that you are not to perform any vascular operations in this hospital." However, his real opportunity to strike arrived in November 1992. At that time, my cancer-ridden mother was painfully winding down. She was living in her own home, assisted by a full-time Russian *babushka*, eating morphine and valium. One night the *babushka* called me: "Your mother has fallen. She's on the floor. I can't lift her." I rushed up the Carmel Mountain to find my mother on the floor with a fractured femur pointing through the skin of her thigh. I lifted her to the bed and called an ambulance — "Take her to Rambam." It was a mistake! My father's old hospital was only a minute away, and had she gone there... but Rambam Hospital was where I was working and where I could always be near her.

In Rambam, the Chief of Orthopedics arranged for my mom to be operated on in the afternoon. Seeing that she was well-sedated and pain-free, I returned to my department's routines. In between, I managed to see my mom before and after the operation. Later on, I was called to the OR where senior resident Gross had managed to completely destroy yet another common bile duct during an elective open cholecystectomy; a standing joke between Ahmad and I was that soon we would be able to publish an entire series based on Gross' botched operations. But Gross was 'protected' by Maccabi, for his father-in-law had been Kodkod's predecessor and, we were told, that Maccabi "owed him a great favor."

Around 8 o'clock in the evening, I left the OR after reconstructing the torn common bile duct. I put on my white coat and went to see my mom. I found her in a double-occupancy room. Her bed was by the door; the one by the window belonged to a young diabetic woman recovering from a foot amputation. The formal visiting hours were over, yet the department was still full of noisy visitors. By then, I had learned that it was impossible to control these undisciplined crowds, who were raised to believe that this country is theirs and nobody could tell them what to do, and that the nurses were resigned to the ongoing chaos.

There were numerous visitors around the bed of the diabetic woman; little kids were shrieking and munching sweeties, running wildly in and out of the room, passing by my mom's bed.

"Son," she whispered, "could you please tell them to be quiet? I can't tolerate this noise and the pain."

She was my mother, and I had to act. I stepped out from behind the curtain surrounding her bed and addressed the crowd. I am not sure what words I used exactly, but it was something like: "Could you please be quiet and stop these kids, she," I pointed to my mother's bed, "just had a major operation. She is in much pain. She needs peace, please."

Yet my restrained statement triggered a mass hysteria. What the diabetic woman said still rings in my ears: "Peace? Does your mother want peace? If she wants peace, take her to the cemetery. There she'll find lots of peace."

One of the visitors, a heavyset elderly woman, started pushing me: "Get lost, and take her with you before we deal with the two of you." The mob was triggered, and its 'delicate' pride was deeply injured; this is how these people had been programmed to respond. I had had enough — I snapped and started to abuse them, referring, not too kindly, to the non-European origin of that scum. I used the term *jachjachim*, referring to the human scum of North African origin, equivalent to 'white trash' in the USA. The commotion alerted my sister, who meanwhile was smoking in the corridor. She dragged me away to the nurses' room: "Don't you see with whom you are dealing with? These people sell vegetables in the market. They are going to burn this ward."

The rabble, once stirred, had to continue — they gathered outside the nurses' room chanting, "We'll kill your mother."

Now, this was not Angola or Somalia — it was Haifa, Israel. Under security guard protection, we transported my mother to my department in the other building.

> **"Deputy Director of Surgery at Rambam Hospital to Family: 'Barbarians, dirty Sephardim, *jachjachim*.'"**

This headline appeared the next day on the first page of Haifa's daily. Below it:

> "These racial slurs were addressed by Dr. Schein, a senior surgeon at Rambam Hospital, to the patient Habiba Amsalem who was hospitalized for amputation in the same room where the doctor's mother stayed. The hospital's management is investigating."

A day later, similar articles appeared in the national newspapers. My friends called from Tel Aviv: "What happened? Are you crazy?" A pamphlet was plastered on the outer and inner walls of the hospital, and also handed out at the gates by a group of women calling themselves "The Mizrachi (Eastern) Women in Israel." This group remained vocally active against me for months to come; I never managed to figure out who had organized them and where they came from. This was the pamphlet:

> **"The cursing doctor**
>
> Primitive *Sephardim*. So said Dr. M. Schein, a physician at the Rambam Hospital, to a patient and her family. Then he called her friend a dirty Moroccan… a doctor like this should not continue holding a surgical scalpel; he should not be left in his senior position… we call on all patients to refuse to receive treatment from Dr. Schein…"

In the afternoon, I was summoned to Kodkod's deputy office. The deputy was Dr Ben-Yishai — Rambam's spokesperson and a TV star. "Come, Schein, we're going to apologize to the patient," the deputy said.

"Apologize? For what? They have to apologize to my mother."

"Details are not important. Look, we are under pressure. You saw today's newspapers and the demonstration, eh? This is only the beginning. Come, let's go, just be nice. Smile, shake her hand, and say 'I am sorry.'"

"But what did I say? I only called them *jachjachim*, and they deserved it. As to the rest — they are lying!"

"So what if they're lying? What's important is what people believe. It'll take just a second. What do you have to lose?!"

So we went to the patient's room, and I mumbled, "I am sorry." This did not stop the onslaught. From another newspaper:

> **"Forty members of the Knesset (Parliament) asked to fire the doctor who cursed**
>
> Dr. M. Schein, the physician from Rambam Hospital, has become notorious after abusing a patient and her family. The directorship of Rambam Hospital forced Dr. Schein to apologize. Still, the organization of the Mizrachi Women in Israel is not satisfied and called forty MPs to act for the dismissal of Dr. M. Schein. A few MPs will raise the case in parliament… the Minister of Health will reply."

Next, I was summoned to appear before the Civil Service Discipline Courts in Jerusalem. I had never been as famous in Israel and would never be as famous again. I was lonely, exposed to a cannibalistic system with almost no backing. The only sign of public support was a lone letter to the Editor by one Marco Kalman, who wrote: "As one who was trice operated on by Dr. Schein, I have to state his excellent attitude, patience, and dedication to me and all the patients in the department. I have no doubt that any hospital would be proud to have him as their surgeon… I believe that his mother, like any patient after an operation, was entitled to her peace and quiet."

In retrospect, this incident exposed me for the first time to the growing tensions in Israel between Ashkenazi Jews (originating from Europe) and the Sephardi Jews, mainly those stemming from North Africa (especially Morocco). Until then, I did not realize the resentment and hatred, fueled by inferiority complexes, against the so-called privileged elite simmering among the latter group. For three years, I served in the Golani Brigade, where more than half of the combatants were Sephardi Jews from low socioeconomic backgrounds. I sensed 'differences' but never overt hostility to us 'white' Jews. But things were changing, culminating in the growing culture clash the county is experiencing as I write this.

Amidst all of this, my mother died (see Chapter 32). For a few months, she had been fading away at the Old Italian Hospital for cancer patients — her tumor-ridden body was crumbling; her mind remained alert and sharp. The beginning of the end was heralded by the usual soft signs: the failing eyesight, the wetting of the bed that had forced her to agree to a catheter, and the occasional bout of confusion.

One afternoon, when I visited her with my youngest son Dan, my mother turned to the wall and started to talk in Polish. A blissful smile covered her face. Her eyes focused on some distant point. She was speaking in a soft but clear voice, pronouncing each of the carefully picked words as if reciting poetry at school: "It was so nice, so nice, he came, it was such a glorious day, he came to me, so much love, and so much love." I do not recall seeing my mother as content and relaxed as in that moment.

Two days later, on the 19th of March 1993, my mother plunged into a coma. My sister and I were standing at her bedside. Her breathing turned irregular, then slower, and finally, two gasps. Life left her body.

Maccabi and his entire crew showed up at my mom's funeral. By then, the tension with Maccabi had escalated. But in Israel, tensions and animosity had to turn into deep hatred to avoid attending funerals.

* * * * *

In the spring of 1993, I was invited for a job interview at the Ben Taub General Hospital in Houston. Why and how I was considered for a position in that prestigious center, and why I didn't get that job, is not why I include this episode in these pages. I do it to describe my meeting with a true giant of modern surgery: Michael DeBakey. At that time, anyone who had anything to do with medicine and surgery knew the name DeBakey, the great surgeon from Houston — the man who pioneered modern cardiac and vascular surgery: techniques, grafts, instruments; the man who operated on the Shah of Iran, and numerous leaders and VIPs around the world.

So after a few days of interviews and hospital rounds, I was brought for a final interview with the great man himself. He was then the Chairman of the Baylor College of Medicine Department of Surgery. His offices were located at the Houston Methodist Hospital — the term 'chancellery' would do more justice to what I found: vast spaces and luxury such as that found at royal suites of grand hotels or presidential palaces. I was welcomed by a middle-aged administrative assistant who led me to DeBakey's inner sanctum. She placed me at the end of a vast oak conference table. "Dr. DeBakey will join you momentarily. Could I bring you some water?" While waiting, I looked around the vast room. The walls were covered with numerous diplomas, awards, photographs, and paintings. I stood up and walked around — the subject of all of this was DeBakey — it was his museum.

Suddenly the door opened. A short, thin man with a Semitic nose, clad in scrubs and a long OR green gown, a green cap on his head, and a white mask hanging down his neck walked in. I noted green shoe covers on his feet (later, I was told that he walked on elevated platform shoes to compensate for his diminutive stature). "Dr. Schein, sorry to keep you waiting. Please sit down," he said with a smile. From the first minute, he made you feel like you were having a good time with an old benevolent uncle who had all the time in the world for you.

"I had a long morning in the OR," he said, "a coronary bypass, a triple A, a gastrectomy for cancer… later today, I will have to scrub in on a thoracic aneurysm."

"A gastrectomy? Are you still doing general surgery?" I asked.

He smiled. "Yes, of course."

"At your age, this schedule has to be quite strenuous," I said. I knew he, born in 1908, must now be eighty-five years old! I felt so relaxed with that 'uncle.' I could ask him anything, I thought.

"I have to carry on," he replied. "You know, patients are coming to see me from all around the world. Today's next case, a woman with an aortic arch aneurysm; she was declared inoperable everywhere she went, Germany, France, New York. I am her last chance. I have to continue. If I don't help them, no one will."

Then he asked me about myself. I was impressed; he took his time to study my CV before we met, unlike most of us who leaf through a candidate's CV while interrogating them.

"So, I see you were born in Poland. What did your parents do during the Second World War?" He listened attentively. When I told him about my father's story on the Eastern Front, Dr. DeBakey spoke at length about his own experience during World War II and the Korean War.

After almost an hour, he stood and led me back to the foyer. We shook hands. I did not get the job in Houston. However, I met a surgical giant.

These days, when I ask a scrub nurse for a "DeBakey forceps," I can tell her who DeBakey was. "You know, I met DeBakey…" I can boast.

Dr. Debakey continued practicing for more than ten years. In 2005, he developed a dissection of his thoracic aorta. He resisted operative treatment. However, when he deteriorated and became unresponsive, a bunch of his pupils — the surgeons he had educated — decided to operate on him, performing an operation that Debakey had pioneered years ago. At ninety-eight, he was the oldest patient ever to undergo the operation for this condition. He survived to live on for two years.

* * * * *

Top: from the newspaper: "Forty members of the Knesset asked to fire the doctor who cursed." Bottom: Heidi, Dudu, Shuli, and Dan.

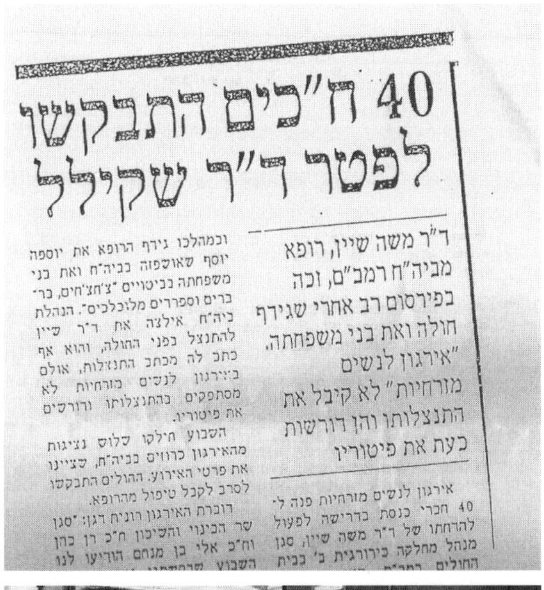

40 ח"כים התבקשו
לפטר ד"ר שקילל

ד"ר משה שיין, רופא מביה"ח רמב"ם, זכה בפירסום רב אחרי שגידף חולה ואת בני משפחתה. "ארגון לנשים מזרחיות" לא קיבל את התנצלותו והן דורשות כעת את פיטוריו

ארגון לנשים מזרחיות פנה ל־40 חברי כנסת בדרישה לפעול להדחתו של ד"ר משה שיין, סגן מנהל מחלקה כירורגית ב' בבית החולים

וכמהלכו גידף הרופא את יוספה יוסף שאושפזה בביה"ח ואת בני משפחתה בביטויים "צ'חצ'חים, כר־ברים וספררים מלוכלכים". הנהלת ביה"ח אילצה את ד"ר שיין להתנצל בפני החולה, והוא אף כתב לה מכתב התנצלות, אולם בארגון לנשים מזרחיות לא מסתפקים בהתנצלותו ודורשים את פיטוריו.

השבוע חילקו שלוש נציגות מהארגון כרוזים בביה"ח, שציינו את פרטי האירוע. החולים התבקשו לסרב לקבל טיפול מהרופא.

דוברת הארגון רונית דגן: "סגן שר הבינוי והשיכון ח"כ רן כהן וח"כ אלי בן מנחם הודיעו לנו השבוע

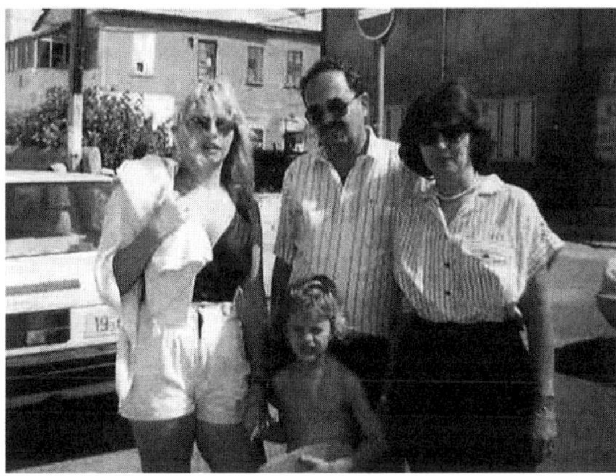

Thirty-two

The story of my mother and the good German

To her now-vanishing generation, the story of my mother's life would not seem extraordinary. She was born in 1920 on her grandparents' farm — a few Jews were farmers like their Ukrainian neighbors — in Eastern Galicia, near Lvov; then Poland, now Lviv, Ukraine. One night, as a three-year-old girl, she witnessed Ukrainian bandits murdering her father, who had been a musician in Austria's Emperor, Franz Josef's, personal orchestra during the First World War.

After her mother remarried, my mom was dispatched to live with her uncle in Berlin. There she attended a German gymnasium, growing up as a Germanized Jewess. As a teenager, she witnessed the ascent of the Nazis — she was expelled from school and gradually lost contact with her German girlfriends. In October 1938, just a few days before *Kristallnacht*, she was among the Polish Jews expelled by the Germans back to Poland. Over the years, my mother used to tell me about her early life in a detailed yet disorganized fashion — many disjointed fragments lacking chronological continuity. One of her tales that left a strong image in my childhood memories was this: returning from school, my mom, a petite sixteen-year-old, black-haired girl with a bundle of books in her hands, saw Hitler's car crossing the center of Berlin.

"I squeezed myself between the crowds… everybody raised their right hand, screaming *Heil Hitler* and *Sieg Heil*, and I saw him, no more than ten meters away from where I was standing. I saw his little mustache. He sat in the black Mercedes, saluting the adoring crowd… you should've seen how they adored him — the old and young, especially the young women; you could see it in their eyes… how they loved that monster."

1939, during WW II and the German invasion of Poland, found my mom in Krakow. There are two versions of her war story. The 'official' one — recounted in a series of anecdotes — and the 'real' version, which we figured out only after her death.

According to the official version, my mom survived in the Warsaw Ghetto. Thanks to her German education, she could work for the German administration, thus sustaining herself and avoiding transportation to the gas chambers of Majdanek. My mum's story continued: just before the ghetto uprising and its final destruction, a 'good' German — a highly placed official in the German railway system in Poland — helped her cross over to the Aryan side. He supplied her with false documents bearing the Spanish name Navara (to account for her dark looks). He sheltered her until the war's end by providing contacts across conquered Europe.

Rarely, when in a nostalgic mood, on Yom Kippur or the yearly Holocaust Memorial Day, Mom spoke about her war experiences: the hungry children of the ghetto and the corpses in the streets. But she dwelt more upon the years after she left the ghetto — about trains packed with German soldiers; German officers flirting, sharing their food and wine with her, boasting that they "can smell a Jew from a distance." The long years of moving from town to town, shelter to shelter, always pretending "I'm a German," always avoiding informers, who would have sold her to the Gestapo for a portion of bacon; these were her favorite tales.

She was the sole survivor among her entire family — not even a second-degree cousin on either side had been left behind, not even a grave. Her survival had left her with many visible and latent scars. Yet, she was proud to come out alive, modestly attributing it to her resourcefulness, cunning, youth, a perfect Berlin dialect, *chutzpah*, and the 'good' German.

Suddenly, in 1974, after my father's death, the good German surfaced from the stories. Herr Herbert Vogt was his name. How and why they met after thirty years is a another story. Herbert and his German wife Inge were now living, in retirement, in Frankfurt, West Germany. From then on, they and my mother would regularly visit each other in Haifa and Frankfurt, respectively. Even after Herbert's death, the two women continued with the mutual visits.

My mother organized for Herr Vogt to be invited to *Yad Vashem* in Jerusalem, where he was honored by the State of Israel as one of the "Righteous Among the Nations." Arranging it required evidence that he had helped save other Jews as well.

Herbert's citation is listed on the *Yad Vashem* website:

https://righteous.yadvashem.org/?searchType=righteous_only&language=en&itemId=4018099&ind=0.

> "Herbert Vogt was born in 1909 in Oppeln/Schlesien (today Opole in Poland). During the war, he worked in the Reich railway administration in Cracow. Deeply religious and opposed to the Nazi racial ideology, he extended help to many Jews, providing them with forged Aryan papers. During the anti-Jewish Aktion, in the second half of 1942, he gave refuge in his house for three days to a Jewish woman, Stefania Kornfeld, and her six-year-old daughter. The young child subsequently remained in his house for six weeks. Another survivor, Anna [Nina] Schein, received regular warnings from Vogt of impending anti-Jewish sweeps. He provided her with two identity cards, one of a *Volksdeutsche* and another of a Polish woman, and thus

she was able to reside in an Aryan neighborhood. In the second half of 1943, when her life was in danger, he traveled with her to a village where she lived for three months as a *Volksdeutsche*. Later, when she returned to Cracow, he obtained papers for her that enabled her to go to Vienna. Vogt also provided her with letters of recommendation to his acquaintances, and they assisted her and made it possible for her to get along in Vienna as an Aryan. She remained in Vienna almost until the Russian entry into the city. On March 25, 1979, *Yad Vashem* recognized Herbert Vogt as Righteous Among the Nations."

I met Herbert Vogt several times during his visits to Israel. I saw a white-haired, slim, elderly gentleman of medium height. The pleasant face and smiling blue eyes betrayed how handsome he must have been in his prime. I found him agreeable, mild-mannered, yet jocular and witty — a perfect older man to share a beer with. He used to, I remember, call my mother "Nina, *mein Kind*." Once, I heard him saying, "*Was ist aus dir geworden Mädchen?* (what happened to you, girl?).

Only after my mother's death we learned about the 'real' version — the true nature of the relationship between her and Herr Vogt. In the depth of her closet, we discovered a bunch of old letters — it was their correspondence from the war years. These were war letters — nothing overt, everything covert — the meaning of things to be read between the lines. Yet it told a love story. Love shared by a German official and a much younger Jewess; their love triumphing amidst a world engulfed in a cloud of burning and smoky chaos. My mom's real identity could have been uncovered anytime — a death sentence for both of them — yet their love went on.

Here is one such letter (translated from German):

November 1, 1941

Dear Anna!

I suppose that fate wanted things to be this way. There is surely no benefit in fighting it. Entrapped in our subjective attitudes we cannot know where to put our steps, and yet subconsciously we choose a path leading us around the abyss.

Dear Anna, it is only sad that we never saw each other here again. But that is how it always goes. Now the roles have changed. You are, hopefully, living in better circumstances now, whereas I find myself in worse as far as my livelihood is concerned. But that does not matter. There are times when one is forced to change roles. Who knows how long my guest appearance here might last. I was there only last Saturday to Monday. Now your letter only reached me today, and so I cannot make any plans at this late stage. I could travel by next Sunday at the earliest…

Please be patient; the reunion will be even more cordial. I imagine that we will have an evening as wonderful as those we used to have, and I am confident that we will consider the interim as something that never happened at all.

What we are experiencing is, in a way, a peculiar thing. If one were to write it down on paper and someone else were to read it, then that person would claim that such things could not happen in life. It is almost like a novel. But, as we know, life writes the best novels. Please, will you wait just a little bit longer, the novel will come alive again, and the characters will talk, and love each other.

Please behave yourself and do not do anything foolish. I wish you all the best for now. I am kissing your hands, your mouth, everything.

Yours Berta*

[* Berta was Herbert's code name]

So this is how it was: they had been lovers. He sheltered my mother in Krakow and then hid her with his family and friends across Germany and Austria, under a false identity of course. That she stayed in the Warsaw Ghetto was her fabrication (she saw it, however, on the outside, from the Aryan side). For how could she, a Jewess, now married to a Jewish doctor — first in post-war Poland, and later in Israel — possibly admit that during the war, which killed her entire family, and a large portion of her people, she had a German man for a lover?!

Herr Vogt's story was remarkable. The man who had arranged the traffic of trains across Europe, including the transport to Auschwitz — had become a 'Jew lover.' Perfect material for a novel, I thought. The story captivated my friend, Chris Meister — a German language scholar at the Universities of Hamburg and Johannesburg.

Based on extensive research and interviews with Vogt's wife Inge and other Jews saved by Vogt (including my mom's friend Steffa), he wrote a Roman à clef entitled *The Man Who Sent Trains to Auschwitz*. One of the questions the book attempted to address was: what motivated that humble German hero, an ordinary young man, to stand out, one among millions, and actively oppose his own nation's murderous system, risking his own life — was it only love?

A paragraph from the book:

"Years later, long after Herbert's and Nina's deaths, I sat opposite Steffa in her apartment in Düsseldorf… Steffa and Nina had been very close friends, yet some of our sources seemed to indicate that, as far as Herbert had been concerned, they had also once again become rivals. 'How was Herbert?' I asked, 'What impression did he make on you in those days?'

> "Steffa thought for a while before replying. 'He was kind. He was so kind, and so polite, so gentlemanly. But the best thing about him was that he was so funny, so cheerful! Oh my God, how we laughed in those days! I have never ever laughed so much in my life again! You know, Nina was always a bit on the serious side, so when the three of us went out together she would sometimes be a bit envious of Herbert and me laughing so much. But we were good friends, that was all — I just liked to be with Herbert because he made me laugh, because he helped me to feel alive again in the midst of all this sadness and fear!'"

Kindness, cheerfulness, a sense of humor, and self-deprecation had been Herbert's antidotes to the ruthless psychopathy which overwhelmed his people and the rest of the world. Herbert's portrait hangs on the wall in my study; in a way, I exist because of him. Herbert died in 1982. His wife Inge passed some twenty years later.

* * * * *

December 1944. The German Eastern front is collapsing; the Russians are knocking on the gates. Here is Herbert's last war letter, the first one that he dared to sign using his real name:

> "Until then I wish you the very, very best, stay healthy, don't forget to eat and look after yourself in every respect. If something should go wrong, you know what to do, and where you have to go. I won't find any peace until I have provided, at the very least, for the immediate future. And that is what is tiring me so terribly at the moment. Once again, all the very best for you, my child of sorrow!
>
> "For now I shall be satisfied if you manage to cope with circumstances for the time being. In any case, my thoughts and worries are with you every minute, and I am struggling, what, how, when, and so forth. Until we meet, fondest greetings and dearest kisses.
>
> Herbert"

They would meet again only thirty years later. My mom kept his letters until her last day.

"It was so nice, so nice, he came, it was such a glorious day, he came to me, so much love, and so much love." Was it Herbert she was talking about on her deathbed?

* * * * *

Top left: mother in Poland after WW II. Top right: early years in Israel. Bottom: Herbert Vogt receiving the title of "Righteous Among the Nations," in *Yad Vashem*, Jerusalem, 1982. From left to right: Herbert's wife Inge, Herbert, my mother, and the German Ambassador of Israel.

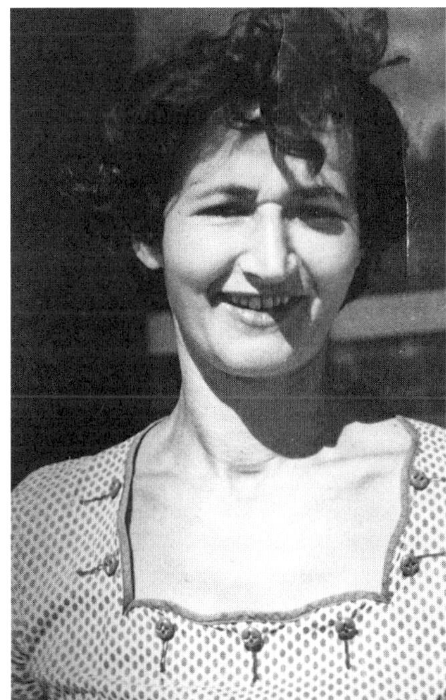

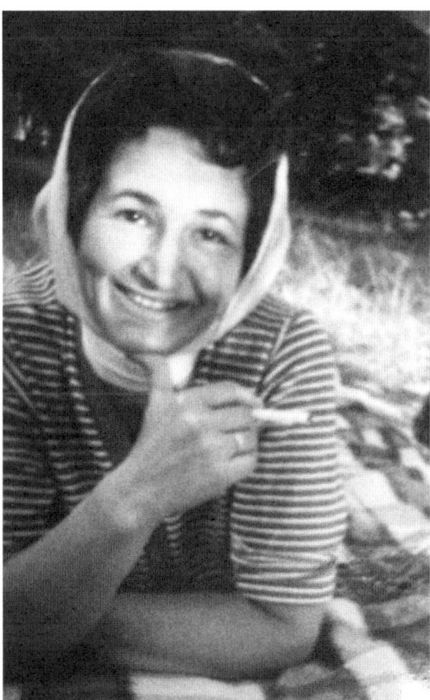

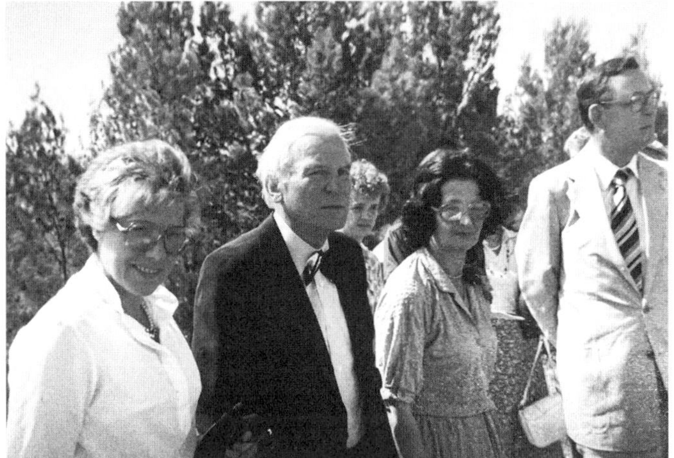

Thirty-three

We bestow tenure only on the very best doctors

Haifa, 1993. The end of my third year at the Rambam Hospital was nearing.

As our rental contract was due to expire, we considered purchasing a home and settling down permanently. A cozy flat, with a sea view, at walking distance from the hospital, had become available. I approached Prof. Maccabi: "Meir, we found a lovely flat, just on the beach. We want to take a mortgage on it. What do you think?" It was as if asking indirectly whether I would continue to work at Rambam — would my contract be renewed beyond the third year — would I become 'tenured'? While describing the desired flat, I noted a change at the bottom of Maccabi's brown eyes — like a shutter closing down behind his pupils. It was fleeting but long enough for me to sense a problem, even before he said, "Moshe, this is a significant decision. Let us clarify your future here before you buy any property near the hospital. By cursing that woman, you didn't improve your position."

"So now you are on their side, eh? As if I was the one to blame? What would you have done if it was your mother?"

"Look, it is *your* name all over the newspapers, not mine — so it is your problem. Wait. Don't sign on any mortgage, and I'll return to you."

During the following weeks, my relationship with Maccabi was courteous on the surface. But below the surface, I perceived an impending change. One day I harshly criticized Dr. Gross — who had just graduated to become an attending surgeon — for doing something stupid in the OR. This time, he replied, "Don't tell me what to do — I only take orders from Maccabi."

"Maccabi's on vacation. In his absence, I'm running this department. I won't let you continue doing what you're doing."

"Really? Your days as Maccabi's deputy are numbered!" *Did Gross know something that I didn't?*

One morning, back from vacation at the beach, deeply suntanned, Maccabi seemed agitated. "Moshe, Kodkod will see you at 9 a.m." He did not look me in the eyes.

I guessed that a decision had been made. It was my second visit to 'Napoleon's' office. The first occurred three years prior when he tried to block my way to Rambam. Kodkod did not stand up from behind his desk this time, nor did he offer his hand. He proceeded frostily: "Look, Schein, we, the management, don't have any complaints against your professional performance. However, we decided not to renew your contract. This decision was based on our perception that your social-personal assimilation within the Rambam family was unsuccessful."

I knew my fate was sealed, and there was no point in arguing further with that military technocrat. But still, I could not just say thank you and leave. "What Rambam family? What are you talking about? I made more friends here than…"

For the ex-brigadier general, however, the meeting was over. He would not let me finish the sentence. "Yes, you made a few friends, but you must understand one thing…" He slowed down, emphasizing each word: "We tend to bestow tenure only on the very best doctors. I would advise you to start looking for a new job, and we will support your applications elsewhere."

We tend to bestow tenure only on the very best doctors. This repeatedly pulsated in my brain as I climbed the stairs back to our department. *The very best doctors — so I'm not one of the very best. Ha? Assholes.* I had a robust surgical ego. Kodkod aimed at the heart; he had managed to hit right on target. I was deeply insulted. It called for revenge. I rushed straight into Maccabi's room. *Coward,* I thought. Couldn't he have warned me about this already a few weeks ago? Now he is hiding behind Kodkod's back. Maccabi appeared reserved; his ceremonial attitude signaled that our brief intimate semi-friendship was now over.

"It was a tough decision, believe me — it was hard," he said. "But please, let us continue to be good colleagues. I would like to ask you to promise me to continue and maintain agreeable working relationships with others until the last day. I will strongly support your application for any job!" Then his face relaxed, and he changed the topic, like switching frequencies on a radio transmitter: "Please, Moshe, no bad feelings — please promise me. You want to go to Hong Kong for the International Surgical Week. Go. We'll pay. Do you want to take Ahmad with you? OK. You two could also visit Bangkok. Did you hear about the massage parlors?"

I accepted his hand. This time his handshake was fleeting.

* * * * *

There is no doubt in my mind that Maccabi sacrificed me to improve his long-term interests. When I joined his department, it had been on the brink of death. I had helped him put it back on the map. And now he was washing his hands of me. So why did Maccabi sacrifice me? He, a tenured professor and chief of surgery, could have backed me. He probably sensed that I had been loyal to him, unlike the previous senior staff that had tried to dethrone him. So why did he forfeit me? The answer, I believe, lay in Maccabi's sexuality which had compromised him throughout his professional life. Because of it, he could not afford 'standoffs' with those who could harm or protect him — like Kodkod. I will touch on it here only briefly — not because I have any issues with gay people but because it has indirectly, but adversely, impacted my career.

So who was Maccabi, the man rumored about in the medical community from Metula to Eilat, the man on whom many had tried to step on and destroy but who always managed to survive?

A brief outline of Maccabi's persona can be reconstructed from what he had told me, from gossip by others, and from the facts. He had arrived in Israel with his parents from Bulgaria after the Second World War — he was their only child. They had settled in Jaffa near Tel Aviv. His parents were poor. "I had one pair of trousers and one white shirt. The shirt was washed each day after school, and eventually, the collar frayed off. As I grew up, my trousers came to the level of my shins, and the kids laughed at me," Maccabi recounted. He had been a studious little chap and possessed an excellent memory. He had been bright enough to be admitted into Jerusalem's Medical School, postponing the obligatory army service. Mind you, while obsessively hard-working, Maccabi was not a classical intellectual. I judged him instead to be an accumulator of information, which he had collected and filed obsessively — he threw out nothing. His collections included many thousands of records — later compact disks — of classical music and operas, and each piece was entered into an elaborate index that was later computerized. Likewise, he had established a fantastic departmental medical library, which I helped him maintain. Not that he read everything, but he loved to have all this information at his disposal — he was an arch-archivist. His other vast collections included albums of travel, nature, and art.

I had been pre-warned about Maccabi's *alleged* homosexuality already when considering the position with him. The evidence for it was sporadic, suggestive, and gossipy. Rambam's old timers spoke about it openly. "Oh, don't you know? Everybody knows. Go to Eli's barbershop opposite Cinema Armon — the barber is the king of *homos* in town, and he'll tell you about Maccabi."

Another source was the deputy battalion commander in which Maccabi had served as a doctor following medical school. Apparently, a few of the battalion's soldiers had complained that Maccabi had 'bothered' them. The military police had been involved in the investigation, but, the deputy commander recounted: "We, the commander and I, liked Maccabi. We saved his butt. He got transferred to a desk job — his record was whitewashed."

After completing his military service, Maccabi commenced surgical training in Rambam. Has anyone reading this ever encountered a gay surgeon? Probably not. They used to be very rare; if they existed, they were well disguised. Surgery, at least at that time in Israel, was a domain of men who undressed and dressed together in OR locker rooms, where they sat in their underwear and told rude jokes — it was a masculine club, like a team engaged in any contact sport. Imagine the fate of a declared gay man trying to be accepted into such a club. Hence, Maccabi had to hide his sexual orientation. He did what gay men do when living in societies — such as India or Africa — that reject homosexuality. He had married, adopted children, and pretended to lead a 'normal' life. However, the basic desires tend to break through, are hard to suppress, and tend to recur.

Maccabi's preferences were apparent to those of us who worked with him.

Twice a week, I attended the outpatient clinic, with five or six residents, where we followed up on old patients and assessed new referrals. Chiefs of surgery in Israel do not tend to waste their time on such clinics — whoever wishes to have their attention has to see them privately and pay. But Maccabi was exceptional — he did not miss a clinic! From my first week, I was familiar with the long-established routine: Maccabi occupied the first room on the right to the clerk's office, and we settled in all the rooms on the left. When Maccabi was on leave, I would inherit the room on the right. The clerk would then drop a bunch of charts on my desk. "Here you are, doctor. You will see twelve soldiers today."

"Why only soldiers?" Soldiers referred to the clinic usually suffered from minor conditions like hernias, hemorrhoids, or non-specific abdominal pain; we had to rule out malingering or GMG, which in our lingo meant *gornisht mit gornisht* — "nothing with nothing" in Yiddish.

"You are Maccabi's deputy, so you take his clinic. Maccabi sees all soldiers; this is routine."

When Maccabi was present, he would often call me into his room to discuss a problem case or to confirm that there was no hernia. I noted that his patients were examined naked. This was a little unusual because when we evaluated a young, otherwise healthy patient for a possible hernia, there was no reason to strip him naked and no justification to do a rectal examination, which he did. Noting my surprise, Maccabi's 'old boys' would smile, laugh, and chuckle — *let the boss have some fun.*

Obviously, Maccabi had a past and a current 'problem' that compromised him. Was this why Kodkod had tried to dump him — an army general disgusted by that homo? To survive, Maccabi had to appease his defenders — a few who wanted my head. He was not in a position to fight for me. And indeed, toward my last months in Rambam, with my revenge campaign (Chapter 34) well underway, yet another scandal reached the newspapers. Now Prof. Maccabi was being accused by three soldiers of sexually harassing them.

Graphic details were published in a leading newspaper under the title, "Does he touch, or doesn't he?" According to soldier A., "He played with my penis for fifteen minutes. I almost ejaculated… I saw him a few times, other doctors never removed my underwear, but he always did and touched my testicles and lower abdomen." Soldier D. told the journalist: "I went to him to exclude a hernia… this started like any routine examination, but then he told me to remove my underwear, touched my testicles and penis, touched it in a few places, moving it from side to side… then inserted a finger in my rectum… he helped me stand up, holding my penis with one hand and my buttocks with the other." The newspaper mentioned, "Fifteen years ago a similar complaint had been filed against the surgeon; the police investigated but the case was closed."

This scandal would smolder for almost two years, receiving sporadic media attention and dying a natural death when the local female state prosecutor — who Maccabi had previously operated on — closed the case because of a "lack of evidence." Why was there no evidence? Because Maccabi denied all allegations, claiming that the soldiers were malingering, asking for "a release from duties" they did not deserve. In addition, "A polygraph test showed that he told the truth when denying homosexual contact with the patients." Of course, some doctors supported Maccabi's practice, like the District Chief Physician, who said, "A thorough examination of the lower abdomen, rectum, and penis is crucial to exclude an inguinal hernia and any discharge from the urethra."

This sexual scandal erupted in parallel with another scandal, which I unleashed as a vendetta against Rambam. However, I never incorporated Maccabi's sexual orientation into my anti-Rambam narrative. When journalists asked me, "Is it true? Is he gay? Does he touch young soldiers?" I refused to answer. To exploit Maccabi's sexual weakness in my revenge against Rambam seemed unfair, hitting under the belt a man whom I had respected.

Ten years after the above events occurred, Maccabi and I resumed polite, albeit formal, communication via electronic mail. Both sides declared that the bitter past should be put to rest and old animosities forgotten. On my side, any resentment toward him has evaporated. I understand why he did what he did. I will remember him as a master surgeon and a good man entangled in the fishnet of life. But before reaching the acceptance stage, I had to try and take revenge.

* * * * *

Thirty-four

The revenge

My revenge was poorly planned, naïve, and thus self-destructive. As with all such acts of revenge, it achieved nothing. Years later, Dr. Wise, my wise chairman in Brooklyn, would tell me, "The perfect revenge should be significantly delayed when those on the receiving end have forgotten what they had done to you. When they can't comprehend who is doing it to them." But Kodkod's words, "We tend to bestow tenure only on the very *best* doctors," continued replaying in my mind — there was no way I could go without leaving scorched earth behind me.

Of course, I could have done what most would have chosen to do — move to another hospital, develop my private practice, provide for my family, and wait. Sooner or later, people would forget about the "racist, cursing surgeon." But my psychological personality or psychopathology called for a different action. I started with the office of the State Comptroller. I knew that that office had already been busy investigating Rambam, so I dropped them a line. I was invited to a shabby office in a gray government building and repeatedly interviewed by a pleasant, soft-spoken civil servant who told me that he was dying of cancer. I divulged all that I knew and handed him hard evidence. I sensed, however, that this official would die soon while Kodkod's corrupt kingdom would survive. This is precisely what eventually happened. I also called the office of the State Ombudsman in Jerusalem and asked for an interview, to which I was invited a year later — a week before we departed for America. I petitioned the Physicians' Union of Rambam — to which I had contributed each month — for legal aid. Their answer: "It's your private problem." At the same time, the Union was paying for Maccabi's lawyers as if his alleged sexual misconduct was a public matter. A year later, the head of the Union became Kodkod's deputy. I hired a lawyer in Tel Aviv but soon realized I could not afford serious litigation. I contacted an organization that declared itself as defending wronged civil service employees. I arrived punctually to the scheduled interview with the organization's president. He did not even show up, nor did he apologize. Later I learned that they specialized in defending Arab citizens — wronged Jews were of no interest to them.

Meanwhile, I applied for vacant positions of chief of surgery in some peripheral hospitals, but Kodkod's influence made such efforts futile. Yes, I know this is boring — "I did, I said, I complained"— is simply unreadable. But I mention it to show how an apparently 'successful' individual can find himself a pariah in his town only because he has fallen out of favor with a few *apparatchiks*. And this was happening in modern Israel — not Stalin's USSR.

Pumped up with resentment, I started contemplating emigration to the US or even returning to South Africa. At that time, I received calls from a few Israeli surgeons with attractive job offers; rumors spread fast within a small country. But I could not face the idea of starting again in another Israeli hospital, under yet another 'Napoleon' — surrounded by a bunch of new adversarial colleagues.

Then the journalist called. He introduced himself as Rami Rosen, a regular freelance contributor to *Haaretz*, the Israeli liberal highbrow daily — a local equivalent of *The New York Times*. "Doctor, my sources told me that the shady Kodkod is busy ejecting you from Rambam, that you know a lot. Would you be ready to talk?" I never learned his sources, but he was well-connected, and I liked his directness. Besides, I was susceptible, and he hit directly on the right spot in my mind — shady Kodkod.

We rendezvoused on an early spring Friday afternoon in a sidewalk coffee house at the center of Mount Carmel. He had a coffee while I sipped a Goldstar beer. He chain-smoked cigarettes, and I puffed on my pipe. He — a scruffy-looking, balding man in his late forties — admitted having just recovered from a heart attack and embarked on a long monologue about his ischemic heart disease. Finally, he asked about Rambam. He was the first person who wanted to listen, and I talked and talked. In my mind, I had nothing to lose. My mind was made up already — I would no longer work within this system.

He listened attentively and said, "This must be a major investigative report. We need evidence. We'll have to verify everything carefully — *Haaretz* is a serious newspaper. Even then, I can't predict how much we'll be allowed to publish. It is a small town in a small country — everybody needs access to healthcare. It may take many months before it'll come to print, if ever."

We stood up. "When are we going to meet again? Oops," he said as he felt in his pocket, "I'm out of change. Can you pay?"

* * * * *

Thirty-five

In the terrorists' camp

Autumn 1993, the Negev Desert, just off the Egyptian border. In Israel, doctors, until the age of fifty, are called up each year for a month of military service. Within such a system, doctors of advanced chronological age and professional seniority, and with the help of *protekzia*, are allocated to serve in the rear or not serve at all. A year after returning from South Africa, I was 'rediscovered' by the Army Reserves' computer. As I had not come up with any excuse or a *protekzia*, I was dispatched to a place no one wanted to go — the notorious military jail of Ketziot. Here, in the middle of the desert (some twenty miles away from the border with Gaza), the State of Israel jailed most of its captured Palestinian terrorists. I would not object if anyone prefers to call them "freedom fighters" or "partisans" because if one looks at things objectively, they have been fighting for their freedom, whatever that may mean. However, among the many thousand inmates, some had innocent civilian blood on their hands, and not a few were probably innocent themselves.

The sprawling jail was a modern concentration camp divided into four separate campsites. Each camp consisted of pens or compounds surrounded by tall fences and barbed wire. Inside each enclosure, a few hundred inmates lived in large tents. On the edge of the camp stood barracks where the camp's sentries slept. The sentries were mainly aging reserve soldiers, too old to serve in the infantry. The permanent staff of the camp, predominantly Arab-speaking Israeli Arab or *Druze* soldiers, resided separately outside the camp.

It was late afternoon when I arrived at Ketziot after a long drive through the rocky desert south of Beer Sheva. I parked near the headquarters and presented myself before the jail commandant, a tall colonel — I think he was a *Druze*. I found him smoking a cigarette and drinking black coffee. "You are the new doctor? What — a surgeon? We never get a surgeon — pathologists, ophthalmologists, skin doctors, you name it — but never a surgeon. Are you a Russian or what?"

"No, I'm not Russian."

"Look, whatever you are, you must understand — the bloody Red Cross is on our backs. They arrive every week and write long, silly reports. I do not need any complaints, human rights violations, or whatever you call this shit, understand? Treat the buggers as if you were treating your patients in Haifa. On the other hand, do understand: this is not a sanatorium, this is not Davos, Switzerland, and they are not *Gandhis*. Most of them would kill you with their bare hands if they could, doctor or no doctor. One more thing: try to solve all the problems and don't send them out. I repeat, do not send them to the emergency room in Beer Sheva unless absolutely necessary. Each time we ship out an inmate, we must dispatch a squad of guards and two vehicles — this is disruptive. OK. That's all. Now go and have dinner, and we'll dispatch you off to camp A."

The jeep maneuvered between the corridors of wire separating the pens. I could see inmates eating, washing their mess tins, kneeling, and praying toward Mecca. I was dropped off at the 'clinic' — a large tent wedged amidst the pens behind tall wire fences — with thousands of inmates on its four sides. A partition separated the tent into two parts: one serving as the clinic, the other as the dormitory for the doctor and his three medics. An obese middle-aged man in a dirty uniform, sergeant's stripes pinned to his shoulders with a security pin, welcomed me.

"*Shalom*, doctor, I'm Motti — a pharmacist from Jerusalem, now your chief medic. Welcome to the Mayo Clinic." Through the thin canvas of the tent, I could hear the inmates shouting, singing, and laughing. Motti lifted the flap, and we exited the tent. A chilly desert night was gathering. Behind the barbed wires, I saw inmates sitting in small groups. "Political sessions," explained Motti. "Those who don't hate us are being brainwashed to do so. You incarcerate naïve kids, and out they'll go as dedicated terrorists, not so naïve anymore."

"What's he doing?" I pointed to a kid throwing something above the tall fence — it flew in the air and fell into the center of a neighboring pen.

"Oh, this is how they communicate — a piece of paper wrapped around a stone. They call it a FAX," explained Motti.

"Is it permitted?"

"Yes, they can do whatever they want within the fences, you'll see. They run their pens under a strict regimen enforced by their *mukhtars*. Each pen gets its supply of daily rations — pitas, vegetables, olives, and meat. They cook and share, like in a happy kibbutz." He giggled.

I shuddered. "Gee, they are so near. Give them a wire cutter or a knife, and they'll find us with our throats cut in the morning."

"Well, doc, everything is theoretically possible, but it hasn't happened yet so…" He shrugged his shoulders. "Come doc, let's go in and have some coffee. Soon they'll start lining up for the 8 p.m. clinic."

"Will it be busy?"

Motti laughed. "Very. Whenever a new doctor arrives, everybody wants to test him." We re-entered the tent, where two medics, in their uniforms, were stretched out on their military cots, snoring lightly. "Hey guys, wake up. Meet the new doc — clinic time!"

"How do the inmates know that a new doctor has arrived?" I asked.

"They know everything. They watch us all the time — what else can they do? By now, they may have already discussed your CV — *nu*, have a *shluk*." He handed me a flat bottle of 777 Brandy. Ahh — it burned my throat.

A long line of 'patients' stretched from our tent back into the gate of the neighboring pen — two poorly shaved reserve soldiers, burning cigarettes between their lips, aimed loaded Galil assault rifles at the waiting inmates. A third guard was 'protecting' the medics and myself inside the 'infirmary.'

The first patient stumbled in and collapsed on the examination bed, groaning loudly and pointing to his buttocks. A handsome, young inmate entered as well. He smiled at me, shook my hand, and said, "I'm Machmud, the translator." His Hebrew was perfect.

"Not only a translator but a major *macher*," said Motti. (*Macher* means a big shot in Yiddish.)

"OK, what's his problem, Machmud?"

"Oh, mister doctor, he suffers from his rectum. He has very bad pain in his rectum. He needs lots of *antibiotica*."

"Tell him please to remove his trousers. I need to examine him." As Machmud translated this, I saw the patient's pupils dilate with fear.

"He says it is very painful, and no doctor touches his insides. He needs *antibiotica*. His supply is finished."

"Ask him how long he has been receiving antibiotics?"

"Five months."

"Tell him no more *antibiotica* until I see his bum. Tell him that I'm a great surgeon from Haifa, a *mukhtar* of surgeons."

After five minutes of negotiations, the inmate stripped off his trousers and underpants to reveal a huge perianal abscess. It was a 'cold' abscess or an *antibioma* — this happens when suppuration is left undrained but is suppressed with antibiotics. This is what happens when internists and ophthalmologists treat pus and do not wish to annoy the authorities by shipping inmates away to a surgeon. "Motti, give him 15mg morphine i.m. and get me some lidocaine and a blade."

To the sounds of screaming, I drained the ischiorectal abscess and packed it with gauze. Now, with the morphine on board, the patient's pupils were pinpointed, and he looked at me with admiration. "I'll see him tomorrow," I told the translator, "Bring in the next patient."

The following patient had a perianal abscess, and so did the next one. "Blease, doctor, he needs Vaseline," said Machmud after I had drained the fourth abscess. Arabs have a problem with the "p" — a "problem" would come out "broblem."

"Why Vaseline?"

"Come on, doctor, where do you come from? Why Vaseline? Why do you think they all have anal problems?" said Vladimir, a tall, skinny blond medic who previously used to be a gynecologist in Ukraine. He spat on the floor. "*Tfu* cholera."

It was 11 p.m., and I continued seeing patients. The line outside was endless. The guards showed signs of irritation. *Fuck it, man, we want to sleep.* Motti said: "Doctor, we have to close shop. We'll continue tomorrow. The word seems to have spread: the new doctor is a surgeon, he cuts and drains pus, no more *antibiotica*. They all want to come now and see you and feel the knife." I looked at Machmud; he smiled enthusiastically, nodding his approval.

"OK, let's see another one, and we'll continue tomorrow after breakfast."

The next guy had a suppurating inguinal lymph node. As I prepared to lance it, the tent flap opened, and a tall, dark officer entered with his entourage. I saw he was a lieutenant colonel — the others were a major and two captains. "What's going on here?" the colonel barked loudly in an Arabic accent. "It's almost midnight. We have to lock up the dens for the night. What are you doing?"

"Are you talking to me?" He was rude, and I did not like it.

"Yes. To you! Send this man away." He gestured at my naked patient and said to the guards, "*Khalas*, the party is finished. Lock 'em up!"

"Would you please leave the tent," I told the officer.

He looked at me in disbelief. "What?"

"I said, please leave. This patient is naked and is undergoing a surgical procedure, and I want you out. And you as well." I pointed to the others. "Just go and let me work!"

"Do you know who I am? I am the Commander-in-Chief of Camp A. This place belongs to me. How dare you contradict me in public. One word from me, and you will be locked up yourself." He was furious. I was irritated.

"Look, I don't know who you are, and frankly, I don't care. I know that you cannot storm into my examination room while I am conducting a surgical procedure. Not even the Chief of the Israeli Defense Forces can do it. Want to lock me up? Please, be my guest, but I promise you that very soon, you will lose your rank. Now please leave and let me finish with this patient."

The officer looked at me silently. He turned around, raised the flap of the tent, and left. His officers followed. We closed the shop and went to bed. An hour later, I woke up to face a blaring light aimed at my eyes. It was the major — the lieutenant colonel's deputy. "Doctor, pack up your things. You are going away."

"Switch this light off, and don't hurry me. Where am I going, to jail?"

"No. We will transfer you to Camp C, changing places with their doctor. No jail."

"Why? I like it here with Motti and the other guys."

"You don't understand. You disobeyed the colonel in front of the inmates. The commandant is a god to them. You have undermined his authority and stature. You have provided the inmates with an example of how to disobey. Understand?"

"No, I don't understand your bullshit, but anyway, Camp C — who cares?"

Camp C was like Camp A — numerous incisions and drainage of abscesses and middle-of-the-night cases of hysterical, hyperventilating young inmates I was treating with generous doses of morphine and valium. It made me, again, very popular. I suspected that many of them had been victims of rape. I got on well with the new commandant and enjoyed treating the 'terrorists' — real terrorists, imaginary or potential.

When reading or hearing about the abuse of prisoners at the US-controlled jails of Abu Ghraib and Guantanamo Bay, I often think about my short stint at the Ketziot Camp. Naturally, it was not a Swiss Alpine sanatorium, but to my knowledge, there was no significant abuse. That the guards were mature civilians from all levels of life, on short-term duty, rather than enlisted mercenaries probably had contributed to the more humane treatment of prisoners. I also learned that we doctors should always take the side of the underdog, whoever they are, even if, in doing so, we must challenge and be challenged by systems that are stronger than us.

Sadly, more than thirty years after the events described above, the Ketziot Camp still exists. In the aftermath of the current ongoing war in Gaza it has expanded drastically. Some say that the conditions in the camp now resemble Abu Ghraib and Guantanamo Bay after the Iraq War.

* * * * *

During my service in the prison, the journalist Rami Rosen called me a few times. After long months of verifying, double-checking, and corroborating the information I had provided to him, he was still busy writing and rewriting his forthcoming masterpiece — according to him, "the bomb which will kill Rambam" — and arguing with his editors and legal consultants about what should not be omitted.

"Schein. When are you returning to Haifa?"

"Next weekend, I will be on leave."

"Well, you'll find a different Rambam. Since yesterday they've been running around like drugged rats in a cage. We sent Kodkod a long list of questions concerning the various cases. They don't know from where the shit is raining on them."

"Oh, they'll guess very fast. I hope my name didn't come up. They are still paying my salary."

"I have told you that your name will come up in the article as one of the many doctors we have interviewed but not as the main source."

But in reality, I did not care anymore. I was on my way out and to hell with them.

On Thursday morning, I bid farewell to my medics and left the camp. I reached Haifa in the early afternoon. Israel is a tiny country — at its widest point, you can cross it in less than an hour. You can drive its length, from north to south, in less than half a day.

Before climbing up to our home on the Carmel — after my mother's death, hers became ours — I decided to stop at Rambam and retrieve my mail. I parked my car. *What should I do with my Galil?* In Israel, soldiers always kept their personal weapons with them, even when on leave. But my gut feeling told me to do the unusual and what shouldn't be done — *what if the car is stolen?* — and lock the loaded assault rifle in the boot of my car. I went up into my department, which seemed deserted at this hour. I approached my office at the end of the main corridor. *Unlocked — why?* I opened the door and found everything in a mess: open drawers, documents on the floor, messy bookshelves. *Bastards.*

I rushed to the nursing station. The nurse in charge smiled embarrassingly at me. Yevgeny, a junior resident, tried to avoid my gaze. "Where is Maccabi?" I asked. "Who broke into my room?"

"Everyone's in the OR."

"Just get Maccabi's ass up here before I break into his room and throw all his expensive books on the floor." The nurse did not reply. She picked up the phone. Meanwhile, I saw the current on-call roster lying on the desk. My name was not included — no calls — no money. *Who did it? What's happening?*

Maccabi arrived: breathless, in scrubs, a mask hanging on his tanned, hairy chest, Dr. Gross behind him. Maccabi's manner was solemn. He spoke to me as one would talk to a mental case. "Dr. Schein, I have to request you, please, leave this department immediately."

"Why? Am I fired? I'm still on contract. And who has broken into my room? Was it you? One is called up for military service," I pointed to my uniform, "and this happens. And why is my name off the roster? Who took me off?"

Maccabi said nothing but picked up the phone. "Please connect me with security." Everything around me moved in slow motion. Everybody was watching the drama evolving between the director and his deputy. No one moved or opened his or her mouth. "Security, this is Professor Maccabi." In

Israel, immediately when you become a professor, you use the title as many times per day as possible and demand that others address you with the title. "We have a disruptive element here on the floor. Yes, Surgery B. Please come up immediately. Yes, I'm Professor…"

"Disruptive element? You little son of a bitch!" I exploded, grabbing the phone's handle from his hand, and slammed it back on the hook.

"You have assaulted me — everybody saw it," Maccabi hissed dramatically, looking around at the bystanders for support.

"I assaulted nobody. I just want to talk to you. You don't want to listen. Why don't you invite me to your office and explain what happened — who broke into my room and why?"

Two security guys appeared and positioned themselves at my sides, each grabbing one of my arms. "*Yalla*, move, or perhaps you want us to get the police."

"Dr. Schein, why don't you leave now? There is nothing that you can achieve by arguing." I do not remember who said it, perhaps our chief nurse. Irritably, I shook off the security men. "Don't touch me. I'm leaving. And you," I pointed my index finger toward Maccabi, "you *will* hear from me."

Beware, Schein. It's a snake pit. Three years ago, I had laughed at the warning, and now — now I knew that my next and last visit to the department would be at night to vacate my tousled office. I unlocked the boot of my car and retrieved the Galil.

"A senior doctor suspected of assaulting a director of department in Rambam Medical Center."

This was the newspaper headline that appeared a while later. It stated:

> "Haifa's police opened an investigation against a senior doctor in Rambam, who is suspected of assaulting Prof. Meir Maccabi*. Prof. Maccabi complained that the senior doctor grabbed a phone handle from his hands forcefully, against the background of tensions and accusations concerning leaking information to the media. A spokeswoman for the police said that there is no evidence that any physical struggle took place. A tense and murky atmosphere continues in Rambam Hospital."

How wise I was to leave the Galil behind — or else the headline could have been different. One never knows.

* * * * *

* Name changed to a fictional name.

Thirty-six

Farewell to Haifa

Haifa, the end of 1993. Following my unarmed encounter with Maccabi, I was forced to stay home on paid leave until the end of the year, when my contract would end.

After many months of preparation, the investigative article about Rambam Hospital was ready for publication. The newspaper sent a draft to the hospital: "You have seventy-two hours to respond…"

Maccabi, surrounded by his wife, adopted daughter, and protégés Drs. Modyin and Gross engaged in a frantic damage control campaign. I was called by a senior physician in the hospital, one close to Kodkod: "Schein, we ask you to abort the article. We know it is due to appear this coming Friday. Tell your friend Rosen to lay it off."

"I don't know what you're talking about."

"Schein, we are not naïve. This is your last chance, we are warning you."

"Or else?"

"No 'or else', but we assume you wish to continue your career in this country. If so — call off this nonsense!"

It was published in a leading Israeli newspaper on November 26, 1993. On the cover — a prominent title in red, "The secret files of Rambam Hospital," along with Maccabi's color picture: wavy gray hair, double chin below a frowning grimace, gray suit over a black vest, white shirt, and a red and white-spotted tie. Above the title, using all the space left on the cover page:

> "When the chopper landed with the injured soldier, Professor Meir Maccabi* was busy with another operation. He should have summoned the other specialist in vascular surgery, Dr. Shlomo Torem, but because of the hostility between the two departments, he did not do so. A few minutes after 15:30, the telephone rang at Dr. Torem's house. The resident on duty from Surgery B asked whether Torem could get immediately to the hospital. Dr. Torem asked whether it was Maccabi who asked to call him. The resident said, 'no.'
>
> "Dr. Torem said that the hospital director had forbidden him to respond on the days when Prof. Maccabi is on vascular call unless Maccabi himself asks him to come. The resident went to check it out. Dr. Torem waited the whole evening by the phone."

* Name changed to a fictional name.

Details about this wounded soldier and many other cases were shared in the article. It spread over six large pages, under a black and white title, "The Bloody Conflict." The young paratrooper, who had sustained a relatively simple injury to his femoral artery, had lost his leg. The article did not mention that I, the other certified vascular surgeon in Rambam, could have come and saved the soldier's leg. It did not happen because of the administrative directive by Kodkod forbidding me to engage in vascular surgery. A copy of the 'timetable' provided by Kodkod's office was included:

Description	*Accumulating time*	
Contact. First aid. Tourniquet applied	0:00	13.21
Chopper advanced to waiting station	0:42	14.03
Chopper flies into contact area	1.11	14.32
Chopper loads wounded and take off	1.39	15.00
Lands in first aid station	1.47	15.08
Takes off to Rambam	1.52	15.13
Lands in Rambam	2.09	15.31
Arrives at ER	2.14	15.39
Beginning of anesthesia	4.39	unreadable
Beginning of operation	5:24	unreadable

That was the official version.

The article continued:

> "A vascular surgeon not involved with this case says: 'The foot is an end organ. It can't survive long hours without adequate blood supply. The muscle can be damaged and die.' The soldier had to await his operation until Professor Meir Maccabi finished another operation."

What was that operation which was delaying the limb-saving procedure? It had been another screw up, as detailed in the article:

> Details about this case which raises serious questions, were shared by a very reluctant Dr. Schein. These were his words: "The patient came in for an elective operation for treatment of hydatid liver cysts caused by a parasite, the *Echinococcus*. He also had gallstones. He arrived with a CT scan showing the cysts and a letter from his physician referring him with that diagnosis. We, the doctors, had discussed this case a few days before the planned operation and decided to operate on the cysts with the possibility of removing the gallbladder if indicated. Gallstones are not an automatic reason to remove the gallbladder. The patient himself (name confidential)

confirmed the above and added: 'They gave me a date for the operation on the liver cysts. I agreed and signed the consent.'"

Dr. Schein continued: "Because of an endemic disorder in the department, the surgeon, Dr. Gross*, didn't even know about the liver cysts and thus removed only the gallbladder. Not only that, but the operation was complicated, and the patient left the operating room in a critical condition, much more severe than usual after removal of a gallbladder."

"What happened then?"

"Three days later, before the patient recovered from the first operation, they realized the error and decided to 'correct' it — risking the patient's life."

"What does it mean?"

"Every doctor knows that one does not rush to perform another elective procedure only three days after a major operation."

"So why was it performed?"

"They told the patient that he suffered from a severe internal infection necessitating an emergency reoperation. But no such infection was detected, and what was done was what should have been done originally — resection of the liver cysts."

We addressed another surgeon in the department that was directly involved. He said: "We have to be careful. Theoretically, one can indeed claim that there were gallstones which would indicate a cholecystectomy and later on suspicion about a liver infection and so forth."

"So maybe this was what occurred?"

"No, the aim was to mask the erroneous first operation. They could have waited until he recovered, then told him the truth and recommended that the originally planned operation was carried out."

"Is this your professional opinion?"

"This is not an opinion. It was stated that there was a need to finish with the missed cysts ASAP; then, a resident was sent to tell the patient that there was an infection."

Professor Maccabi reacted: "After the first operation, the cholecystectomy, during which no liver cysts were observed, the patient deteriorated. A CT was performed showing pockets of collections in the abdominal cavity, some suspected as cysts, so we had to reoperate and, indeed, found infected fluid, and we drained the abdominal cysts."

About this, the patient told us: "I had CT scans in the past, and I know what a CT is. I had no CT in Rambam and none after the first operation. I came to Rambam with CT films from the beginning."

Dr. Schein: "As already stated, I saw the CT with liver cysts before the first operation."

* Name changed to a fictional name.

Enough. I will not tire you with the other cases or stories of hospital political intrigues and personal vendettas disclosed by that article. Whereas many laypersons enjoy reading, often in great detail, stories about lawyers — by Grisham, for example — people are not as enthusiastic, perhaps uncomfortable, hearing doctors' medical horror stories.

But here is some follow-up: two weeks later, the journalist Rosen published a sequel: "Rambam. The Military Connection," accusing Kodkod, the ex-general, of using his military ties to whitewash the hospital mistreatment of soldiers. He wrote:

> "Following the recent revelation..., Prof. Kodkod* assembled a general meeting of all senior personnel in Rambam Hospital, during which many condemned those who had leaked information to the newspaper. A senior physician cited in our ears the words of one of the heads of department, who had said to that assembly, 'There's a need to catch the leakers and kill them.'"

Meanwhile, the mother of the soldier who had lost his leg spoke to the journalist:

> "The military report implies that my son's operation started at 5.24 in the evening, but I arrived at the hospital at 7.00 p.m. and was told that the operation would start soon... then at 7.30, General Mordechai, the chief of the northern command, arrived, he told me not to worry because Maccabi would be the surgeon... by 8.30 my son was still waiting. At 9.00 I saw Professor Maccabi emerging from one of the operating rooms and entering another. The delay was almost six hours, double than reported."

After reading the articles, the Minister of Health appointed a committee to investigate the "alleged dysfunction of Rambam Hospital." The three members of the committee, a medical administrator and two senior surgeons, Professors Klausner and Ayalon, arrived from Tel Aviv and questioned the key players. Twice I was invited to appear before them. They were hostile to me. I could sense how nauseated they were with the 'whistleblower' (we have to eradicate this phenomenon... *imagine if somebody like this would expose our own problems in our own hospitals and departments* — this, I guessed, they were thinking). When I said, "You treat me as if I were the chief criminal — as if you came here to investigate me, not Kodkod and his hospital...," the committee's chairperson said: "Schein, who do you think you are? A Don Quixote?"

Other key witnesses were intimidated. Even my good friend X did not dare to tell the truth. "Did you tell them everything you saw?" I asked him

* Name changed to a fictional name.

when he came out of his hearing. He looked pale, "I told them that I know nothing. Look Moshe, you can find jobs anywhere, but I'm stuck here with them. What did you expect me to do — to commit professional suicide?"

So how did it end? As often is the case with inbred systems of limited size, the scandal continued gathering momentum and then died spontaneously — evaporating. A few years later, Rosen wrote:

> "What we described then was a series of shocking cases of negligence and malpractice in Rambam, which cost lives. Responsible for all of this was Professor Kodkod, but neither he, nor the others were punished for their carelessness. In better functioning societies, hospital directors would be going home for much less. And the internal investigative committee was appointed only to whitewash and help the key players Kodkod and Maccabi to stay in place."

It seems that the joint struggle against the enemies had bonded Brigadier General Kodkod and Prof. Maccabi, for after I left Rambam, the two, previously hostile to each other, continued to cooperate and 'protect' each other. Maccabi retired from public service ten years later, but not before surviving yet another highly publicized scandal that erupted after he removed a young woman's uterus for suspected cancer — which proved to be endometriosis.

Kodkod continued his dictatorial, mediocre reign over the institution and retired a few years later. The journalist Rami Rosen died in 2019. I read in his obituary that originally, he had been a physicist and later wrote plays and comedies. Two professors from Haifa's medical school received the Nobel Prize (in chemistry), which made everybody proud of "our excellent medical system."

* * * * *

When we let the curtain fall on the Rambam Medical Center scene, some readers may ask: what about Schein? What did the narrator accomplish during those few years, except criticizing others? Academically, we were pretty prolific — including randomized clinical studies — leading to a long stream of publications in prominent international and local journals (see PubMed for those years). As always, a few others climbed on my academic wagon — some enthusiastically, some as parasites — while others observed it from the sidelines, cynically or virulently. For example, whenever any of my cases would develop an actual or alleged complication, I could hear, on our rounds, senior resident Dayag murmuring from behind, "This is what happens to a surgeon who writes too many papers!"

One day, the *British Journal of Surgery* unexpectedly invited me to join the Editorial Board. A month later, my photograph and a 'bio' appeared on the opening page of that notable journal. That was a great honor — never before bestowed on an Israeli surgeon. Maccabi congratulated me warmly. The others, especially those in the competing department, looked at it suspiciously: how did he manage to arrange it? What contacts does he have in the British surgical establishment?

On the clinical side, I think I brought some fresh surgical air to the stagnant local dogmatism. I introduced them to new concepts in treating trauma and abdominal infections, including the 'open abdomen.' I showed them that patients with infected pancreatic necrosis are not condemned to a slow death in the ICU but can survive with multiple operations and dedicated care. Overall, I believe I converted, at least those who were open-minded, to some modern surgical concepts.

At the same time, I was a little too bold and enthusiastic, which must have irritated not a few. For example, one of the first cases I operated on in Rambam was a woman with a giant retrosternal thyroid goiter. To remove it, I had to split open the upper portion of the sternum. It went smoothly; I had performed numerous thyroidectomies and thoracotomies in Johannesburg. But the repercussions were immediate: "How dare he? He is a 'cowboy'!" For in Rambam, thyroid surgery was the sole domain of the ENT surgeons, and thoracotomies belonged to the thoracic surgeons. Encroaching the territory of others was considered a sin.

Or take the case of the old Russian woman who repeatedly presented to the ER with brisk bleeding from a scar under her left clavicle. They contacted Dr. Torem, the Head of Vascular Surgery, who said it was not his problem: "Call the thoracic surgeons." The thoracic surgeon on call claimed that it had to be addressed by the vascular surgeon. Arterial blood continued pumping from a hole in a scar under the clavicle, so they called me, the general surgeon on call. I immediately realized the situation: many years ago, the woman had undergone a mastectomy for breast cancer in Russia, followed by radiotherapy. The scar from which she was bleeding represented the skin damaged by crude, excessive radiation, which also destroyed the subclavian artery. She was hemorrhaging from a false aneurysm! I took her immediately to the OR. I had to open the left chest to control the origin of the left subclavian artery at the arch of the aorta. At that stage, I summoned the Head of Thoracic Surgery. It was a wise move, for we decided that the only option to save her would be to tie the artery, amputate the arm, and use the healthy skin and muscles of the shoulder to reconstruct the chest wall defect. Predictably, the same vascular surgeon who refused to treat the patient now criticized what we did: "Why did they have to amputate the arm…" Sharing responsibility with the thoracic guy shielded me from further attacks.

We did 'crazy' things as well; like using vascular grafts for palliative biliary-enteric bypass in patients with malignant obstructive jaundice — at that time, methods of palliative endoscopic stenting were just emerging.

First, we experimented on large dogs, ligating the bile duct and bypassing it to the stomach with a Gore-Tex graft. It worked. The dogs survived. No complications. However, the outcome was not as favorable when performing the Gore-Tex bypass in a few humans, all with end-stage pancreatic cancer. Humans do not always behave like dogs… Yes, they would have died anyway within a few months, but such 'experiments' were inappropriate. They were, however, possible in an otherwise poorly controlled and chaotic, 'cowboyish' milieu.

And, as always, the patients I 'killed' in Rambam, or contributed to their demise, are etched in my memory. Like the middle-aged guy presenting with deep obstructive jaundice whom I took for a Whipple pancreatic resection. He developed a leak and died. Pathology showed only a tiny obstructing benign adenoma in his common bile duct. It was not cancer. I remember talking to his wife… and the pathologist… trying to justify myself. Or how can I forget the older Russian man who was busy dying for a week — looking at me pleadingly with his sad black eyes — his wife and daughters holding his hands? The man developed recurrent stomach cancer a few years after a partial gastrectomy. Maccabi had seen him with the oncologists and agreed to 'explore' him. He appeared on the OR list when Maccabi was on vacation. Senior resident Gross was performing the operation list on that day. And so he started 'exploring' the patient. I was summoned for help when Gross was confronted with a large tumor occupying the gastric remnant — what to do? I should have told him to abort. I would not have agreed to reoperate on such a case from the start. But here we were, the abdomen open, and the tumor appeared mobile. We proceeded.

We divided and tied a tiny artery. We thought it supplied the stomach. It was the superior mesenteric artery — the main artery supplying the intestine, which had been glued to the tumor by the scar tissue from the previous surgery. Devoid of blood supply, the entire gut started dying, together with the patient, who continued staring at me with accusing eyes. *Each surgeon carries in his mind a personal graveyard.* There are not a few variants of this aphorism attributed to the French surgeon René Leriche.

Amidst that stressful and chaotic period in my career, I failed to appreciate the surgical revolution that was occurring in the early 1990s — the gradual introduction of laparoscopic surgery. Around me, people, including Maccabi, started experimenting, purchasing equipment, and traveling to France or Germany to "see how they do it."

I was skeptical. I saw how they struggled to climb on the 'learning curve,' — producing complications and how simple open procedures became more complex. Thus, I did not rush to acquire these new skills. The process of emigration and settlement in America further delayed my training in laparoscopy. Ultimately, I adopted laparoscopy but never became an expert advanced laparoscopist. Somehow, I missed the bandwagon.

Finally, what happened with Maccabi's Three Musketeers? Dayag, the fisherman, became a director of vascular surgery in another hospital. Modyin, the canny ex-intelligence officer, immediately, enthusiastically replaced me as the second in command to Maccabi, later to become a professor and head of surgery in a peripheral hospital. Gross, the surgeon who habitually used to injure common bile ducts, became a dedicated breast surgeon. I suspect he was made aware that botching breast operations is less morbid than screwing up abdominal procedures.

* * * * *

In January 1994, I became an attending surgeon in another public hospital in Haifa. My late father had developed and led this hospital for many years. The Chief of Surgery was Shmuel 'Shmil' Eldar, a large, relaxed, smiling man — unusually benign and benevolent for an Israeli head of department.

Shmil's department was well organized and controlled, and patients' care was adequate. The Bnai Zion Medical Center, formerly the Rothschild Hospital, was clean and neat. Even its director, who appeared to be a humble public servant, welcomed me wholeheartedly. However, Shmil had his own 'boys,' the most visible among them was Ibrahim. He was a Christian Arab who had studied medicine in Greece and then trained in surgery under Shmil to become Shmil's right-hand man. Shmil would sit in his office and read while Ibrahim managed the department. I found Ibrahim knowledgeable, technically excellent, and friendly. But very soon, I realized that with Shmil and Ibrahim around, my role in their department would be marginal. So I made a real effort to shut up and let them conduct the show. I kept a low profile, operated on my cases, took a few calls, and smiled at everybody. This, for a change, was a pleasant situation.

The hospital was precisely three minutes' walking distance from our home. I came and left whenever I wished. My private practice at that small HMO, which I had managed to gain access to, was gradually increasing. Heidi and the boys seemed happy. We had friends, and the country was beautiful. Europe was so near — I often wonder what would have happened had we decided to stay. But I was obsessed with the greener grass beyond the ocean.

All I had in the USA was a promise of a visa and a temporary, poorly paid job. What would happen afterward was unknown — would my surgical training be recognized without a US residency or a board certification, the latter not obtainable without the former? I didn't want to stop, think and reconsider; in my mind, the Israeli system wasn't for me — it was time to move on. But what about Heidi? What was her perspective? I had dragged her from Switzerland to Israel, then to South Africa with a toddler on her hands, then back to Israel, where the Scuds had nearly fallen on her head, and now? Did she complain: why do you keep taking us to the unknown, with three boys in school? With almost empty pockets… No, she didn't complain. Like most of us, Heidi has her rich internal monologue that she, quiet and not overly extroverted, tends to keep mostly to herself. For many years she accepted her destiny to be schlepped from country to country and town to town: packing, unpacking, always organizing a cozy home, looking after the family, and the often disastrous finances. Years later I asked her: "Heidi, what did you think back in 1994? Would you have preferred to stay in Israel then?"

"Well, I liked Haifa, the friends; the boys were doing just fine. But at the same time, I hated them for what they did to you in Rambam… and, you were the breadwinner, and it was your career."

In retrospect, my intermediary four years in Israel, between South Africa and the USA, significantly hindered my surgical career. I had arrived in Israel at the age of forty — a confident do-it-all surgeon — and instead of further consolidating my skills and gaining recognition in a named field, I wasted my best years on political wars. Now, at my father's age, when he had brought us from Poland to Israel, I was going to take my family from Israel to America — to start yet again from an even lower starting point.

* * * * *

In the summer of 1994, we packed our belongings and shipped them to Wisconsin; this consumed most of our savings. We divided what we did not want to take between friends and family. Liquidating your old family home is a painful affair, mainly if you are leaving the country, have no place to store things, and cannot take everything. The little old family house, serving generation after generation, so typical in 'stable' countries that had suffered no recent wars or migrations: you climb to the attic and discover the books of your great grandfather; you let your children breathe the environment which had surrounded your parents. But this was impossible in our case, and most of my father's vast library, which had arrived with him from Poland — many volumes of early 20th-century anatomical and surgical German texts, first editions of Russian and Polish classics — ended up in the municipal garbage dump.

Ibrahim was keen to rent our house, as it was so near to the hospital. We stored the few remaining things we decided not to take with us or discard in boxes in the attic above the kitchen. It included mainly family memorabilia and old letters. In my mind, I hoped that we would come back one day to this house, at least for retirement.

Three years later, Ibrahim contacted me with an attractive offer to purchase the house. I agreed. "Just keep the boxes in the attic," I pleaded, "we will empty them when we visit next time." A month after Ibrahim bought the house, the attic collapsed into the kitchen. My boxes were thrown in the dump with all the rubble. My parents' letters, and other family treasures, are all gone. Ibrahim continues to live in our old house. He is now the head of the department. I do not know the details of the yarn, but it appears that Ibrahim managed to dethrone his boss Shmil, well before the latter was due to retire. Shmil's mistake was to give everything to Ibrahim and establish him as the uncontested crown prince rather than follow the rule "divide and rule." Shmil Eldar suddenly died in Haifa, April 2024 at the age of seventy-nine. He was a good guy!

We were to travel to the US on tourist visas — the Milwaukee Hospital promised to arrange H-1 visas on arrival. Thus, up to that point, we were spared the well-known saga associated with any dealings with American embassies abroad; we could not guess how many immigration sagas this would create in the future. Heidi and the boys left for Switzerland, leaving me to finalize all the little matters, such as selling our car. But just then, our Subaru Wagon got stolen from under my nose. A few days later, the police found it severely damaged near Nazareth. I had it towed to a car shop; the insurance paid 75% of the damage. A few days later, with the car already placed on the market, it broke down with a burnt-out engine. I rushed to the garage: "You didn't fix it properly; a three-year-old car doesn't die suddenly!"

"Sorry, doctor, this has nothing to do with our actions. It'll cost you 3000 dollars!"

I went to the insurance company and spoke to the director — he, and his father before him, had been my family's insurance brokers for thirty-five years. Knowing that I was leaving the country, he became elusive: "Well, we just spent $4000 for the last repair; we are not responsible for a faulty repair."

I had to sell the car immediately, so I paid the fee to the garage. A potential buyer showed up three days before my planned departure day. I remember him well: a short guy with a white shirt, a *yarmulke,* and a pregnant wife. I had to disclose that the car was in the garage, having its engine replaced, and he sensed that I must sell — he bought the cheapest 1991 Subaru Station Wagon in history. But the few thousand dollars he paid were not mine yet: arriving in Israel as newcomers, we had been entitled to a tax-free car — on the condition that should we sell the vehicle within seven years, the tax on it would have to be fully paid. It was entered in my passport; I could never have left the country without paying the tax. What was left in my pocket would eventually be enough to buy a shabby 1987 Dodge in Milwaukee.

I went around bidding farewell to people. Hitler had seen to it that I had no real uncles, but there was Uncle Yaakov, a widower who had been married to my father's cousin. He had been an old pioneer, arriving in Israel in the 1920s; he "paved the roads, dried the swamps, and..." — a common phrase from Israeli books of history. Yaakov was an autodidact who had directed the National Electrical Company for many years. In 1957, when we arrived at the Port of Haifa, he was there to receive us. He sat with me in the ICU's waiting room when my father was announced dead: "It's finished," he gasped; I noted the shudder of pain descending at the back of his eyes. Such tiny flickers of empathy are registered in one's mind forever. Now, in his late 80s, after a few strokes, he was fading away in his home on Mount Carmel.

I found my uncle sitting by the window in the large living room, thousands of books on the shelves. "Uncle Yaakov, I came to say goodbye. I'm leaving the day after tomorrow, you know. I told you, America."

"Yes, America… drink something. There is orange juice in the fridge. Here, take a chocolate." We sat, looked at each other, and said nothing. I knew what he was thinking: why is he going to America? We came here and built this country for him, provided him with everything he needed, and now… what would he find in America that he doesn't have here?

After some ten minutes, I stood up. "Uncle Yaakov, I have to go. There are many things I still have to arrange."

"Yes, go," he stood up, supporting himself on his cane. We hugged and kissed. "Sit down, Uncle Yaakov, sit," I said, "I will help myself out."

As I closed the door behind me, I heard a loud shriek, a desperate howl, as if somebody was dying. I turned around and saw the old man shuffling towards the door. "Moshe, Moshe," he shouted and cried, "I will never see you again, never, never." He stumbled towards me and hugged me tightly, "I love you, Moshe," he sobbed.

I was six years old when I met Uncle Yaakov for the first time. Thirty-seven years had passed, but this was the first time I saw him crying. I helped him to his chair and walked away. I closed the door lightly behind me. I descended to the scorching midsummer street, where I could not suppress my tears. He was right: I never saw him again.

* * * * *

Yaakov Khousy.

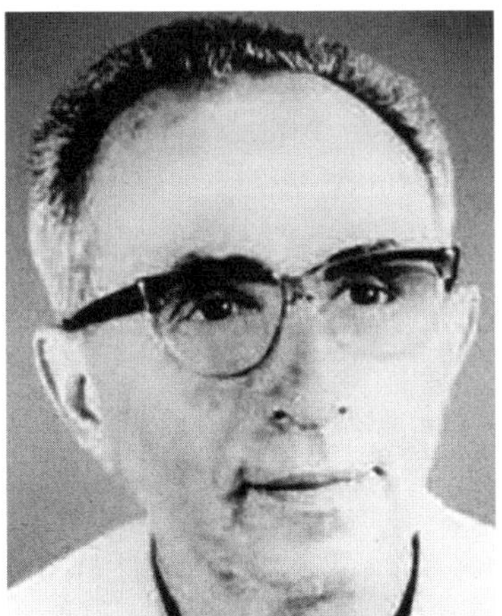

Thirty-seven

The taxi driver

On Friday morning, a day before my departure, I took a taxi to the Bat Galim beach to meet with my friend Avi R. We had some hummus and a Goldstar beer for lunch at a beachside Arab joint. Then we walked to the nearby railway station, where Avi took the last train back to Tel Aviv just before the Sabbath. I caught a taxi back home. It was the usual Israeli taxi, a Mercedes diesel; the driver was an Arab. According to regulations, his name — or was it the name of the taxi's owner? — was engraved above the rear door.

As usual, I sat in the front passenger seat, not at the back. "Golomb Avenue," I said to the driver, "near the Bnai Zion Medical Center."

"Meter or fixed?" the driver asked. He was obese, with a large black mustache. Sweat dripped from his brow.

"Fixed, please." In Israel, drivers ask whether you want them to activate the taximeter or pay a pre-arranged, mutually agreed sum.

"Thirteen shekels, OK?"

"Sure. Why don't you start the air conditioner?" It was a hot and humid mid-summer day.

"A/C down," the driver replied.

The driver turned on the radio to an Arab station with music of wailing quality — the sound of a tortured cat. I looked at the first page of the *Haaretz* as the taxi proceeded up the slopes of the Carmel. In the narrow and curving streets of Hadar — the midtown — we encountered heavy Friday traffic. The driver cursed in Arabic under his mustache, drummed on the steering wheel, and continued sweating. "What's the problem?" I asked, "You shouldn't have taken this route early Friday afternoon."

"I thought it would be a ten-minute drive. Now it's thirty minutes, thirteen shekels. I'm losing money." He cursed again and hit the steering wheel with his fist.

"Well, you asked me "meter" or "fixed." We agreed on a price. The risk was yours, not mine. Anyway, how long have you been driving taxis in Haifa?"

Taxi drivers in Haifa, especially the Arabs, were usually polite — what is wrong with this nervous one? *Let him curse and sweat — he'll get his thirteen shekels and fuck him,* I thought. Finally, after passing the steep Balfour Street — steeper than any street in San Francisco — the traffic eased, and we approached my home. "Here, please stop here," I pointed to a parking bay.

"Here you are," I handed him a note of fifty shekels. "I would advise you to fix your A/C. This may improve your mood."

"No change?"

"No, I have a few coins and this note."

"I don't have change."

"So, what do you want me to do?"

"Go home and get me the exact change."

"Nobody is at home, and I don't have the exact change, I told you."

"Go to the neighbors and ask for change." *This is too much,* I thought. According to local regulations, taxi drivers were responsible for always giving small change.

"Look, dear friend, it's Friday afternoon, everybody is napping, and I'm not going to disturb my neighbors. Anyway, the change is your responsibility."

He said nothing but drove on while my door was open and my legs were outside the car. "Are you crazy? I shouted, "Stop!"

"We find a shop, and YOU get change," he barked.

A small supermarket was two hundred meters up the road, just beyond the hospital. The driver stopped at the curb with the engine running. I saw the shopkeeper gathering his vegetables, closing the shop for the Sabbath. "*Yalla,* go inside and get the change," the driver commanded rudely and handed me the fifty shekel note.

I had had enough of this asshole. "I'm going nowhere. The change is your responsibility. Here, take my fifty shekalim, just move your bulk, go over, and get the change. I stay here."

"What!? You..." he uttered a series of well-known juicy Arabic profanities, "You won't get the change... I'll show... you..." He shifted into 'drive' and shot forward; he took a violent and noisy U-turn, speeding at 80kph down to where we came from. Until now, I was calm, but now, sensing trouble, I started to worry. My window was open, and I wanted to shout. But on this Friday afternoon — siesta time — opposite a busy hospital, on a main artery road, there was no human being around. A second passed, and we were half the distance between the hospital and my home... *where is he taking me... I have to stop him.* I lifted my left foot, forcefully brought it in front of the driver's right foot, and slammed it on the brakes. "*Kos omak*" — your mother's cunt — the driver cursed when the car stopped with a jerk, and the tires screamed just ten meters from the bridge leading to my home's front door.

I opened the door, "Have a nice weekend. It was nice meeting you..." I started saying but had to stop as a pair of heavy and robust hands compressed my neck from behind. As the hands plastered my neck against the back of the seat, the driver leaned in front of me and closed my door. "*Yalla, yalla, udrub,* let's go…" the owner of the two hairy hands shouted in Arabic as he continued choking me. I knew that they were taking me away, I was fighting for my life, and my brain was multitasking like a mega computer — processing information, ideas, and options.

The taxi sped down Golomb Avenue and the curve opposite the Bahai Temple. In that instance, I thought how absurd it was to be kidnapped in my street, opposite my house, near my hospital, in daylight, in my town and country. How silly it would be to die a day before leaving for America. What would Heidi and the boys say when the news arrived in Switzerland? *Who do these choking hands belong to?* I could not see his face, but he sounded like an Arab.

Was he the driver's friend? Impossible. What was he doing here, walking down Golomb Avenue as I pressed the brakes? Most likely, he was a bystander, an Arab construction worker walking down to the nearby subway station; he saw the car stopping — an Arab driver having problems with his Jewish passenger. *Yaala,* let me help my brother and teach the *yahud* (Jew) a lesson. He had opened the back door and jumped into the seat behind me — *Yaala, yaala, udrub,* let's go.

The taxi continued speeding down the narrow, meandering Arlozorov Street. *Where are they taking me? To their village? To the municipal garbage dump? To the deserted beach in the industrial section of town?* I tried shouting, but the pressure on my throat increased. Another two seconds and then, a hundred meters down the road, I saw a police car, a blue Ford Escort, its hood lifted and two police officers leaning on it.

Seeing the racing taxi, one of the cops jumped forward and lifted his hand: halt! As the cab stopped, the two hands left my neck. The cop leaned forward and looked through the taxi's window: "What's the problem? Are you out of your mind? Driving double the speed limit? Driver's license, please!"

"Mr. Boliceman, actually I was speeding because I was taking this mad passenger to the bolice station downtown… he refused to pay… and assaulted me."

"Who is the gentleman at the rear?" asked the policeman.

"Oh, he's from my village. He works in construction. When he saw what the passenger was doing to me, he helped me to restrain him."

I massaged my neck and left the car. "Now listen to me," I told the cop. I'm a surgeon from the Bnai Zion Medical Center. I live here on Golomb Avenue." I recounted the rest of the story.

"Well, we saw nothing, and there are no eyewitnesses. All we can do is ticket him for speeding. But if you insist, we'll take you all to the police station. You'll be able to lay a formal complaint."

Police station, formal complaint; there were no eyewitnesses, and tomorrow I was leaving. Useless, What for?

I removed my beach bag from the taxi. I looked at my watch — only an hour ago I entered this taxi, but it seemed like an age — and said to the policemen: "Thanks, but let's forget it. I'm off. Thanks for saving my life. *Shabat shalom*."

"No problem. *Shabat shalom*." They didn't believe me that my life was endangered.

"Hey, hey, where's my money?" asked the driver. One of the cops handed me five notes of ten shekels and took my fifty.

I handed the driver two notes of ten shekels each, "Here you are, keep the change."

Let him have the extra seven shekels. After all, I survived. All I wanted at that moment was to go home, shower and leave this town behind me.

"Doctor, why don't you let him drive you home?" asked the policeman.

"Thanks, I want to walk."

* * * * *

Saturday 4:30 a.m. I sat half-naked on the verandah and let the cool sea winds please my skin. Below me, Haifa was still sleeping, a light mist assembled at the bay's far end; the lower Galilee lights flickered in the distance. Some morning birds chirped on the olive trees in our garden. Soon the town would wake up, early worshipers would walk to the synagogue, worshipers of the sun would drive to the beach, and I had to take a cab to Tel Aviv and later to the airport.

Behind me, the house was empty: with the furniture and carpets all gone, the polished stone floor of the living space leading to the balcony shined in its emptiness. I had never realized how large it was. The bottle of vodka was almost empty, with the help of Ahmad and other friends who had come to say a final goodbye. I poured the last drops into a glass and added an ice cube. I lifted the glass — *lechaim*. I guessed that I would never sit on this veranda again, my family's favorite veranda, and look from here down on the vista that had become a part of my life.

I emptied the glass in one gulp. I took one last look at the sea, turning blue as the sun shined on it from the east — a patrol boat steaming into the port. Soon, the wind from downtown would carry the muezzin's *Allahu Akbar*. I closed the balcony shutters, dumped the empty bottle of vodka into the bin, and washed the glass. I looked back when the taxi drove me away — the yellowish-white house with a bridge leading to it.

* * * * *

Thirty-eight

The back door to the USA

The vast majority of international medical graduates (IMGs) — a politically correct term invented in lieu of 'foreigners' — can practice surgery in the United States only after having completed an accredited US surgical residency program. For many of them — fully qualified and experienced surgeons in their countries of origin — this represented a second, repeated surgical training. The graduates of US surgical residencies are considered 'board eligible' (BE) — eligible to take the board examinations by the American Board of Surgery. Those who pass, and most do, become 'board certified' (BC). BC — this is the magic word used to define well-trained specialists; it is a term used to select prospective employees ("we look for a BE/BC surgeon"), or to guide patients ("be sure that your plastic surgeon is board certified"). However, a very small minority of surgeons who practice in America have managed to enter the system without having to go through, or repeat, a local residency. A selected few, internationally renowned experts in a specific field — 'academic stars' — are imported by university hospitals — "come and lead our hepatopancreatic service" or "we need you to establish our surgical molecular biology laboratory." Another tiny bunch of IMG surgeons enter the US surgical system through the 'back door.' This is how I did it.

Notably, without a US residency one cannot be BC or BE, period — one is simply not allowed to take the examination. The foreign surgical gurus sitting in one of the ivory towers are not bothered too much about not being BC, but surgeons like me, who entered through the back door and practice within the community, are often asked: "Hey doc, how come you are not board certified? Couldn't you pass the examinations?" Now go and explain to them that you were not permitted to sit before the examiners. But let me tell you more about my 'back door' to US surgery.

The back door was opened to me by a German surgeon — I will call him Wolfgang — who himself had entered through the back door some seven years before me. I had first met Wolfgang at the International Surgical Week in Stockholm, 1991. I approached him at the end of a session dedicated to 'abdominal sepsis' — a topic in which both of us were interested. From his multiple publications I knew that he had previously worked in Hamburg and was now stationed in Milwaukee. He looked down at my nametag, attempting to retrieve my name from his memory:

"Ach, zo, you are that Dr. Schein who writes so much, but we never see you, vhere vere you hiding all those years?" He spoke perfect English, with a pronounced German accent, which he tried to conceal with forced American cadence. He was a large and powerfully built man, with graying blond hair, blue eyes, and small teeth — altogether handsome — about ten years older than I. He smiled pleasantly and placed a heavy hand on my shoulder, "Can I call you Moshe? Yes? I'm Wolfgang, let us forget those silly old European formalities, after all, I'm American now. Zo tell me, what did you think about the session, silly, ah? They talk nonsense, what do they understand about abdominal infections... all their old concepts. Look, Moshe, we must get together, we have to cooperate, to do something together, but I have to leave tonight, first to Hamburg, please come and visit me in Milwaukee. I mean it, you'll stay with us."

A year later, I decided to use Maccabi's department travel budget for an American tour, the first station of which was Manhattan, New York, where I attended an international breast symposium organized by the Long Island Jewish Hospital.

The Chairman of Surgery at that hospital, someone called Leslie Wise, opened the symposium at the posh Waldorf Astoria Hotel. From my back seat I saw a short, chubby man, his pink cheeks hanging down over a short neck. He lectured in a heavy foreign accent — Hungarian? I could never guess then, that in a few years, this man would become my boss in Brooklyn (he will 'star' in the following chapters). From New York I traveled to Milwaukee. It was February; the town was immersed in dirty snow and ice, under a metallic, gray sky. Wolfgang and his wife picked me up at the airport — she was a stout blonde woman, pleasant but proper in the German way — and took me to their new, white carpeted, imitation-Tudor mansion in Brookfield.

I stayed with Wolfgang for a few days. Between tours in his hospital, formal and informal dinners, I listened to his life story — more layers to it were to be added in the coming years. He was born in 1940 in the Rhineland, a child of the War. His father was sent to the front and his mother moved to France with a Frenchman — never to reunite with the father. Instead of going to high school, the young Wolfgang had been sent off to labor in a French flourmill where he lost some of his hearing. In his late teens he had returned to Germany to enlist into the new *Bundeswehr* where he also completed his secondary education. He continued with medical studies and surgical training in northern Germany, and spent a few years on a surgical mission by the German government in Algeria. Finally, he became an *Oberarzt* at the Altona Hospital in Hamburg. Here Wolfgang got himself involved in clinical research on surgical infections. Unlike most of his German colleagues at that time, he was fluent in English — learned on long visits to England with an old Jewish German family friend — a fact which helped him to publish in international journals and to establish academic contacts abroad. A shrewd promoter and eloquent speaker, Wolfgang had become closely associated with the antibiotics industry, whose drugs he advocated, and from which he had learned to squeeze out funds. In 1988, he co-created the Surgical Infection Society Europe and organized its first meeting in Hamburg. Among the invited guests was Professor Robert E. Condon (REC), the Chairman of Surgery at the Medical College of Wisconsin. REC was the one who had offered Wolfgang the back door entry to American surgery. At that time, Wolfgang's relationship with his own boss was deteriorating. He was accused of being too cozy with the drug industry, and in general too outspoken for one who was not as yet a *Chefarzt*. In Milwaukee, Wolfgang joined the section of trauma and emergency surgery, first as an associate professor but was rapidly promoted to a full professorship.

From my visits to Wolfgang's trauma unit, I remember seeing a young patient treated with a chest tube inserted for a simple pneumothorax. He was attached to numerous monitors and tubes. I was not impressed. *God,* I thought, *they are over treating everything, what a waste… in Johannesburg such a patient would be already exercising in the hospital yard…* However, I was impressed with the digital radiography they had; X-rays appearing on the computer screen, no need to put up the cumbersome celluloid. *Those Americans are advanced…*

At the end of my first and brief visit to Milwaukee, Wolfgang drove me back to the airport. I was relieved. The few days of semi-imprisonment in his huge white-carpeted mansion, driving around frozen gray lakes, and icy and empty streets, had a claustrophobic effect on me — I longed for the temperate Middle East. We bear-hugged at the airport: "Zo, Moshe, you could come and work here with us," Wolfgang said.

"Thanks, it is very kind of you, but we are very happy in Haifa." At that stage, the honeymoon between Professor Maccabi and I seemed everlasting.

A year later the situation had changed and my mind as well. During the 1993 International Surgical Week in Hong Kong, I met Wolfgang again and discussed the prospects of a position in Milwaukee. His boss, REC, had been there as well. He gave me a three-minute standing interview in the corridor and promised: "We'll see what we can do to accommodate you."

* * * * *

Thirty-nine

New immigrants in America

August 1994. One remembers best the first and last day of any period. And so I remember that steamy Chicago morning at the airport, the rented minivan to take us to Milwaukee, the boys exhausted, stretched out on the floor around the mountains of luggage; Pimpush the dog and Goofy the cat (both South African) howling in their small plastic cages.

An afternoon thunderstorm darkened the sky as we approached Milwaukee on the elevated lakeside highway. On our right Lake Michigan: foamy waves rushing to shore, an empty expanse of gloomy water from horizon to horizon — no sail or ship chimney to be seen. This is how we would see this lake from now on, during the freezing winter or scolding summer, sunny or foggy — always vast, endless and absolutely empty — lifeless.

Just before downtown Milwaukee we turned into highway I-94 West towards Madison, then taking the exit to the suburb of Brookfield: private houses on large plots, parks, trees, and flowers — a typical affluent Midwestern suburb. We parked the Chevy Astro van at the driveway of a semi-detached house and retrieved the keys from the mailbox. We had rented this house two months prior, during a brief scout visit from Israel. Our half of the house consisted of three tiny bedrooms, a small living room, a wood-paneled kitchen, which included a cozy breakfast nook, and a light-deprived basement converted into a family room — here the wood burning stove was situated. A double car garage (without one, one cannot survive the Wisconsin winters) opened directly to the basement. The back door led to a small patio and an expansive lawn, surrounded by tall oak trees. The next house was a third of a mile away. The rent was $950 per month — more than a third of what I was to be paid by the Medical College of Wisconsin.

After the storm, the night turned warm and muggy, aggressive mosquitoes buzzing around the garden. We drove to a nearby supermarket to buy some food for dinner. We munched on it sitting in a circle on the carpet in the living room. The kids drank Coke and I opened a bottle of red wine. We fell asleep on the soft carpets. Our first night in America.

The following day we started to roam around, procuring the essentials: beds, mattresses, kitchen table, chairs, tools, and a TV — to keep the boys entertained. Late in the afternoon, in some department store, Heidi suddenly collapsed onto a chair: "I can't walk, the whole world is spinning around me." "You must be tired, the flight, and all the running around," I said and took her home. But an hour later in a food store, between aisles loaded with cereals, suddenly everything started to gyrate around my head and I fell onto the ground. I tried to stand up but again the floor seemed to be in the ceiling and all the boxes of cornflakes and Cheerios appeared floating upside down. I collapsed again. By the next morning both Heidi and I had recovered our sense of balance; the acute vertigo was probably a combination of a prolonged journey, intensive and constant movement, and stress. Who said that immigrating to America was easy?

A day later, I visited a car dealer. I had to get rid of the rented car that was eroding our budget. For a few thousand bucks I got myself a 1987 Dodge Lancer hatchback. For Heidi, to drive the kids around, and for the out of town journeys, we desired a newer and safer car — a minivan. We lacked enough cash for an expensive car, but we knew that in America it's simple — here you could lease everything. Are you poor? Doesn't matter — enjoy and pay later. The Plymouth Voyager was the best minivan we knew about, even in Israel. So we called the Brookfield Chrysler dealer who assured us that they would lease us a Voyager for as low as $299 per month.

The clean-shaven, square-faced, white-toothed young sales clerk — from the start, we were pleasantly surprised by the jovial outgoingness of the Wisconsinites — took us on a test drive.

"Smooth, ah? Enjoy the ride? This is a Grand Voyager, the bestselling minivan in the country! You will love it… have any pets, doc?"

We returned to the sales room — not one of those shabby car shops like in Israel, but like an airport lounge — and sat opposite the car dealer. "Well, doc, your lease, with the basic accessories will come to $370 per month."

I looked at Heidi and she looked at me: the house rent, and now this lease, add in the car insurances, and half of my prospective salary was gone. But who cares — this is America, the highways are wide and endless; we have to move around comfortably. Otherwise — why did we come here? I read in Heidi's eyes something like "it is too expensive, let's look for something more modest," but I ignored it and said: "OK. We'll take it." *After all, am I not an American surgeon now?!*

"Great," said the smiling dealer, "your van will be ready on Monday. Please sign here, and here, and initial here. Thank you Sir. This is an application for a lease, and please bring with you on Monday your social security number, a letter of employment from your hospital, a letter from your bank… do you own a house? No? No problem, please bring your last electrical bill."

Alone with Heidi in the Lancer, driving home, I said: "We must find out about that stupid social security number."

"Whatever it is, the question is whether we can obtain it; don't forget that we are here on tourist visas." Wives are always more cautious and skeptic.

Armed with all the necessary documentation — it proved that anybody could get a social security number — we presented at the car dealership to pick up our brand new silver Voyager 1995. The radiant salesperson intercepted us at the entrance: "How're ya doin doc, Ma'am... please come this way, the manager is awaiting you." The manager, an older and heavier version of his junior, beamed at us above his reading glasses. He shuffled through a mound of papers on his pine desk: "Folks, there's just a tiny problem. Unfortunately, our bank declined your lease, um, you see doc, you have no credit history and no US-based assets, but," — a big smile — "fortunately we managed to locate another leasing bank which is ready to take the risk, um, and this of course would translate to a somewhat higher monthly payment, eh, it would come to $465 per month for thirty-nine months."

Heidi seemed devastated, ready to stand up and leave, but I kept my cool — I had brought her to America and I wanted her to drive the new shiny minivan. "OK, no problem," I said dryly, "and how much would the total advance be?"

The manager punched vigorously on his calculator — the type with a roll of paper feeding into it. "Here you are Sir, sorry, doc." He handed me the long slip, which amounted to $3900. Heidi was silently shouting at me but I continued to ignore her. I signed and initialed, signed again and again, wrote the check, took the keys, and we rode home — Heidi in the sparkling Voyager, me behind in the old Lancer.

This was the beginning of our slide into poverty. During the next year and a half in Milwaukee we would have to live and eat from the remains of my South African pension fund and whatever my late mother had left. It was also our introduction to the concept of a credit history; lacking one, as we did — the important thing is your US credit history, not the previous foreign one — you are simply a non-entity, forced to buy everything in cash or pay more. The Milwaukee Bank, noting my low income, limited our credit card to $500. Thus, only two years later, in New York, I could afford to buy a personal computer; meanwhile I had too little cash and no computer store would let me take one on credit or monthly payments.

August in Milwaukee was hot, wet, and steamy. Our container arrived from Haifa and we settled into the house and neighborhood. During the days we explored the surrounding lush green, lake country; at night we sat around a small Cadac charcoal barbecue. I could not start working until my work visa arrived, but it had not arrived. "Doc, you have to be patient," I was told every few days by a junior administrator at the Medical College of Wisconsin, "we placed a petition for your H-1B visa. We'll contact you as soon as we receive it from our legal office, they should get it shortly from the INS." (The H-1B visa is used by employers to 'import' and hire foreign workers with specialized skills.) Meanwhile, our dollar reserves were plummeting to the red line.

September. The mosquitoes disappeared, and yellow leaves were already gathering on the lawns. The boys started to attend school. Where is the visa? "Doctor, we're so sorry, but it appears that there's a backlog at the INS," said the junior administrator. Heidi called her pensioner father in Switzerland: "Papa, we need some money." He sent a few thousands Swiss francs. "Our tourist visas will soon expire, why don't you speak directly with the legal firm?" suggested Heidi. I did: "Oh, doc, the INS approved your H-1B visa a month ago — didn't you get it?" I rushed to the College: "Sorry doc, your file must've been misplaced, we found it. Your visa has been approved."

"When can I start working? Tomorrow?"

"No, doc. According to the immigration laws you have to leave the country and get your visa stamped into your passport by a US consulate in your country of origin."

"What?!"

After a few phone calls, we learned that any US consulate would do; we decided to try Canada. We left the boys at home under the command of their older brother Omri, who was already fourteen years old, and drove to Toronto. When we woke up early morning, in a shabby roadside motel in upper Michigan, the windows of the Voyager were coated with ice — the winter arrived early that year.

We reached Toronto before midnight and found a semi-deserted lakeside hotel. Over the street there was an all-night Chinese food store that provided us with chop suey and a bottle of wine. "We'll have an early breakfast and then walk to the US consulate," said Heidi, looking at a Toronto City map, "it should be a few blocks away, business hours 8.30 a.m. until 3 p.m."

The following morning. Cold wind was blowing from Lake Ontario when we walked to the consulate, where, at 7.30 a.m., the line of visa applicants stretched from the gates well into the neighboring street. I positioned Heidi in the line and went on reconnaissance: there were at least two hundred people in line — Indians, Pakistanis, Russians, Asians and East Europeans of questionable origin, and of course, numerous Arabs. Many were dressed as if exiled to Siberia, some sat on folding chairs, munching on some food and drinking from thermoses. At the head of the line I found a young Indian who was friendly enough to communicate, waggling his head: "Well, Sir, on average, they'll see a hundred applicants per day, I camped here last night."

I loitered a little at the gates — any chance to sneak in? In Israel it was always possible to bypass the queue, to squeeze in; but here — no chance. I returned to the tail of the line where Heidi was standing obediently — the Swiss would stand in a line until the Messiah arrives.

"Come, let's have a second breakfast. If we want a visa we'll have to camp out tonight," I said.

"You'll camp out. It's you who wanted to go to America."

That night I did not lie down to sleep. At midnight, wrapped in whatever warm clothes I had, armed with a flat bottle of Johnny Walker, I took myself to the consulate to spend the night standing between a Ukrainian and a Jordanian — I was number nine in the line. Heidi arrived at 6 a.m. with coffee and doughnuts. At 10 a.m. we had an H-1B visa stamped in our passports. We were euphoric. In great spirits we embarked on the same 700-mile trip back to Milwaukee. Our saga of immigration was only just beginning.

And so here I was, forty-four years old, starting my new job as a surgical care fellow under the leadership of Professor Wolfgang who had just been nominated the Director of the Accredited Fellowship Program. The Fellowship Program was to last one year — "and what would I do later?" I had asked Wolfgang already in Hong Kong. He replied: "Don't worry, just come and prove yourself. REC is influential and well connected. He's a friend who will never let us down."

* * * * *

Forty

Fellowship in Milwaukee

Armed with my working visa and a Wisconsin State license, I moved into a comfortable private office at the Section of Trauma in the dark and damp basement of the old John L. Doyne Hospital. I was lucky to obtain a Wisconsin license because, at that time, they did not require previous US training; nowadays, a prerequisite for licensing in most states is at least two years of US-based training. Wolfgang's office was on my right; the one opposite belonged to Charlie, the Director of Trauma. Charlie, in his early sixties, a bear of a man — tall, large, very dark, of Armenian descent, was well known in the American trauma community. The main Department of Surgery was situated at the newer Froedtert Memorial Lutheran Hospital; to reach it, one had to trek a long tunnel and a mile-long corridor.

Wearing a new white coat with a name tag, "Moshe Schein, M.D., Surgery, Critical Care Fellow," I presented myself before Wolfgang. I found him busy pounding on the keyboard of his computer with one index finger. "So Wolfgang, finally, I'm here. I'm now your fellow. What do you want me to do?"

"*Vot* do you mean *vot* do you want me to do? You're the SICU [surgical intensive care unit] fellow, *ne*? This means you're practically running the SICU — the bridge between the residents and the attending surgeons. Until today each team of residents cared for its own SICU patients, reporting to the responsible attending surgeon, but from today they will report to you. *Zo* go up and start working." Wolfgang's attention returned to the computer.

"But, I don't understand. What exactly should I be doing in the ICU?" I persisted. "You see, this is my first day of work in America. I know very little about the system, the chain of command, and who does what, and I have never seen an American hospital patient's chart. And what if a patient needs an abdominal re-exploration — who would decide about this, and who'll do it? Who is my boss — you or the individual attending surgeons?"

Wolfgang gazed at me irritably. I could see the long hair growing at the tip of his nose. I had a sudden urge to pluck at them. "Moshe, look, you were a senior surgeon, right? You saw everything. So, walk up to the ICU and start to manage the patients — and show some leadership!"

"Don't you want to introduce me to the residents and ICU nurses?"

"No need. Introduce yourself. Ach, *scheisse*, one more thing — as of this week, I want you to organize the residents' ICU weekly symposium."

I sensed that something here was not *kosher* — bizarre. But I had no choice but to obey, and play the game. "OK, well, I'll try the role of the ICU fellow, but I have to warn you that my last close involvement with the science of critical care was six years ago."

"Ach you'll manage. By the way, I want you to look at our experience with *Etappenlavage, ya* planned reoperations, this would be a great publication, you'll write it with me, *ne*? And I want you to get involved with the pilot study funded by Mayer… *und*… what I wanted to say, yes, start to prepare a lecture on the advantages of cefotaxime in severe intra-abdominal infection. For the Bermuda meeting next month."

"But, but, I have never used cefotaxime, I know nothing about its advantages, so why don't you let me start and function as the ICU fellow and find somebody else for the lecture?"

"Moshe, Moshe," Wolfgang laughed, "for a Jew, you are *zo* innocent. Some Jews I knew were so much cleverer. It doesn't matter what you know or don't know about cefotaxime. Just prepare a lecture about its advantages and let the Mayer Company of Basel fly you to Bermuda, together with that cute little Swiss wife of yours. Now do leave and let me finish this chapter; *scheisse*, suddenly everybody is asking for a chapter from me. This is what happens if one is famous. Listen, I won't be able to finish it. The day after tomorrow, I have to leave for Bogotá, *ya*, the South Americans love my talks, so perhaps you could go over it, see what's missing, and polish it. Jessica will give it to you on a diskette." Jessica was Wolfgang's secretary.

I navigated the long tunnel to the Froedtert Hospital. I had to stop a few nurses and ask for directions. I took the elevator and climbed to the second floor — or was it the third? I entered the SICU. It was a typical surgical intensive care unit in a large university hospital: at least twenty patient cubicles surrounding a vast central space, where numerous people — mainly females in different types of uniforms — were involved in some hectic activities around elevated desks. A few young, tall doctors in scrubs and stethoscopes hanging around their necks were running around.

You are the ICU fellow. You manage the place. Show leadership. But to whom should I speak? I approached a senior-looking lady in an impressive uniform — surely she had to be the head nurse: "Good morning, my name is Schein, and I'm the new ICU fellow. You must be the head nurse?"

The lady lifted her head from the chart and smiled politely. "Sorry, but I'm one of the nutritionists. The nurses sit there." She pointed in that direction.

I repeated my introduction to a group of nurses, drinking coffee and chatting around a few monitors. They looked at me with amazement and little interest; who is this guy? What does he want from us? One of them bothered to say: "Welcome, doctor. I think you should speak with one of the attending surgeons."

"Where are they?"

"Oh, they have already rounded. They'll be back tomorrow."

Show leadership. I noticed a group of young doctors entering one of the cubicles. "Hi guys, you must be surgical residents, right?"

"Yes, we're the blue team," one replied.

"Well, my name is Schein, and I'm your new ICU fellow. Do you mind if I join in your rounds?"

In their eyes, I read something like *who the fuck is this clown? Doesn't he see that we're busy?* But I had to persist. "What are your names, and which year of residency are you doing?" I asked and shook their hands. "Would one of you present this patient to me, please," I said.

They looked at each other, silently noticing they had no choice but to comply. "OK," said one of them, a tall, blond, beanstalk of a man, "this is Mr. Jones, ten days after blunt trauma to the chest and abdomen; status post-splenectomy. His flailing ribs were wired…"

"Operative fixation of a flail chest? Is this still done?" I asked. "To my knowledge, all studies have showed that non-operative treatment is as good, if not better."

The beanstalk shrugged: "This is the policy of our thoracic surgeons."

I saw a large plastic bag connected to the patient's intravenous line with milky contents. "What's that? Why is he getting parenteral hyperalimentation?"

"All our trauma patients receive hyperalimentation. They are catabolic, you know," said a shorter, baby-faced resident.

"Can't he eat?" I asked. "He's two weeks after a laparotomy, right? I bet that his gut is functioning, so use it. Stop unnecessary intravenous nutrition, which is costly and risky. Feed him. Use his mouth!"

Silence.

"What medications is he on?" I asked.

One of the residents lifted the patient's ICU chart and read: "Vancomycin, cefotaxime…"

"What?!" I interrupted him, "Why does he need these big guns? Is there any evidence of infection? He seems all right to me — no fever, no elevated white cell count. Why do you poison him with antibiotics, inducing bacterial resistance and wasting money? Stop all antibiotics!"

"Doctor Schein. The vanco was ordered by the thoracic surgeon. He likes to keep such patients on long-term prophylaxis."

"He likes it, but where is the evidence? There is no evidence. Just stop the silly drugs."

Silence.

I dragged them on for a few more patients — more unnecessary hyperalimentation and antibiotics were noticed and stopped. And then they deserted me: "Sorry, but we've got a seminar." Satisfied, I returned to my shadowy office. *Good, I showed leadership and did some good. After all, this enforced year of fellowship could be fun.*

The next day I returned to the ICU; the nurses still ignored me, and I ignored them. I saw no residents around — I didn't know where to find them. The entire system was alien to me. I rounded alone, writing notes in the charts and changing orders. Back at my office, I met the few attending surgeons in the trauma team. They shook my hand, said hello, and from then on, over the next year and a half, only spoke to me if I addressed them first.

Charlie, the section's chief, invited me to his office and warmly welcomed me. When I complained that I wasn't sure as to what exactly I would be doing, he smiled and said: "This is Wolfgang's problem; he wanted this fellowship program, he organized it, he convinced the Chairman, he's the program's director — you are his baby. To tell you the truth," he smirked, "there was and is an opposition in the department to the idea of having an ICU fellow; for many years each of us managed his own ICU patients — we are all ICU experts, ha, ha — so no one understands, except our dear Wolfgang, what your role will be. Where's Wolfgang, anyway?"

"In Bogotá."

"But he just returned from Korea! Listen, Moshe, do whatever you wish. Enjoy your time here, and come to me if you have any problems." Charlie was a great guy, indeed!

* * * * *

That year the winter arrived prematurely, covering the town in snow, ice, and sleet. I retired home for the weekend, not expecting to be disturbed. Even though Wolfgang had declared bombastically, "Moshe, the ICU fellow is always on call" — I was never called. But this Friday after midnight, the phone woke me up; it was a nurse: "Dr. Schein, Dr. Wolfgang wants you in the SICU asap." I jumped into my Dodge; the roads were packed with fresh snow and the visibility was poor — it took me forty-five minutes to cover the otherwise fifteen-minute distance. I parked and rushed to the ICU. I immediately noticed the frantic activity in one of the cubicles. On the bed lay the patient: his scalp wrapped in blood-soaked bandages, his face looking as if it had been through a meat grinder, an endotracheal tube in his mouth, a gastric one in what used to be a nose, his neck in a collar, chest tubes emerging from both sides of the thorax — connected to bottles full of blood. His abdomen was bulging like a giant balloon, and was covered with blood-soaked dressings; both lower limbs were in splints. Blood was on the floor.

Hovering around the bed, I counted at least seven people: Jack, a junior trauma attending, three residents, three nurses, or whoever they were. *For God's sake — why do they need me here?*

No one acknowledged my presence. I put on disposable gloves and opened the patient's eyes to look at his pupils: maximally dilated. I took a flashlight from my pocket and shined it at the pupils — no response — fixed and dilated. *Why are they still working on him? Trying to save his organs for transplant?*

Wolfgang entered the cubicle, his scrub shirt tight over his bulging girth, and stained with clotted blood. He noticed me immediately: "Moshe, this guy was airlifted two hours ago from up north, an unrestrained driver. I laparotomised him: a shattered liver, we packed it, took out his spleen, a large perinephric hematoma, we did not touch it, flail chest, both femurs gone, Glasgow Coma Scale 3 on admission…"

Wolfgang reported like a German general in a Hollywood WW II movie: slowly, carefully, clearly, in short sentences — this was the first time I saw him in surgical 'action.' "Moshe," he continued, "I want you to learn from Jack on how to use the heart-lung bypass machine to warm up this guy. He's hypothermic, you see."

Heart-lung machine — is he fucking crazy? "But, but, Wolfgang" — I was searching for words, not wanting to oppose my new boss in public — "what about his head? He has fixed dilated pupils. Did you scan his head?"

"Ach Moshe, how could we scan his head? His abdomen was blowing up in front of our eyes, and we had to rush straight to the OR, and now he's bleeding from everywhere. We've got to warm him up to improve his clotting. Jack is conducting a pilot study on using the heart-lung machine for rewarming. I want you to help him and learn how to do it when he is unavailable."

A pilot study, my ass; the guy's brain is dead. I shrugged and said nothing. I watched Jack trying to insert a large tube into the patient's femoral vein. But the patient's EKG line became flat, and it was the end. I took off my gloves, washed my hands, and drove home. By now, the highways had been cleared, and our slumbering neighborhood looked like a Siberian village at dawn. I lit the fire in the basement and poured myself a whiskey. It was to be my first and last night trip to the hospital during my 'fellowship.'

* * * * *

A month or so into my fellowship, I realized that this was a bogus fellowship. Nobody desired a critical ICU fellow except Wolfgang. It was clear that REC, the Chairman, had approved it only to satisfy the latter and perhaps, or most probably, to accommodate me.

"Moshe, were you writing notes in ICU patients' charts?" Wolfgang asked me one Monday morning. "People are complaining about it."

"Of course I did," I said — I was angry. "You want me to round and see patients, right? So I'm rounding and writing notes."

"The other surgeons are unhappy about you stopping TPN [total parenteral nutrition] and antibiotics. You should have asked them. I must also say this: from now on, you can't scrub in with me anymore. The residents went to REC and complained that you're taking away their cases, their experience."

"OK. I don't care. You wanted me to be a fellow. I tried…"

"Relax, Moshe. You desired to come to America, and you are here. As to the future of your fellowship and American prospects in general — why don't you consult REC. By the way, is the talk on cefotaxime ready for Bermuda? Do you have it with you? Please hand me the manuscript in a Word file and the PowerPoint presentation. I'll let Beatrice present it. She and her boyfriend will fly to Bermuda with me." This is how I learned that our tickets to Bermuda had been transferred to his daughter — a first-year medical student.

* * * * *

Forty-one

The rabbi and the surgical god

One morning I was summoned to the office of the Chairman of Surgery. I ran across the long corridor and was ushered into the Chairman's spacious chamber. REC shook my hand and sank his impressive bulk into a leather recliner.

REC was considered one of the 'last Mohicans' of American surgery. In his late sixties, he was a relic from a generation of 'giant' surgeons who had dominated academic American surgery during the second part of the twentieth century — people who had risen to fame based on their surgical clinical and educational leadership — not only their fundraising skills. Of Irish, Upstate New York stock, previously a Captain in the Marines, REC had — in addition to his intimidating frame and a sizeable plethoric face crowned with white, rich hair — a loud and forceful voice, which dominated lecture halls. He was famous in America and abroad — there was no surgeon who had not read one of his books.

"Well, Moshe," he started, "how many months have you been with us? Three, four? My sources and I think you need a little help adjusting to this new environment, eh? You see, to get on better with people in America, you need to *schmooze* them. I was thinking about it and… well, yesterday I called a big shot rabbi here in Milwaukee. I talked to him and told him to teach you how to charm and *schmooze*. Take this phone number. Call him, go see him, and report back to me. I want to see results."

I was surprised. *What does he want from me?* "Did I do anything wrong?" I asked.

REC fiddled with a paper-knife — his fingers, like the rest of him, were large and pink; he was a gourmet cook and a wine aficionado — and smiled: "Wrong? No, you did nothing wrong. You find yourself in a difficult situation and on unfamiliar ground. As to the fellowship, I understand that there are problems. But do not take it personally. Just enjoy your time and spend it as you wish. Write with us — I know you are a writing machine — and do not worry, we'll find you a suitable position at the end of this year. Consider this a year of adaptation to America. Now go and see this rabbi."

The rabbi, a bearded and bespectacled dark man, received me in his small office at a local Jewish cultural center. We spoke in Hebrew; his was grossly Americanized.

"Tell me, who, for God's sake, is this Dr. Condon? Last week, a man I had never heard about called my office and commanded me to educate one of his doctors! 'Teach him how to *schmooze* Americans, make him a *mensch*.' Who is he at all? Does he think he is God?"

The rabbi and I had a long chat over black coffee. "Look," he said, "I've served as a rabbi around the Midwest for over twenty years. I know these Americans well, Jews and Gentiles — he pronounced the gentiles like genitals — alike; they are tough within but sweet and polite outside. We are the opposite, but here you must behave like them: smile, smile, and smile — always, but think what you think. Understand? That is probably what your boss wants me to teach you."

At the door, the rabbi added: "You know what? How many years have I been a rabbi? Um? I do not remember a Jew being referred to a rabbi by a *goy*. Condon is not a Jewish name, ha?"

Two weeks later, I was summoned again by the Chairman. "So Moshe, how was the rabbi? What did he say? Learned any good *schmoozing* techniques yet?" A big and hearty laugh.

At the end of the academic year, the graduating chief residents organized a party for the surgical faculty, during which the latter were subjected to imitations and ridicule. They mocked Wolfgang as a large German. I watched him during the show: he pretended to laugh and enjoy it, but his sweaty red face showed otherwise. One by one, each attending surgeon was subjected to different measures of 'abuse' except, of course, the almighty Chairman. The Chairman was not ridiculed but worshipped. When his pre-recorded, commanding loud voice blasted from the ceiling, all residents fell to their knees — the Lord has spoken. For the residents, he was a god, I thought — the rabbi should have seen it. To me, this god also proved to be a *mensch*.

* * * * *

Milwaukee was submerged in a cruel, arctic, icy winter from November to late April. Even when the sun appeared, and the sky turned blue for a few hours, fierce winds continued howling from the frozen Michigan Lake.

I took REC's advice and buried myself in the gloomy basement office, writing papers and book chapters. Nobody spoke to me — except Wolfgang, Charlie — the Chief of Trauma — and REC. It was like in the UK again, but eight years later. Again, I learned that if you do not have a meaningful clinical position, you are ignored — you are nobody, and people do not waste their time on you — whoever you were or are. Gradually I perceived that being imported into the system by Wolfgang was one of the problems. A foreign protégé of an unpopular foreigner — he a protégé of the boss — is in a severe predicament. I detected that Wolfgang was unpopular from casual remarks behind his back, making fun of his Germanic persona and attitude. "The man is out of touch," I overheard one of the other surgeons say, "does he ever read an American newspaper?" Of course, the residents adopted the attendings' scorn against the surgeon who did things 'differently.'

Partially, Wolfgang brought it on himself with his supercilious, proud attitude. I remember him standing up in one faculty meeting, smiling his arrogant smile, proclaiming: "In Germany, we would have done it differently. We would have no such problems..." It drove the Yanks mad. Didn't he know that Americans do not care — nay, they hate hearing about how things are done elsewhere, and above all in Germany — from that Kraut.

So, from Wolfgang's clinical fellow I unofficially became his research fellow.

Until then, I had always been a one-person publishing team. I used to write for myself, not for somebody above me; but here it had to change. One day Wolfgang, after returning from some national meeting, told me proudly: "I flew first class with Dr. Nyhus of Chicago. He invited me to write a commentary on the treatment of intra-abdominal infection for the next edition of his book, *Mastery of Surgery*. Would you start working on it? I will be leaving tomorrow for New Delhi."

Mastery of Surgery was considered a prestigious and internationally acclaimed surgical text. I was happy to have been asked to coauthor the commentary with Wolfgang. The latter did not utter "coauthor" but asked me to write the piece. I naively assumed that in academia, when you write something, you deserve to put your name on it.

When Wolfgang returned from his India tour, the 2000 plus word commentary — a mini-chapter — was ready on his desk with a floppy disk. "Thanks, I will look at it," he said. A few weeks later, I asked, "Did you like the commentary?"

"*Ya, ya*, not bad. I made a few changes; it has already been submitted. The book should be out in three months."

"Am I the first or second author?" I asked, predicting that he had put me second but I was already resigned to such a fate.

"Moshe, I am the sole author," he replied. I did not notice any embarrassment in his demeanor, as if this was the standard of academic conduct. "You see, it was a commentary, not a formal chapter, *zo* more than one author would not be appropriate." I was stunned but said nothing — he was my only friend and protector in this frigid Midwestern wilderness. Later on, I saw the fresh copy of this book on Wolfgang's desk; my commentary — he added a few words to it — read well. It was then that I understood and decided that if I wanted my name to appear in surgical books, I had to write my own books.

But despite this 'confiscation' of intellectual property, not an isolated phenomenon, Wolfgang proved a kindhearted and concerned person. With Wolfgang, I traveled to my first national surgical meetings. I remember driving the night away to Louisville, Kentucky, in his minivan: I drove with him snoring in the back with his long legs stretched forward. We shared the hotel room for which he could be reimbursed — me not.

Quite often, Wolfgang invited us to his home for dinner. After which, he routinely would drag me to his study, leaving the wives over coffee in the living room to show me his new PowerPoint slides. Wolfgang was an excellent public speaker and enjoyed popularity internationally — less so on the national surgical lecture circuit.

Sitting at his side, I observed that preparing a surgical lecture was not a science but an art: accurate data were less important than the beauty of PowerPoint slides. If he did not have exact data or any data at all, he could create it with the mouse. A color graph looked more attractive when larger figures were included. So if a specific operation was on only 23 patients, why not add a zero to make it 230?

A lecture had to impress, to capture the audience — fiction often helps, *nicht wahr*?

* * * * *

In the middle of May, the spring arrived in a great hurry. Over a week or two, the trees were covered with leaves, and the vast grass meadows turned yellow to green. And just when the flowers began popping up in the gardens, the summer emerged. We watched these revolving Southern Wisconsin seasons as outsiders, realizing we were not here to stay.

Yes, we were outsiders. Obviously, the boys developed a few friendships at school, but we, their parents, suffered the fate of adult immigrants in a foreign land — social isolation. So we lived amongst ourselves, walking the lovely neighborhood during the scented sunsets, eyeing the lakeside properties — old Wisconsin mansions with outlying brown, red barns — toying with the idea of possessing one but knowing that this land was not ours.

Heidi spent her energies at the gym, where she taught aerobics classes, and I at the computer — a black and white museum piece, DOS, no Windows — donated by Wolfgang. In the gloomy basement room, I started to associate with SURGINET — an international surgical discussion forum on the internet — just then founded by Tom Gilas of Toronto. For me, it began serving as an outlet for my surgical voice, which was muted locally.

Invitations to American homes were so rare that each event is easily recalled: a superb dinner with Wolfgang and his wife at Charlie's — the Chief of Trauma — high-quality wines and brandies were poured liberally, and the atmosphere was relaxed and pleasant. A dinner — was it during *Chanukah*? — at a riverside mansion of a Jewish pediatric surgeon. Here the mood was chilly, and no wine was poured. Again, I could sense the condescending attitude of the wealthy and well-established local Jews to the Israeli immigrants, who were not members of their beautiful Jewish Community Center (JCC) and did not attend their magnificent *shul*.

I mustn't forget to mention Barb, who was Wolfgang's personal assistant. She was a Greek American girl in her late twenties, a college graduate wasting her years in Wolfgang's office, accommodating his tyrannical ministrations. Barb had that Greek look: petite but plump, with an ample bosom; she had a soothing soft voice, a ringing laugh, and was well-read. In the prolonged darkness of that subterranean office space, Barb, with her Greek soul, had become my antidote to loneliness and depression. Later, she moved to New York, finished a higher degree, became a professor, and married.

Looking back, I realize how traumatic the sudden dislocation to a completely different existence was for me, and how stressful it was for a senior surgeon to play the role of a humble, unrecognized trainee. In the first winter of our stay in Milwaukee, I developed severe herpetic esophagitis, rendering me ill and dysphagic for two weeks. This condition typically develops in immunocompromised individuals — in my case, the cause of immunosuppression most probably was the overwhelming stress.

* * * * *

My fellowship year was ending. As hard as I looked for it, I could not find another job. Simultaneously and acutely, the new dean of the medical college manipulated the great Chairman REC out of his position. So the man who had brought me to America, and promised to help arrange my future, was moving out of his chancellery on his way to retirement — while my contract was expiring. I had no Green Card, our Visa was dependent on continued university employment, and whatever we had in the bank would not suffice for more than a month's survival. Was this to be the end of our short-lasting American dream? Where should we go now? Back to Haifa? No, I wouldn't give those bastards the pleasure of seeing me coming back defeated, begging for a job. I wrote to my friend Roger in Johannesburg, asking for a position in his Baragwanath hospital and a loan to buy flight tickets back to Africa.

Robert E. Condon (REC) retired and moved to Washington State to spend his energy on gardening and cooking. He died in 2015 at the age of eighty-six. Wolfgang, after having lost his protector, was forced, in 2000, into early retirement despite his tenure. He contested it in court but failed.

He lives in his dream house on the west coast of Florida. The Wikipedia page he wrote for himself describes his professional accomplishments.

* * * * *

Robert E. Condon (1929-2015).

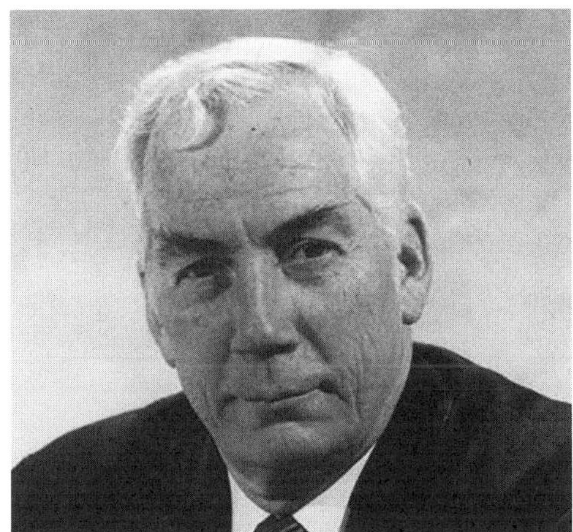

Forty-two

From Milwaukee to New York

Spring 1995. My so-called fellowship was ending. To extend my US visa, I had to find a job. But how naïve was I, thinking that because I had trained in South Africa, could perform an extensive range of operations, had ample clinical experience, and had published over a hundred papers — that because of all these reasons, I would be a hot commodity in the United States. Initially, I responded to advertisements for any surgical vacancy published in surgical journals; I sent numerous copies of my CV each week: California, New York, Florida, Texas — no reply. I mailed my CV to remote spots in Alaska — surely they would appreciate my experience — silence. I frantically FAXed my CV to Maine and North Dakota, even Wyoming — *nada*.

Then one day, I got a phone call from Seattle: "Doctor, thanks for sending your CV. Listen, I'm familiar with many of your publications. You're a famous guy." The caller sounded very enthusiastic, but when I started talking, I detected a change in his tone, as if a gush of wind had blown away the candle of his gusto.

I immediately understood: *it was my accent* — until that moment, I was a 'famous' surgeon he had read about in the *American Journal of Surgery*, and now I was just another foreigner. "Let me talk to my partners about you. I'll call again." I knew he wouldn't, and he didn't. Consequently, I had started using Jessica for preliminary calls in recruiting hospitals or licensing bodies. But why was I surprised and upset? What was my reaction to phone calls by black-sounding voices in South Africa or the Russians' heavily accented Hebrew in Israel? While local accents are soothing to local ears, foreign accents irritate many.

Guilelessly, I had assumed that my 'thick' CV, which I had mailed around like Christmas cards, was alluring. But academic positions tend to be filled from 'inside' or through a network of chairmen; academic positions are advertised, but most jobs eventually go to in-house trained surgeons or those directly referred to the chairman by his buddies around the nation. Years later, with 400 publications and many books on my record, and a past full professorship, I knew better: that when applying to positions in the community, all such academic accomplishments constitute only a burden and raise suspicion — what does this 'academician' (almost a derogative term, like a 'liberal') want among us? We do not write but we work. Or, he probably spent all his time writing and not operating.

Roughly, the following is a taxonomy, as perceived by me, to delineate, unofficially, American surgeons:

Local geniuses: this is the crème de la crème who follow a predictable path; top colleges, scholarships, ivy league medical schools, residency in leading ivory towers, fellowships of their choice under well-known masters; positions, academic or private — the distinction between the two has blurred over recent decades — in the hospitals of their choice. Many of them eventually land in leadership positions. Included in this category are members of minority groups who were born in the USA (children of immigrants) — when they talk like Americans, they are Americans! Being a bright Asian-American, Latino, or black is a plus. Females included in this group might have a considerable advantage.

Local average guys: this is the majority group, dispersed in the community and academia nationwide. They take priority for jobs: when a vacancy opens in an academic teaching department, the tendency is to give it to "one of our graduates," irrespective of how academic they are or plan to be. Occasionally, a local average guy would be imported from elsewhere, but generally, the trend is not to contaminate the atmosphere with some 'otherness.'

Locally trained international medical graduates (IMGs): with the declining numbers of US graduates seeking a surgical career, more and more IMGs (the leading source for them being India) find their way to US surgical residencies, mostly not in the ivory towers but in community-based teaching hospitals. Wherever they come from, the US residency makes them board-eligible or certified 'American' surgeons. After completing US training, IMGs tend to practice in inner city enclaves, where they dominate some hospitals; some drift into rural underserviced areas, which are shunned by American graduates (for many, working in an 'underserved area' is a pathway to obtaining a Green Card). Not a few, however, the talented ones, find their way to prestigious fellowships, landing finally in the ivory towers.

Not belonging to any of the above groups, I had to find my own way.

* * * * *

Manhattan, May 1995, late afternoon. The taxi dropped me off in front of the University Club at the corner of 54th Street and Fifth Avenue. I remember the breeze and the budding trees on the sidewalks — in Milwaukee, it was still winter; here in Manhattan, it was early spring. I paid the driver, took a receipt, and stepped into the majestic all-marble lobby of the University Club. A uniformed valet checked my name in his registry, and another valet showed me to my room on the fifth floor, a spartan, vast, high-ceilinged space.

I showered, changed into my only dark suit, white shirt, and tie, and took the ancient elevator back to the grand, calm, and dimly lit lobby. I awaited the man who had invited me to New York for a job interview. The posh venue he had chosen for this banal occasion was characteristic of that man, as I would find out in the ensuing years.

At the reception desk, I was approached by a tall, trim man in a well-tailored, stylish dark blue three-piece suit. "Hello, you must be Dr. Schein. Moshe?" I noticed his shiny black brogues and the white handkerchief peeping out from the breast pocket of his suit.

"Hi, nice to meet you." I offered him my hand.

"I'm Jim, Jim Rucinski. I'm working for Dr. Wise. I'm responsible for the residents' education. The boss will be late. He's coming from Long Island, rush hour, New York rush hour." He had a pleasant, educated American accent, definitely not the typical Brooklynese. "Meanwhile, let me show you around the Club. Yes, I'm a member. I'm on the squash team."

He led me across the lobby. "The Club was built in 1899, modeled after British, London clubs; you could say that this is New York's grandest clubhouse. Its deep rustication, grand proportions, and superb craftsmanship make it the city's finest Italian Renaissance palazzo-style structure."

"Really!" Renaissance or palazzo, my mind was focused on the expected arrival of Dr. Wise. It was to be my only 'real' job interview. I knew that I must do well. Or else we were doomed. (In fact, the only other interview that I had managed to arrange took place a month earlier, in Hinton, West Virginia. It was a poor, depressed little railway town, surrounded by majestic nature. I didn't get the job.) "Come and see," continued Jim enthusiastically, like a professional tour guide, leading me into a giant hall: "This is our reading room. Impressive, eh?" I saw a few suited elderly gentlemen reading *The New York Times*, *The Wall Street Journal*, or slumbering in one of the deep, antique easy chairs.

"OK, it's 6 o'clock. Let's have a drink," Jim said. We rode up the elevator to a cozy wood-paneled bar room. A few men stood at the bar. We sat at a table. Portraits of old members decorated the walls. "Are you a Scotch drinker? Yes? Great. Tom," Jim addressed the bartender, "two of the usual, make it a double please, yeah, on the rocks." Two crystal glasses arrived, almost full of ice and a yellowish liquid. "This is my usual," Jim said, "it's Laphroaig, single malt, taste how smoky it is? Cheers." We drank. I had tasted Laphroaig before. It was too smoky for my taste. "Can I smoke here?"

"Oh sure, whatever you like, let me tell you more about the Club. Perhaps you wish to know that women were admitted only in 1987, not to this bar but to the dining room."

Jim seemed like a nice guy, and the venue was awe-inspiring. Now we had to survive the encounter with the boss. With each sip, I started to enjoy New York more. "Oh, here he is," exclaimed Jim excitedly. He jumped to his legs, rushed toward the bar's doors, and led the boss toward our table.

"Dr. Wise, this is Moshe. Moshe, this is Dr. Wise, our Chairman," Jim tried to be formal. And indeed friendly in a formal way he was, as I would see during the next five years.

I stood up. "Nice to meet you, Dr. Wise," I said, suddenly feeling the pleasant warmth of the single malt rushing in my veins.

"Leslie Wise," the boss mumbled and offered me a soft hand for a brief and weak handshake.

"What will you drink, Dr. Wise?" Jim asked.

"As a matter of fact, I will drink nothing," he remained standing. "In fact, I'm famished." He spoke with the same marked mid-European accent I had noticed during that breast symposium a few years ago.

"Great, let's eat," said Jim, and louder to the barman, "Tom, put it on my tab, please add five bucks for yourself." "Thanks, doc," nodded the bartender. *Five bucks! Gee, these New York guys are generous*, I thought.

In the corridor, while Jim continued lecturing me about the glorious history of the Club, I silently observed the Chairman: in his mid-sixties, about 5′5″, corpulent, pudgy, big-cheeked face, thick Semitic lips, a plump nose burdened with an oversized pair of glasses, thinning gray hair, and short neck. He was immaculately dressed in a dark, expensive-looking suit, white silk shirt, pearled sleeve cufflinks peeping below the suit's sleeves. These guys dress well — I'll have to upgrade my attire, I made a mental note to myself.

From the elevator, we entered the magnificent third-floor, triple-height dining room that stretched the length of the building's side street frontage. Again, there was wood paneling, heavy chandeliers hanging from the decorated ceilings, ancient portraits of long-dead club members looking from the walls — the good old world at its best. The vast dining space could easily accommodate a few hundred diners and was virtually empty. A group of businessmen in one corner; at the other, an old man dining alone, reading a novel.

We were seated. Jim maintained a steady pace of small talk. The Chairman said almost nothing, immersing himself in the study of the leather-framed menu — he held it an inch away from his inch-thick lenses. "What will you drink, gentlemen?" asked the sommelier.

Jim looked quizzically at his boss, "Dr. Wise?"

"Oh, let us have a bottle of red." To me, he added: "You drink red wine, don't you?"

"Of course."

Dr. Wise looked above his glasses at the sommelier: "Get us a bottle of Bordeaux, yes, St. Julien." To us, he said: "As a matter of fact, 1978 was a good vintage."

Jim appeared satisfied with that astute decision but considered it his duty to warn the boss: "Do you know how much it costs?" Dr. Wise ignored such a trivial comment and focused on a freshly baked roll, which he carefully halved, smeared with a thick layer of butter, and stuffed it in his mouth.

The wine arrived. The boss allocated the task of sampling it to Jim. Food was served, and Jim elegantly dissected his filet mignon and maintained the flow of small talk. Dr. Wise slurped, with great enthusiasm, his bouillabaisse — he brought his mouth to the plate rather than the spoon to his mouth. He maintained silence, short of a few isolated questions aimed at me: "You served in the Israeli Army, uh?" or "How is my friend Bob doing?" Bob was REC, the recently evicted Milwaukee Chairman who connected Wise and me.

A little Italian waiter appeared, pushing a dessert cart loaded with mouthwatering cakes, tarts, tortes, mousses, fruits, and ice creams. I saw Wise's eyes sparkle with delight: "As a matter of fact, I have had enough, but please let me have some fresh strawberries, a spoon of cream, um, add a tiny sliver of the Kirschtorte, and a double espresso, thank you very much," he ordered the waiter. To me, he added: "I need the coffee. We live in Long Island, you see, a forty-five-minute drive. This is New York, not Milwaukee. As a matter of fact, I used to live in the Midwest. We stayed a few years in St. Louis, at the Barnes Jewish Hospital. I couldn't endure that town and the Midwest; New York is the place to live, as you will probably find out."

"Dr. Wise, a small cognac?" suggested Jim. "Moshe?"

"Sure," I replied enthusiastically. I predicted that the cognac would not be American or Spanish brandy — I realized that the products are magnificent when Jim orders and the boss pays. After a few seconds of pondering, the boss said: "Jim, as a matter of fact, I have changed my mind. I won't be driving to the Island. I'll sleep in my flat." He turned to me: "It is just around the corner, the Trump Tower, you know; in fact, Moshe, I'll be able to pick you up tomorrow morning and drive you to the hospital. Jim, would you please cancel the limousine. Listen, didn't we once have a wonderful Armagnac here? It was 1968, I think, yes, let's have it."

After dinner, Jim made us stroll through the enormous, two-level, vaulted library, an accurate copy of 19th-century libraries in Oxford or Cambridge. A large Churchill portrait hung on one wall. We descended into the lobby where both men collected their light trench coats — Jim's black and smooth, Wise's gray, baggy, and crumpled. I saw that Jim carried a black umbrella and wore a 1940s bowler hat on his head — he looked like a British diplomat. Wise shook my hand, "Good night. I'll pick you up tomorrow at 6.30 a.m. Please wait here on the stairs. I'll be in a white Mercedes Sport."

He rolled down into the street; like Mr. Smiley from John le Carré's novels, I thought — a Jewish, central European Smiley.

I do not remember which model of Mercedes it was, for in the successive five years, Dr. Wise frequently changed his sports cars: Jaguar, Porsche, Lamborghini, a Benz again — often keeping a few of them simultaneously. But now, early in the morning, after an evening of drinking, he looked amazingly fresh and well-groomed, his sparse hair smoothed over his bald spot. Henceforward, I would be impressed at how resilient this older man was: late to bed, early to rise, a busy surgical career constantly intermingled with social events and, hence, steady but never excessive consumption of alcohol. However, he always appeared rested, tidy, spruced up, and in a good mood. He seemed like a man who constantly enjoyed himself. Probably he did — this being one of the secrets to his success.

I buckled myself in as we merged onto the FDR Drive, southbound. "Are you going to buckle up?" I asked him.

"No," said Wise, "I never do. This is an accident-proof Benz." Crossing the Brooklyn Bridge we drove directly onto Ocean Avenue. It was my first glimpse of Brooklyn, and I looked at the colorful and confused shabbiness with interest. It reminded me of the southern part of Tel Aviv. Wise navigated his car at sixty miles per hour, made a right turn onto Fourth Avenue, a left turn onto Fifth Street, and here we were, at the doctors' parking lot of the New York Methodist Hospital (NYMH).

* * * * *

What do I recall of that spring day many years ago?

I recall a midsize hospital, a hybrid of 19th-century red bricks and modern concrete, in the heart of Park Slope, a block away from Prospect Park.

I recall Wise showing me a spacious, high-ceiling empty room on the sixth floor: "This could be your office…" I looked out of the wooden framed window: blue sky, New York waterways, ferries leaving a long wake, and directly ahead, the Statue of Liberty. An office with a view of the Statue of Liberty — isn't this the American dream? I was in awe. Only later I learned about the surgeon who Wise had just fired to vacate the position and office…

I recall the tour with Jim around the hospital. In the operating room's scheduling office, near the coffee machine, we came across a short surgeon in full scrubs. He was leaning against a Xerox machine, a polyester cup of coffee in his hands. "Moshe, please meet Dr. Rahman," Jim introduced us in his habitual formal fashion, "Dr. Rahman is our Chief of Vascular Surgery." We shook hands — yet another spongy handshake.

Rahman studied me with amused dark eyes and said in what I perceived was an Irani accent: "So this is the professor recruited by Wise?" To my sensitive ears, the "professor" sounded sarcastic. It was the first hint to what I would comprehend soon — the low-key war of attrition conducted between the local Iranian surgical gang and Chairman Wise.

Next, I recall, Jim took me to the hospital's roof for a topographical lecture, describing accurately the vistas in all directions. To the south, he pointed to the Verrazzano-Narrow Bridge glistering in the midday sun. "What is that green hill?" I asked.

"That is Staten Island, Todt Hill. Many of our surgeons live there."

It is how and why we ended up living on Staten Island.

After a teaching session with the residents late afternoon, Wise took me into his elegant corner office. His secretary — I forgot who she was, for so many were replaced over the ensuing years — served us tea in decorated porcelain cups and Italian dry cookies.

Wise sat at my side on the black leather sofa and squeezed my left elbow: "Moshe, do you have any questions? The taxi should be taking you to LaGuardia in thirty minutes."

"Well, what, um, are my chances of getting the job?"

"As a matter of fact, it appears to me that the job is yours. I spoke at length with Bob, and I trust Bob very much, he's a friend," — which probably meant to him a good *goy* and not an anti-Semite, "and we did our homework," — a smile — "we have our resources overseas as well."

"What about my visa? I am on an H-1B visa. A New York license would require permanent residence, a Green Card?"

"Leave this to us. We'll organize something. I'll talk to the hospital lawyers to transfer the H-1B to our hospital. You will have to apply for a license and a Green Card. It may take some time, but, as a matter of fact, meanwhile, you can start functioning on a temporary license."

"I'm delighted and flattered, but how would I contribute to this department?"

Wise pondered briefly: "When I took over the department two years ago, it was in shambles. I had to fire a few full-time attendings. I'm changing the culture. Before I arrived, how should I say it, it was definitely not academic. I need you to help me shape the residency program. I need somebody I can trust. As a matter of fact, there is a small dispute going on here with some elements that don't welcome any of the changes I brought with me. I need an ally, and what I hear from Bob — you seem suitable."

Money. Ask about money. "And how much would the pay be?"

"As a matter of fact, I talked yesterday with the hospital president Mr. Musk; he has agreed to pay you a base salary of $150,000. In addition, like the others, you will be billing your patients, getting forty percent of the income; twenty percent goes to the departmental fund, your books, meetings, and so on; forty percent goes to the hospital."

I could not hide my satisfaction. To me, currently earning $25,000 per year, the $150,000 seemed an immense sum — unbelievable, and the end to our miseries and tribulations. Wise sensed it, adding, "It wasn't so simple to obtain such a generous sum from Mr. Musk."

"Thank you, Dr. Wise, it's a very generous offer," I replied. I did not know, of course, that Wise's salary was astronomic and, in addition, he kept a hundred percent of his billings.

Wise accompanied me through the long corridor of the Department of Surgery. He grabbed my left elbow with his right hand and guided me into the elevator.

Over the subsequent years, he would prove to be the most agreeable and humane boss I ever had — almost until the bitter end.

* * * * *

My mood was elated when the Midwest Express airliner approached the Milwaukee Mitchell International Airport. Light rain was falling on the dismal pre-spring expanses. I saw a few patches of old snow, but in my mind, I still felt the exciting air of spring in Manhattan.

Yes, New York is where I wanted to be, New York is where we were going to, the Statue of Liberty — our liberation, finally — New York, we were coming!

Heidi picked me up in her minivan. Driving back home, I recounted, enthusiastically and excitedly, like a child returning from his first visit to Disneyland, my New York adventures: the University Club, Brooklyn — the numerous ethnic restaurants surrounding the hospital, how lovely Wise is, and of course, the financial offer. At home, I told her about the encounter with the vascular surgeon in the OR and his sarcastic comment.

"So that Wise has opposition, right? How secure is his position?" Heidi asked. I told her what Jim Rucinski had explained to me: that a small group of old timers, private surgeons, mostly of Iranian extraction, who previously had dominated the scene, were not satisfied with Wise; that Wise was a shrewd politician and very well connected — he knew how to deal with them and was winning.

"Didn't you have enough political wars in Israel? Is this what you need now? Do you know what they'll say? A Jew is bringing in another Jew to fight against the Iranians."

"But Heidi, what other options do we have? It is the only real offer I have after a six-month search. Without a Green Card, I'm a lame duck. Politics or not, it is either back to South Africa or Israel, or forward to New York and Brooklyn, and $150,000."

"And where would we live?"
"Well, either in Brooklyn or Staten Island."
"Who is living in those places?"
"I don't know. We'll find out."

* * * * *

January 2, 1996, on the way from Milwaukee to New York: me with Pimpush, our South African Dachshund, leading the convoy in the rattling Dodge hatchback; Heidi, behind, in her leased Voyager with the boys and two cats. On the frozen interstate approaching Cleveland, a stone flying from under a passing semi-trailer shattered Heidi's windshield. We stopped for the night, dining on a family-size serving of Kentucky fried chicken and mashed potatoes.

A tremendous rainstorm accompanied us throughout Pennsylvania into New Jersey the following day. A snowstorm was gathering when we settled for the night at a roadside motel. The distant horizon to the east was bright, illuminated by the great city. We crossed the Hudson River in the morning and entered our promised land.

* * * * *

The author with Dr. Wise (left) at a dinner. (The overfed faces reflect New York's life style.)

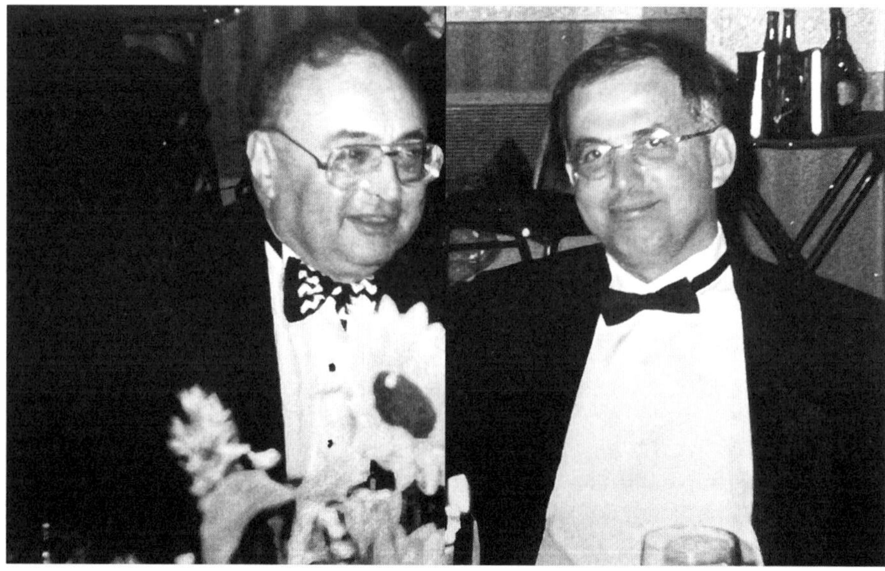

Forty-three

The New York Methodist Hospital, Brooklyn

January 1996. A gray winter morning. We crossed the Goethals Bridge to find Staten Island digging itself out of the "snowstorm of the decade."

We drove directly towards our rented house on Sinclair Ave, at the island's southern tip. A tall mountain of garbage bags — many split, discharging decaying contents into the white snow — blocked the entry to the driveway. As pre-arranged, we found the house keys in the mailbox; the house was relatively clean but had the aroma of a cheap curry joint in Bombay.

We had rented it from an Indian who had introduced himself as Captain Choprakumar. Initially, we assumed that "Captain" was his first name, but it turned out that he had been a ship's captain in the Indian merchant navy. It was a typical cheaply built pseudo-Tudor, two-story wooden Staten Island house — the front shrouded with a thin layer of red bricks. It consisted of a small landscaped gravel garden, four bedrooms, a spacious basement, a study on the landing, a wooden stairway in the front, an alternative winding metal staircase at the back, a roomy living room, polished wooden floors — not bad for $1600 per month in New York.

Thus started our ten-year sojourn in New York City — a long ten-year period: we lived, raised our sons, and had good and bad days. But looking back at those years, I mainly see a single hazy picture: an endless commute to work and back and neverending wars with the 'enemies.'

Trying to sum up our New York saga — to recapture the atmosphere — I will borrow, in chronological order, brief segments from the Roman à clef I penned, under a pseudonym, in 2001— *Life Means Nothing Behind the Green Wall*. For many of the protagonists mentioned, fictional names have remained.

* * * * *

September 1998. My black 1991 Caddy de Ville reaches the top of the Verrazzano-Narrows Bridge and rolls on toward Brooklyn. It is misty as the sun rises from Coney Island. I relish the sight, for the upper deck of the Verrazzano offers a magnificent vista. In front is Brooklyn, on the right I see Coney Island, on the left, I can make out the southern tip of Manhattan and the Statue of Liberty. And behind me, Staten Island and the house we bought last year: a well-built 'colonial' on a quarter of an acre. It had cost us 400,000 dollars, of which eighty percent had to be borrowed. But it is a pleasant house, only ten minutes by bicycle from South Beach. Unlike the routine rush-hour bumper-to-bumper morning crawl to Brooklyn, today's drive is agreeable.

Driving is the only time I can think properly. Sometimes my thoughts embrace me so tightly that I end up in front of the hospital without knowing how I got there. I plan my day. First, I have to do an appendectomy for acute appendicitis, which had been admitted at night; if not performed before 6 a.m., it will have to wait until the end of the elective cases — usually in the evening. Next, at 8 a.m., we'll have the weekly morbidity and mortality meeting. I wonder how stormy it will be as the war with the Iranian 'mafia' carries on. They control everything: the Medical Board, the Board of Trustees, admissions, referrals, and committees — CEO Musk is under their boots. Only Wise and I stand up against them. Are we going to win? Wise is extremely rich and powerful and will survive, but what about me — *how long will I last in this hospital?* In 1996, after I had joined the department, the Iranians, who were dominating the hospital's credentialing procedures, found a loophole in the bylaws to prevent me from treating patients and entering the operating rooms — "he cannot be an attending surgeon on a temporary license," they claimed. When I eventually received the Green Card, and thus a permanent New York license, they blocked my clinical privileges by repeatedly canceling the meetings of the credentialing committee. I was limited to teaching residents and writing papers for an entire year.

Brooklyn. I snap back to the present. I take the Thirty-Eighth Street turnoff and start bouncing over the potholes anchored like landmines in the roadway. I turn right off Fourth Avenue onto Ninth Street and into the hospital doctors' parking lot. I insert the electronic card, and the railing opens up. The lot for the attending physicians is empty now, but only for a short time. It will soon be filled with cars, branded Mercedes Benz, BMW, Lexus, and the customary large jeeps and SUVs whose farthest off-road will be crossing a grassy median.

* * * * *

Main auditorium, 8 a.m.

"I present the case of M.J., a ninety-year-old female patient. Diagnosis: right carotid stenosis. Complications: stroke and mortality. Procedure: right carotid endarterectomy. Surgeon: Dr. Mantzur. Resident: Dr. Ed Johansson."

The weekly morbidity and mortality conference, known to everybody as the M&M meeting, is starting. It is the hottest ritual in the life of any teaching surgical department in the country. The purpose of the M&M meeting is to discuss all so-called 'adverse' outcomes generated by any member of the department. At the Methodist Hospital, we always had a long list of cases to discuss; a waiting period of a couple of weeks between the actual event and its eventual analysis was not unusual. But then, of course, the patients concerned no longer stood to benefit from those discussions. It was the future patients who might benefit. The aim of the M&M meetings is to educate the responsible surgeon and help him learn from his mistakes. The best we can hope for is that repeatedly exposing members of staff to the mistakes of others will prevent them from making similar errors later on. The least we can hope for is the prevention of complications by intimidation. "If I know that all my mishaps will be routinely exposed to my colleagues," this line of reasoning goes, "I will be more cautious." To achieve such ambitious goals, the M&M meeting has to be objective. The rules are simple: all complications and fatalities in any patient treated by any member of the department should be presented. A complication is a complication, regardless of whether the eventual outcome is a triumph or a tragedy. Whether or not the M&M meeting is objective and accomplishes its objectives depends mainly on the local chairman and the political environment.

Today, Dr. Leslie Wise is conducting the meeting. The resident who shares the stage with the Chairman and is presenting the case is Dr. Johansson — his tall frame dwarfs Wise's comparatively diminutive, though not small, frame.

Wise peeks above his glasses at the printed summary of the case: "Please tell us what happened, Dr. Johansson."

"This elderly woman presented to the vascular service with transient ischemic attacks involving the right cerebral hemisphere. An arterial duplex scan demonstrated a seventy percent stenosis of the right carotid artery. After obtaining medical clearance, the patient underwent a carotid endarterectomy under general anesthesia. A shunt was used. The operation was uneventful."

There is a hush in the auditorium. The tense silence is not unusual during a weekly presentation of one of the habitual complications of Dr. Mantzur, the New York Methodist Hospital's 'godfather.'

Dr. Joseph Mantzur, in his late sixties, fragile-looking, is a typical 'do-it-all' Brooklyn surgeon. You name it, and he'd do it: general surgery, vascular bypasses, and chest operations. Born in Iran, he had immigrated to France with his aristocratic family well before the downfall of the Shah. He completed medical school in the Sorbonne, Paris. He did his surgical residency at the Methodist Hospital long before "New York" had been added to its name. He has been considered the leading local private surgeon for thirty years — gathering immense influence and wealth. The showpiece of his wealth is an oceanfront mansion and a large boat on the tip of Long Island. It is where Dr. Mantzur escapes each Friday night after a strenuous operating week, far from his dying patients and their anxious families. To appease the Iranian mafia, Wise recently nominated Mantzur as the Vice Chairman of Surgery.

Mantzur has a hearing aid but is not using it. Instead, he cups a hand behind his right ear and appears to listen attentively. He sits in the center of the second row.

"What happened then?" Wise adopts his characteristic calm and objective tone.

Johansson talks into the microphone: "In the recovery room, the patient failed to wake up from anesthesia. She was observed to suffer from a dense left hemiparesis, weakness of the left side of her body. We rushed her back into the OR. On re-exploration of the neck, we found the artery pulsatile, without a thrombus. A postoperative CT revealed a massive stroke of the brain on the side of the operation. The patient expired the following day."

I cannot bear to listen. In my mind, I had long since nicknamed Mantzur "Terminator One." We are presented with a similar case of his every week, and yet even he is outperformed by long and far by "Terminator Two," Dr. Mahmud Sorkhi. Sorkhi is the almighty President of the Medical Board, the second surgeon in the ruling triumvirate at the New York Methodist Hospital. A son of a Persian Ayatollah, he had studied medicine in Iran and trained in surgery at the Methodist Hospital under Mantzur's wings. He had married a local Irish nurse and established himself in private practice. He had been a real 'cowboy' surgeon for many years, considered the 'top knife' by the hospital medical community. Unlike his mentor Mantzur — always calm, controlled, and poker-faced — the gray eminence of the Methodist Hospital — Sorkhi is loud-mouthed, macho-like.

My lists are full of their cases; I know their patterns. Full names are never mentioned during the M&M meeting, but I can present Mrs. M.J.'s story in full detail without looking at her chart. By now, I know how they manage to terminate their patients.

Dr. Johansson finishes his brief presentation. He dries the sweat from his face. Dr. Wise looks at him: "What can you tell us about this complication? Was it preventable, avoidable?"

The resident shrugs. "Dr. Wise, the operation was uneventful. We had no problems."

Wise leans over and pinches the resident's left elbow: "Whaddya mean no problems? The patient died. This is no problem?"

Loud laughter erupts from the audience, stirring the slumber of many junior residents. They look around briefly, quickly lose interest and start napping on their other hand. Just about everyone else appreciates the Chairman's sense of humor. They know that Johansson is not terribly bright, that he is digging his own grave. "In fact, we were very fast. We cleaned the artery in forty-five minutes. We used a shunt to perfuse the brain," Johansson says, moistening his lips.

"Were you happy at the end of the operation?" asks Wise.

"Yes, we were happy!" Johansson almost screams.

The audience knows what to expect; this is a part of the weekly ritual — slightly funny but predictable unless someone dares to open his mouth. I look around. Mantzur hides behind his poker face. In the back, David Glass is sulking. Dave is a private vascular surgeon. He abhors Mantzur. I doubt that he would speak up.

Wise addresses Dr. Rahman, the Chief of Vascular Surgery, a Kurdistan-born private surgeon. "If this were your patient, would the results have been different?" It is Wise's famous gimmick. It makes the M&M meetings allegedly more objective.

Rahman, a short, thin man in his early fifties, completely bald, is known as a technically solid surgeon of very good judgment. His comments at the M&M meeting are usually informative and balanced — unless the discussion involves his friends, mentors, or partners. Rahman pronounces his words with precision. "Dr. Wise," he says, "I had the opportunity to read the duplex scan. It showed a seventy percent occlusion in the right internal carotid artery. It was a significant lesion, which indicates the need for an operation in a symptomatic patient such as this lady. Indeed, we are told that she had suffered from transient ischemic attacks. As you know, recent prospective randomized trials from this country, as well as from Europe, have demonstrated that the operation would have been appropriate even in the absence of any symptoms. Therefore, the indication for surgery was appropriate. As to this unfortunate complication, we know that the combined mortality and stroke rate after such operations is five percent in the best hands, even at the top centers. I believe that Dr. Mantzur took all the usual precautions, including administering heparin and inserting an intra-luminal shunt. Yes, the outcome is sad, but I do not see how it could have been prevented or better managed. Operating on these old patients is risky. We have to take risks like these. We are surgeons."

"Anybody want to comment? Does anyone think the complication could have been avoided or better handled?" asks the Chairman.

Silence. The few vascular surgeons present stare at their hands. Dave Glass winks at me but doesn't open his mouth. *Screw Rahman. What a bullshitter.* To operate on a ninety-year-old bedridden woman is crazy.

Rahman himself would not have touched her, but he is prepared to lie in public to defend his old mentor. Another kill for Terminator One.

I raise my hand and begin talking before being acknowledged by the Chairman. "Dr. Johansson," I say clearly, "could you please tell us a little about the exact nature of the patient's symptoms? Could you be more specific?"

Wise shoots a look of mild irritation at me as if to say: "shut up and let me close this case." But Johansson responds anyway: "Mmm, I guess she had TIAs. I can't tell you more. I never talked to the lady before the operation. She arrived at the OR directly from Medicine, and then she died."

Faint laughter is heard from fellow residents. One should not say such things. Residents are supposed to know the patients they operate on. An essential requirement stipulated by the American Board of Surgery is that the operating resident evaluates his patient before the operation and actively participates in postoperative care. Everyone knows this is sometimes impossible and that the resident may first meet the patients when they are already deep under anesthesia, but admitting to it frankly is daft!

"Dr. Mantzur, do you have anything to add?" Wise addresses Mantzur himself, the attending surgeon responsible for the operation.

I stand up this time. I will not let this one slip so easily. *Fuck 'em.* "Dr. Wise, I asked Dr. Johansson for information on the symptoms displayed by this patient. Could I have an answer, please?"

Wise ignores me and looks at Mantzur, who responds in a low voice, whispering and swallowing words. "Dr. Wise, this is an unfortunate case — a pleasant old lady with a significant carotid lesion. The operation was routine. The shunt went in and out with no problems. I could not do it any better. Very unfortunate."

"Dr. Mantzur," I blurt out before Wise can take over. "The symptoms? What were the symptoms? Was she symptomatic at all? What was her functional status? Could she walk?"

The *Padrino* — so we call him behind his back — turns around and looks in my direction. There is a hush in the auditorium. No one had ever directly questioned the great Mantzur about indications. For Mantzur, the indication for surgery is the mere desire to operate. He speaks with belabored patience. "Dr. Schein," he says slowly and methodically, "the patient suffered from headaches and dizziness. She had significant stenosis. Why didn't you listen to Dr. Rahman?"

"Because these are non-specific symptoms, not TIAs. This ninety-year-old lady was bedridden, is that not so? I do not think there was any reason to operate on her."

Wise holds his hand up. "Let us move to the next case," he says, pointing to Dr. Jim Rucinski, who takes minutes of the meeting: "Dr. Rucinski, what is our conclusion for the minutes?"

* * * * *

Ten a.m. The grand round lecture, which follows the M&M meeting, is over. No one bothers to ask questions. I stuff the printed M&M case summaries into the pocket of my white coat. This is confidential department material to be collected and destroyed after the meeting. Only one copy is kept by the department. I'm nevertheless collecting the papers for my files. I see others doing the same. An "insurance policy," we call it, against potential enemies — only as a prophylactic measure. In the corridor I bump into Dave Glass. He puts his arm around my shoulder: "Moshe, very brave, very brave. Did you notice the silence? They were astounded. To ask the old fart about indications. Unheard of at the old Methodist Hospital!" Dave has a pleasant, smiling face, a well-trimmed brown mustache, and a perfectly matching curly brown hairdo. Our residents claim it is a wig that had recently been spotted sliding down his wet scalp after a difficult repair of an abdominal aortic aneurysm. We walk towards the elevators. "Hey, Moshe," he continues, "I watched Sorkhi's face during the discussion of the Padrino's case. Boy, he suffered. Watch your back, though. You know Sorkhi and Zalzer are buddies. I can tell you, Fat Brian has some rough connections in this part of town." Dave is referring to the third in the aforementioned triumvirate — Dr. Brian Zalzer: a half-Jew, half-Italian, born and bred in Brooklyn. A graduate of a Caribbean medical school, he completed an internal medicine residency in the Methodist, where he met and bonded with Sorkhi. Energetic despite his immense size, Zalzer became a clinical professor of medicine with two publications on his curriculum vitae. He and Sorkhi, both in their late fifties, are as close as brothers. They socialize at top Manhattan restaurants, the Bahamas' casinos, and with women in Atlantic City. Zalzer is known to have a connection with the 'family.'

"Dave, don't get carried away. This is just a hospital in Brooklyn, not a mobster's joint. But look, I've been here for almost three years now. Mistakes and errors happen everywhere and to everybody. But what these guys are doing is appalling."

Glass laughs. "I've known them much longer than you. Before your arrival, the Padrino attempted to remove my vascular privileges for nothing. Wise managed to save my ass. I need to make money; you know how much my ex-wife gets? You have to pay the mortgage as well. So let's be careful."

I nod. "I wonder how Wise will react."

"He will give you shit for opening your big mouth. Just shut up, listen to him, and swallow it. Whether you like it or not, he's the boss. Leslie is a good guy, but he has to coexist with these guys."

* * * * *

Back on the medical floor, I see a few consults. The first one is a semi-comatose, post-stroke octogenarian. I am requested to insert a stomach tube — a gastrostomy. I place the old man in a sitting position and bring a spoonful of water to his mouth. He swallows nicely. He doesn't need an operation or even an endoscopic gastrostomy. All he needs is to be patiently spoon-fed. And what is wrong with a small diameter, soft feeding tube from his nose to the stomach? "No indication for gastrostomy," I write in the consult note, knowing that a few days later, somebody — like Sorkhi or one of his buddies — will perform the gastrostomy anyway — another *unnecessary operation*. Similar patients are presented frequently at the weekly M&M conferences nationwide. "How could we let him starve?" is the usual justification, or sometimes it is: "The nursing home won't admit him, or her, without a gastrostomy."

The next patient I see is even more depressing. Three months ago, I bypassed her stomach and bile duct for a widely spread pancreatic cancer. I injected her celiac plexus with alcohol, eliminating the intractable back pain. Now she is lying moribund in bed with an infected venous catheter. It was implanted elsewhere for the administration of chemotherapy. I talk to her daughter. "Didn't I tell you that chemotherapy is useless in her case?"

"Yes, but they told me it may prolong her life."

I will need to remove the infected portacath. Another futile procedure. Do all terminally ill patients need to be decorated with feeding tubes and poisoned with costly and mostly ineffective chemotherapy? One of Dr. Wise's habitual jabs to the residents is: "What is impossible to find in any hospital?" Answer: "An oncologist who refuses to administer chemotherapy."

Another consult: a ninety-five-year-old, totally demented lady lying, contracted in a pool of fresh feces; the obligatory stomach tube in place. Her acute surgical problem is two large trocanteric bedsores for which she receives intravenous antibiotics. I prescribe 'local' treatment and recommend the cessation of the antibiotics, hoping the disease will take its natural human course. I have seen similar patients subjected to major plastic reconstructive surgery, most likely motivated by Medicare coverage.

Today I decided not to stop on the fourth floor. Moving around on this floor would not enhance my mood. The fourth floor is dedicated to chronic ventilator cases — patients who have partially recovered from a severe acute illness but still need artificial breathing through a tracheal tube. After a prolonged and costly stay in the intensive care unit, they are transferred to this section for long-term ventilation at a lower daily cost.

Our residents call the floor "Cape Canaveral" because it is from here that cases are launched into eternal space at night. It is predictable. The tracheal tubes require dedicated suctioning and cleaning to remain patent. However, this service is seldom provided, and definitely not at night. You see your patient during evening rounds smiling and well. The following day you may be informed that he or she has expired.

"What happened?" you ask. It is a rhetorical question because you know they suffocated, drowning in their tracheal and bronchial secretions.

"Poor old Mrs. Santiago," the resident would say. "She was launched." No further explanation is needed. We often exchange the tracheal tube in such patients, knowing how dirty and clogged they can get. No use to complain. No one is interested.

Next, I have to go to a hospital committee meeting. I dread exposure to a team of administrators in gray suits and nurse managers in high heels, talking a neologistic jargon spiced with words such as "proactive" and "prioritized." According to them, we are doing well, meaning the budget is positive. Every launch at Cape Canaveral, each of the unnecessary operations by Sorkhi, Mantzur, and friends eventually translates into numbers in black ink, often in the shape of zeroes.

* * * * *

Previously, in South Africa and Israel, I had encountered corrupt and greedy doctors; I had seen serious errors committed and hushed up. I knew that some surgeons are like vultures — that they love to operate and need to operate to make more money. But what I had found here in New York was beyond description. The overcrowding of surgeons and other specialists, the extreme fee for service system — actually, you were penalized for not operating — the 'balkanization' of doctors based on their ethnic origin all led to a constant cutthroat struggle for even the most minor hernia case. The corruption, malpractice, and political intrigues I encountered at the New York Methodist Hospital were astounding when observed through my relatively naïve eyes of those days. This situation seemed to prevail, at least in the medical jungle of the boroughs, away from the few ivory towers of Manhattan. But I'm not sure that this was, or is the case…

Meanwhile, the months and years passed by. The 'cold war' between us — Wise and his boys — and them — Mantzur, Sorkhi and their private mafia — was occasionally interrupted by hot skirmishes, which continued incessantly at the M&M meetings, at hospital committees, and in the background. As Wise's right-hand man, I was drawn into the struggle with which I had gradually become obsessed — my personality seemed to enjoy combating forces perceived as evil and dangerous. In the interim, supported by Chairman Wise, I was climbing the academic ladder at Cornell's Medical College, with which we were affiliated. I was teaching residents, helping them to publish, and writing and editing a few books. My clinical practice, however, never grew to be busy enough, as most elective referrals from the hospital and community were channeled by our enemies to themselves, away from us. We, the full-time surgeons, were fed on the 'leftovers' — the emergencies and indigenous patients. The latter were obviously of no interest to Mantzur and Sorkhi *et al.*

Otherwise, in retrospect, at least, our life was satisfying. Our previously dire financial situation improved, the family was reasonably happy, and we traveled extensively — nationally and abroad. Staten Island restaurants offered the best Italian food. Only the daily commute was horrendous and nerve-wracking. But, hey, what do you want? This was New York!

* * * * *

Forty-four

Brooklyn — the beginning of the end

Winter 1999. Staten Island.

Naked, I run to the open-air spa in our backyard. The fresh snow feels soft and frosty under my bare feet. I remove the cover and plunge my frozen body into the hot water. It is one of the pleasures of winter – soaking in the hot tub, with snow-covered trees all around, the starry sky with the constant, soft hum of Newark-bound airplanes emerging from the ocean. I sip from a glass of brandy. The glass is almost frozen. The liquid remains fluid and pleasantly burning. I close my eyes.

Heidi arrives from the house, removes her bathing robe, and lowers herself into the water. She watches as I take another quick sip, "What are you thinking about?"

"The usual, you know, the hospital, the department."

"You are obsessed. You come home and sit at your computer, then you eat your dinner, and all you talk about is Mantzur, Sorkhi, and Wise and… who's the fat one again?"

"Zalzer."

"Whatever. And after dinner, you go back to the computer, and now you think about the same crap. It's not healthy."

"What do you want me to think about?"

"I don't know. Rub my foot. I hurt it at the gym today."

"Okay, where is it?" I feel for her foot in the dark water. "I wonder how I can liquidate those bastards? They are much too powerful to be eliminated through conventional, civilized channels. Now, with Wise romancing them, they are untouchable. I have only one remaining option. I have to report them to the State."

Heidi bolts upright, creating waves in the small tub. "You are going to report nobody. They will destroy you!"

"I could do it anonymously. The New York State Department of Health encourages complaints from anybody with valid or invalid criticisms or complaints. Remember that case of mine from two years ago? When I performed a colostomy on the wrong loop of the bowel… on that black woman with advanced cancer? The poor woman died. What an awful disaster! I had to appear before the OPMC. I never learned who reported me."

"You know, I forget all these acronyms. What is the OPMC?"

"The Office of Professional Medical Conduct — or, I suppose, it should be called medical misconduct. I was lucky. I was only admonished. It could have been much worse. Anyway, I could report the bastards, both Mantzur and Sorkhi. It would trigger an investigation. They'd relish landing two big fish simultaneously."

"What about Wise?"

"That is the problem. Wise would welcome the downfall of Sorkhi, but he has a soft spot for Mantzur. I don't know why. Perhaps he senses the growing friendship with that old fart is the secret to his survival. My action could start a domino effect. If they find out that Mantzur is a bad boy, they could ask why Wise did not control him. A journalist writing for a newspaper or magazine is another possibility, for example, Jennifer, that lady who writes about health issues for *The New York Times*. You saw her articles, eh? But that might create more problems."

"Absolutely. Never trust a journalist. Once you start with them, your case is their story. The more you suffer, the more they thrive. They are whores. Remember what happened in Haifa?"

"What's new, Heidi? Quite a few professionals are whores to some extent."

Heidi's usual soft manner adopts a hint of anger: "I won't tell you what to do," she snaps. "But before committing yourself to any crazy move, understand that we cannot survive without your salary. I pay the bills, and I know. We've been through this before. Don't do anything without Wise. He is not an angel. Nobody is. But he likes you, and he is on your side. Get that into your head."

Heidi climbs out of the water and shuffles toward the house. I empty the last drop of the brandy, wishing for more. *Perhaps she's right*. Take Wise, for example. He is making big bucks. Nobody knows his financial arrangements, but cautious estimates are that he rakes in up to a million a year. On the surface, his residency program runs smoothly and is developing some reputation reflected by a better quality of candidates applying each year. I am sure that Wise likes me in some fatherly way. He respects me and perhaps is even proud to have me around him. Sure, he needs me for the residency and enjoys boasting about his growing list of published books. But what about hospital politics? He knows that I am controversial and physically unable to keep my mouth shut. He also knows I depend on him and am still awaiting a full professorship. I am a newcomer to the US, with house payments eating into my cash flow. I could apply for another job, but even then, I would need the unequivocal support of the Chairman as a credible reference. On the other hand, he knows I have the 'lists.' Wise is shrewd, no doubt about that. He can afford to be — with his contract, it would cost the hospital a couple of million to dispose of him. Not likely.

And me? I am on three months' notice. Heidi is right…

* * * *

Summer 1999. I find Wise in his office, deeply immersed in several open texts on his desk. It is Thursday, and he is preparing for the Friday morning professorial rounds with the residents. Wise is an excellent teacher; his excellence comes through systematic and thorough preparation. "Good morning, Dr. Wise. You wanted to see me?"

"Yes, Moshe. Sit down." He motions me to a chair opposite his desk. "As a matter of fact, I was looking at these books, searching for guidelines, whether mesh should be used to repair hernias in the presence of contamination, but I can't find anything decisive."

"Textbooks tend to be hazy about such matters."

"Shouldn't we include this controversy in our next volume?"

"We could, why not? A great idea." An awkward silence follows. "You know that I am going to the State — the OPMC (Office of Professional Medical Conduct), today in the afternoon. I have been invited to discuss anonymous complaints submitted to the OPMC against Mantzur. Yesterday I went to Mantzur's office and told him that the OPMC had invited me to discuss his cases. I assured him that I was on his side." Only I know who that anonymous source was.

Wise fidgets with his red silk tie, well matched with the white shirt and the dark blue blazer. "Yes. Mantzur told me about your visit. You did well, Moshe. Perhaps you will become a politician one day."

"I'm learning from you, Dr. Wise." He likes to be flattered. He hasn't realized that I am learning to manipulate people, too. Or maybe that's what he means.

"Moshe, I was thinking a bit about this. Sorkhi is a big problem. One cannot reason with him. He constantly parades across the hospital, threatening to get rid of all of us. We have to do something about this, and I was thinking that perhaps you…"

"Dr. Wise, do you want me to take Sorkhi's folder with me to the OPMC?"

"No, no, no. Don't do that! Please let me finish. You know that he and I share the bariatric clinic. Did you notice that the number of gastroplasties I did last month was almost zero while Sorkhi does them like crazy, three or four a week?"

"Of course. He is stealing your patients. Didn't you know that he controls the whole hospital?" *He wakes up only if his interests are at stake.*

"Moshe, I haven't decided yet what to do about him, but let us keep all options open. When you meet today with that guy at the OPMC, why don't you ask him… why don't you — you know what — tell him that we have this small problem with one of our leading local private surgeons. Tell him what the problem is. You do not have to be specific, you know. Ask his advice on what should be done or could be done. Do you understand what I mean?"

"Absolutely." Until now, Sorkhi had been 'murdering' patients, but bringing him to justice seemed to be a crazy idea to Wise. And now, approaching the State about Sorkhi would be okay because Wise's pride and personal well-being had been disturbed. Mantzur is still useful to Wise, so he can continue his rampage as he sees fit.

I head to my office and gather a few documents into my briefcase. I replace the white coat with a blue blazer and walk out of the hospital towards the subway station.

* * * * *

The steamy Manhattan daylight strikes me when I climb out of the humid subway station on 34th Street, soaked in sweat. The contrast between this street and the one I left in Brooklyn twenty minutes ago always amazes me. I buy a water bottle from a street vendor and proceed towards 5 Penn Plaza. The OPMC offices are on the sixth floor. The elevator opens to a spacious waiting room.

"Dr. Schein?" A white-haired man in a plain gray suit calls me from the door. "I am Dr. Carducci. Please come in." He shakes my hand vigorously — an honest handshake. We enter a large meeting room; behind a long table stands a woman. "This is Mrs. Thompson. She will be present during the interview."

We sit down, and Carducci starts. His voice is deep and warm, tainted with a Staten Island Italian accent. "Dr. Schein, you know why you are here. It may take a few hours. To start with, here, take this form and read it." It reads:

> "Complaints: OPMC receives complaints from various sources: patients, family members, friends, other healthcare professionals, hospitals, medical societies, government agencies, and out-of-state agencies. Every complaint is investigated.
>
> "Investigation: some complaints are dismissed due to lack of jurisdiction. Others are resolved by OPMC staff. Some are administratively closed after an investigation fails to find evidence to support a charge of misconduct. Some are referred, after thorough investigation to an investigative committee of the Board for Professional Medical Conduct."

I skim through the rest of the document. "Okay, I am familiar with all of this."

"Very well then." He removes his reading glasses, "Let me introduce myself to you properly. I'm a medical coordinator of the investigation committee that will assess Dr. Mantzur's case. As stated in the form in your hands, this committee will examine all the evidence. We will then have a few options, ranging from dismissal to a hearing referral. We could also recommend to the State Commissioner of Health to summarily suspend the physician's license."

"That is extremely rare, eh?"

"Correct. This occurs very rarely, indeed. The offending physician has to literally rape the patient or execute him. This has to be clearly evident, of course. The OPMC cannot risk any counter-litigation from the accused physician."

"I understand."

It is much easier for a surgeon to kill a patient than for someone to prove it was a killing.

"By the way," continues Carducci. "I am a retired surgeon so you can talk with me surgeon to surgeon, okay?"

"May I ask why me? Why did you invite me and not the others?"

"Dr. Glass — your friend? He gave us this list that I believe has been prepared by you. A very detailed list. Congratulations. It saves us a lot of homework." He places a copy of my Mantzur's list of complications on the table.

Over the next half hour, Carducci questions me about the structure of our department, who is doing what, and who is friendly with whom. "You have to understand," he explains, "that we are cautious not to be involved in personal vendettas between physicians. Your friend Glass, for example, is a vascular surgeon like Mantzur. They must be competing for referrals and patients. Therefore, we evaluated his complaint very cautiously. Your list, which he provided us, impressed us, however. Here's a copy."

"I know this list by heart," I respond. "Did you notice the ongoing reckless pattern? The guy operates on anything he can lay his hands on. Did you see the results?" *Be cool. Don't give the impression that you hate the man. Be academic and detached.*

Carducci listens patiently as if he has the whole day for me, which is probably the case.

"Moshe, please understand something. We cannot talk about patterns. Yes, your list is long, and if we go back another five years, we could find another fifty similar cases. He has been doing this since he started practicing. I know these characters. I was a chairman myself. Going over each case and studying the pattern is beyond our means regarding time and resources. It would be an expensive process, which the State cannot afford. You have to select the worst ten to twelve cases. Take this red pen and circle what you think are the most terrible cases — they will become our focus of investigation."

I study the list, holding the red marker in my hand. It is easy. I talk as I highlight the most nightmarish cases. "Eighty-five years old, asymptomatic carotid stenosis, a technical mishap during endarterectomy. He tied the artery, which is unheard of! The patient stroked out and died. A tiny aortic aneurysm with prohibitive risk factors, no indication for operation, death. Another asymptomatic carotid was in a patient who couldn't swallow because of an undiagnosed esophageal carcinoma. Death. Distal arterial bypass, horrendous graft infection, failure to manage appropriately, death. Diagnostic thoracotomy in a patient with brain metastases. Death."

I look up at Carducci to see whether he is as horrified as I was. He shakes his head solemnly. "Please continue."

"One more carotid in a terminal Alzheimer patient. Death. Thoracotomy for an unresectable cancer. Death. Esophagectomy and radical nephrectomy for advanced esophageal cancer and small renal cancer — why the nephrectomy? Mortality, of course. Another aortic aneurysm — intra-operative urokinase infusion, bled to death — can you believe it, injecting a thrombolytic agent during such an operation? Distal splenorenal shunt on an advanced cirrhotic, technical mishap. He had never done such a case before and did not know where to place the shunt. Death. Bilateral, staged, axillary-femoral bypass, unnecessary on one side, bled to death from an anastomosis on the unnecessary side." I pause to take a sip of water. "Do you see the pattern? The wild negligence?"

Carducci nods. "Leave the pattern alone. Please go on."

I highlight the twelfth case and hand him the list. "I hope that this will remain confidential. Everybody knows that I was called to see you. Perhaps you could also interview a few of my colleagues. A smoke screen?"

"Whom should I see?"

I mention a few names.

"Will they talk?"

"I think they will. They know Mantzur well and are abhorred by his practice."

"We will have to invite the Chairman, of course."

"Dr. Wise asked me to talk with you about another confidential matter."

Carducci is beginning to show signs of impatience. "This is all confidential. What does he want?"

"This does not concern Mantzur. It is another matter I prefer to talk about only with you." I look at Mrs. Thompson, who remains expressionless.

"Let's finish with Mantzur. We need your help. We are still waiting for Mantzur's charts and X-rays."

"They're locked in his office. He is working on them."

"They are all the same," Carducci sighs, crashing back in his seat and removing his thick glasses only to toss them on the desk. "They're always trying to add notes, delete data, and tamper with evidence. Do you have access to the departmental M&M summaries?"

"Of course. It is filed."

"You have the list of the twelve cases, then. Please send us anything you have about them."

"Sure. What happens next?"

"First, we have to gather all the evidence. It takes time. The hospital could be more helpful. Then we will send the evidence to external experts, according to the individual case, be it vascular, general or thoracic."

"Who are those experts? Are they independent, objective?"

"Yes. We use out-of-town surgeons. We pay them to review the cases. It is an expensive process, as I said."

"And then what?"

"The experts will decide with me whether or not this deserves a hearing. A hearing is like a court case, with a judge and lawyers on both sides."

"What could be the end result of a hearing?"

"There are a few possible outcomes. A reprimand, or administrative warning, is the mildest form of discipline. Then there is probation, and there could be actual license suspension — from a few days to six months or longer. The most severe form of discipline is a permanent license revocation, which the physician may contest or accept. Of course, a physician who wishes to save himself the expenses and humiliation by public disclosure may voluntarily surrender his license."

"What do you predict will be Mantzur's fate?"

"This is unpredictable. I guess he'll be referred to a hearing and I've told you about the possible outcomes. How old is he?"

"Almost seventy."

"Impaired a bit?"

"He may be impaired now, but he was doing the same things years ago."

"I guess we'll offer him the last option — surrendering his license. It could save him a lot of money with the outrageous fees lawyers charge." Carducci looks at his watch. "You wanted to tell me something else?" He nods to Mrs. Thompson as a hint to leave the room. "What's Wise up to? What does he want?"

I tell him about Sorkhi and his practice and provide him with a copy of my Sorkhi's list. I describe the association between Sorkhi and Mantzur and their brethren. "They are the President and Vice President of a Medical Board in a large New York Hospital," I conclude.

"I read in *The New York Times* that your hospital was named one of the top ten hospitals in the city," Carducci says. "Tell me. That Wise, wasn't he at the Jewish Island Hospital before?"

"Yes, he was."

"Didn't he receive millions for leaving?"

"Yes, he did."

"Correct me if I am wrong, but according to what I hear from you, Wise wants us to persecute Sorkhi but is friendly with Mantzur, and more than that — he made him a vice chairman."

"There is a special bond between the two of them. I do not understand why."

"This doesn't sound kosher to me. Your distinguished Chairman wants to destroy Sorkhi and spare Mantzur, eh?"

It is late afternoon when I emerge from the building and join the crowd of people rushing to get home. I feel good. I had crossed the river. I had blown the whistle on the 'terminators.' To celebrate the occasion, I treat myself to a small glass of draught beer at one of the Irish pubs on the way to the subway station.

Five p.m. I emerge from the Fourth Avenue station in Brooklyn. At this time of the day, Park Slope, revived by the yuppies returning from across the East River, looks like Manhattan. I pass through the emergency room to assess a patient with an acute abdomen. I tell the resident to book her for the OR and go up to my office. David Jacobs, one of our interns, comes towards me.

"Dr. Schein, I was looking for you." He seems a bit upset. "Could we talk in your room?"

I close the door behind us. "What's the matter?"

"I just finished a case with Sorkhi. He performed a lumpectomy on a nine-year-old girl."

"What? You must be kidding." I had had enough of Sorkhi and Mantzur today, but I can't ignore this. "You're not talking about a breast lumpectomy?"

"Listen," Dave says seriously. "There was this nine-year-old girl, apparently a daughter of Sorkhi's secretary, the blonde woman from the Medical Board. I had to assist Sorkhi. When I entered the room, the girl was asleep. Even under the drapes, I noticed that the chest wall and breasts belonged to a child. So I asked Sorkhi, like: 'What are you doing?' and 'How old is this child?'

"He said, like, 'She is nine and has a breast lump. We have to remove it to exclude cancer.' I told him that the likelihood of cancer at that age is negligible. He said the girl's mother — his secretary — drives him crazy. He then made an incision and grabbed the lump with a Kocher clamp. I think it was the girl's breast bud, the tissue from which the breast would grow. He took the knife and was ready to chop it off, but I stopped him. I said, 'Hey, Dr. Sorkhi, why not only take a portion for biopsy?' He said, 'Okay,' and removed half of the bud."

I am busy changing into my scrubs. I have a case in a few minutes. "Dave, the man is crazy. He cuts half of this poor girl's normal breast. He may have disfigured her forever. You saved her half a breast, maybe. Congratulations!" I slap him on the shoulder. "The man is fucking mad, manic, and almost unstoppable. There's only one way to end his stranglehold on this hospital."

"I trust you know the way?" he asks cautiously.

* * * * *

Forty-five

Brooklyn — the going gets tough

The State investigation of Drs. Sorkhi and Mantzur spilled well into 2000 and continued for over a year. They hired expensive lawyers, manipulated, and procrastinated, but at the same time, stupidly continued to damage patients, events that I immediately reported to Dr. Carducci — thus tightening the noose around their necks.

Meanwhile, Dr. Wise was under immense pressure to abort the case against the two surgeons — which he obviously could not do. Simultaneously, our caseload continued plummeting as the Department of Medicine had been pressured not to refer any patients to us. The emergency room had similar directions. But the primary efforts of the Iranian mafia and their collaborators at all hospital levels were concentrated against me — calling on Wise to eliminate the 'virus' that had contaminated the hospital and altered the long prevailing status quo.

March 2000. The Chairman's room. Wise picks up a document and says: "As a matter of fact, this is very serious. Let me read you from a letter I was handed by Dr. Statinsky just a few minutes ago." (Statinsky, an aging Jew, was the hospital's Director of Medical Affairs, second in command after the CEO.) Wise reads from the letter in a flat tone devoid of emotion: '"We have defined a need to develop a trauma center… we have urged you to proceed in a concerted, timely effort to recruit the surgical team that will be needed for this program… as previously discussed, we are quite concerned with the current economic status of the Methodist Hospital and find it necessary to make staff reductions to decrease our expenses. Reductions in personnel have already occurred in management and non-management positions. Unfortunately, we have concluded that our physician organization must also be reduced and that Dr. M. Schein's position will be terminated on July 1, 2000. Similar reductions in salaried physician staffing are currently planned in the hospital for this summer. Kindly inform Dr. Schein of our intentions.'"

Wise puts the letter down and studies me.

"I was waiting to see this," I say.

I have only three months left. I have miscalculated. I did not believe they would dare to fire me. Where exactly did Wise stand? Is he playing their game now, trying to save his butt? I have to start looking for a new job ASAP. What will Heidi say?

I stand up to leave, but Wise calls me to stay. "Moshe, Moshe," he's trying to comfort me, "in these places, a person is considered fired only if he does not arrive at work the day that follows the day of termination. You know I will not allow this to happen. Let us continue functioning as if nothing happened."

* * * * *

In the afternoon, I see Mantzur shuffling along in his scrubs. He looks pale, unshaven, exhausted. A few minutes later, I learned why. While operating on yet another asymptomatic carotid stenosis, the endarterectomy thrombosed in the recovery room. The patient became aphasic. Disaster follows a disaster. What is the difference between him and Dr. Harold Shipman, the British country doctor, a mass killer of older women? Or the notorious Dr. Michael Swango, the good-looking doctor from the Midwest who got his 'high' from poisoning patients? A few of our residents call Mantzur Dr. Kevorkian behind his back. But Kevorkian did what he did out of compassion for dying patients. Mantzur is not another Kevorkian. Looking today at the Padrino's drained face, I feel sympathetic towards him. Is this how one loses hatred and contempt against a defeated enemy? *But is he defeated?* Time to call Dr. Carducci.

"Dr. Carducci, our friend Mantzur continues to eliminate a patient per week. Last week, he excised the hemorrhoids of a patient who then bled to death from the colon above. Two weeks ago, he sat on a patient with a huge leaking aortic aneurysm for two days. The guy had excruciating back pain, but Mantzur decided to schedule it on his elective operative list. The patient decided not to wait. His aneurysm ruptured, and he died. Dr. Carducci, are you there?"

"Yes, I'm listening."

"You want more? Three weeks ago, he performed an elective arterial bypass on a terminal cirrhotic patient — tense ascites, jaundice — he could not survive the anesthesia."

I sense Carducci's voice softening. "The reports from the external reviewers about Mantzur finally arrived. Tomorrow, we'll meet to decide whether to continue with the hearings."

"Why don't you suspend his license immediately?"

"The cases are not so clear as you indicate. Most patients were old and sick anyway. It is not like an operation on the wrong side of the brain."

"Come on, Dr. Carducci," I interrupt, "what about his impairment, that ninety percent of his cases are presented at the M&M meetings?"

"Your friend Wise has to stop him. He is the Chairman. Unfortunately, he is defending him instead."

"Wise can't do anything. Sorkhi obstructs him. Dr. Carducci, you have been in this business for a long time now. What do you predict will happen to them? I have to know."

"They will both lose their license. Give me another six months."

"This is what you told me more than a year ago. Did you know that I have been fired?"

Silence. And then, "No. Who did it?"

"The CEO and Statinsky, the medical director. They obey Sorkhi."

Silence. Then: "Just hang in there, okay?"

"I'm trying."

Six months. A patient per week could perish at the rate Mantzur was going now. Twenty-four more deaths rested in the hands of the OPMC.

A month later, Wise managed somehow to convince the management to rescind their letter of my termination. I knew, however, that this was a temporary measure.

* * * * *

The final, face-to-face standoff between Sorkhi and myself — it had been simmering now for three years — had to take place eventually. Until now, despite the mortal enmity existing between us, we had avoided a frontal clash. At the Morbidity & Mortality meetings, we engaged in a seemingly civilized discourse through the Chairperson. At social departmental gatherings and dinners, we would share a shot of vodka and a coarse laugh — obeying the oriental rule of laughing cordially in the face of your enemy. The stab in the back would come later. Now the two gladiators were under pressure: I was threatened by losing my job; he was under the State's investigation…

The hospital's auditorium. Tuesday's Morbidity & Mortality meeting. I don't know what motivates me to sit so far back, just behind Sorkhi. He notices me and seems to be covering up his nervousness by joking and laughing loudly with Radmunsen, the big pink Swedish neurosurgeon. *What's he doing here?* Sorkhi is probably thinking. *He never sits at the back. What's he up to?* I see Dr. Wise entering the auditorium and sitting in the front row. For some reason, he decided not to chair the meeting today. Why?

The third case presented by Jim Adams, our fourth-year resident, is a classical case in Sorkhi mode. Jim reads from the handout. "Mrs. S.H., eighty-nine years old, was admitted for poorly controlled diabetes, severe respiratory and cardiac failure, and arrhythmias. On admission, she was disoriented…"

"Zalzer's patient, a bedridden wreck," whispers a junior resident in my ear.

"On hospital day fourteen," Adams continues in a monotone voice, "due to the inability of the patient to tolerate any oral intake, she was scheduled for a percutaneous gastrostomy by the gastroenterological service. Seven minutes into the procedure, it had to be terminated due to desaturation to seventy-eight percent and an arrhythmia." Adams pauses as if waiting to be asked a guiding question by Dr. Bachus, our intensive care unit's director, who is chairing the meeting today. None arrives, so he continues: "The medical attending then requested an open gastrostomy. Four days later, the patient was cleared for the procedure by the primary medical attending, pulmonary attending, and cardiology attending."

"What type of anesthesia was given?" asks Bachus.

"Epidural. The open gastrostomy was performed without difficulty. The patient was transferred to the recovery room and then discharged to the floor with a PCO_2 of sixty and O_2 saturation of ninety-two percent. Two hours later, a resident was called because the monitor had no tracing. She was found unresponsive and in asystole."

"What was her arterial blood gas before the operation?" asks Bachus, not looking up from the handout.

"O_2 saturation was ninety-five percent, PCO_2 was eighty-two."

Clearly, she was in respiratory failure when taken for this elective — and unnecessary — procedure. Let's see who'll dare to say anything.

Deep silence. Bachus looks around. "Dr. Wise, any comments?"

The Chairman stands up and clears his throat. "In general, I don't have an issue with the indication for gastrostomy in this case. But the timing was wrong. Gastrostomy is, at best, a semi-elective procedure. This patient was not in the best condition to undergo the procedure. I would have wanted to prepare her for the operation, to improve her respiratory status. Meanwhile, I would have fed her via an alternative route — a nasogastric tube, for example."

"Any further comments?" asks Bachus. "Anyone? Dr. Rubinstein?"

The retired Rubinstein is afraid of nobody. His words are clear to everyone: "I don't know what the hurry was. Why not feed her intravenously or place a feeding NG tube? It was the wrong time to operate. Gastrostomy was unnecessary — not in a septic patient in respiratory failure."

"A nasogastric tube could not be passed. She had a large tongue!" exclaims Sorkhi.

Rubinstein raises his voice again. "Nonsense. If you can pass a scope, you can pass a tube."

"Dr. Rubinstein, why don't you switch on your hearing aid? I told you the NG tube would not go down."

Rubinstein is obstinate yet again. "I do not accept this."

Sorkhi looks around. "You can accept it or not but I'm telling you that this poor patient needed the gastrostomy to provide her with drugs, antibiotics, and nutrition."

"Dr. Sorkhi," says Rubinstein. "You could have placed a soft, tiny feeding tube with an endoscope. You could have fed her via this tube and given her antibiotics."

"Three attending physicians cleared this patient for surgery, and you tell us that she was not ready. Why didn't you invite the gastroenterologist to this meeting? He'll tell you that endoscopy would have been difficult. And where is the anesthetist who agreed to the operation?" Everyone can now hear the anger in Sorkhi's voice.

Reflectively, I stand up, walk to the aisle, and raise my hand. Bachus ignores me, mumbling the closing words. I approach Sorkhi until I am two feet from him. Then I speak up: "I have two questions for Dr. Sorkhi. First, I want to know how the patient was fed during the fourteen days in the hospital before the operation? I see here that her pre-operative albumin was 3.9g/dL. She was not malnourished. And second, Dr. Sorkhi, why do you habitually operate on patients who are busy dying?"

Silence descends yet again. "Dr. Schein, would you please repeat the last question?" says Bachus.

"I asked Dr. Sorkhi why he habitually operates on patients who have already died. We know that this is not the first case."

Sorkhi shouts: "I don't agree to discuss this case further. This was not my case. I was asked to do a gastrostomy, and I did. We need to have the anesthetists and referring physicians here to discuss it properly!"

"Why do you always blame others?" I inquire loudly. "You were the surgeon. It was your responsibility. This is not the first time that you have inserted gastrostomies in dead patients," I say.

We are so near each other — I am ready for a fistfight. Almost five years ago, when we first met in this auditorium, I knew that I had met my archenemy, my moral antidote. My nemesis. Now, our mutual loathing explodes. Sorkhi points at me and then points his index finger at his brain. "He is crazy, absolutely crazy." He stands up and raises his hands, gesturing at his friends. Then, he walks toward the doors of the auditorium.

"Why can't you have an open academic discussion for once?" I shout at his back. "I asked you a question! Answer it. Tell us why you operated on this dead patient?"

Sorkhi's face twists with contempt. "Ha!" he laughs. "An academician is what you are. An A-C-A-D-E-M-I-C-I-A-N." At the door, he turns and spits out: "Why don't you report me to the State, also for this case?"

I take a deep breath. Finally, I have accused him of murder in public. I see that the meeting has been disrupted with surgeons standing in small groups and discussing the events. I hear a voice saying: "This is unacceptable. This is not how to address a colleague at the M&M meeting." Wise exits the auditorium without looking at me.

I find them all in Wise's office a bit later. Wise attacks me as soon as I enter. "Why? Why? Why did you do it? This was a grave mistake!"

I shrug. "Well, he operates on dead patients, no? So I asked him why. Big deal. What's the problem?"

"No, no, no!" his voice is rising, "This is a big problem, Schein. I can't protect you if you continue this way. I saved you once. I made them rescind your termination, but I won't be able to do it again. You can't be emotional at the M&M meeting. Scientific — yes, emotional — no!"

"Dr. Wise," I exclaim, "I can't be emotional? I have to get permission from the Chairman to be human? Please forgive me, but I suffer from an unfortunate psychological disturbance. I become emotional when observing how patients are being killed at a rate greater than one per week."

"Jim," Wise urges. "Talk to him, explain to him. Make him understand."

"Moshe, the private surgeons are very upset," Rucinski says, "forget about Sorkhi's friends. The private guys are afraid of you. Each of them has a few skeletons in their closet. As they watched you attacking Sorkhi, each of them was thinking: this is not unusual, I did a few gastrostomies on dying patients. Everybody does. They think you are crazy, that after you 'do' Sorkhi you may turn your fury on them. So now they are definitely against you. They wish you would leave this hospital. You are a threat to them."

"Jim's absolutely right. While the OPMC is dealing with Sorkhi you grant him an aura of martyrdom. A grave error," says Wise.

I see I had exhausted my usefulness to him in the depth of Wise's blank eyes. More than that, I am a burden. Each of us has a role in Wise's puppet theatre. My task was to liquidate Sorkhi, and spare Mantzur. But my fire is now consuming Mantzur. It seems to have threatened too many bystanders. It has become so uncontrolled that it may even endanger the boss himself. My role as Wise's marionette is over.

Back in my office, I change to scrubs and climb into my white Swedish OR clogs. As always, my father looks at me from his black and white portrait on the wall: in a white coat over a white shirt and a dark, striped necktie — a burning cigarette in his right hand, the smoke ascending to his face, causing his left eye to squint. Why can't he provide me with any advice?

* * * * *

My father's portrait on the wall.

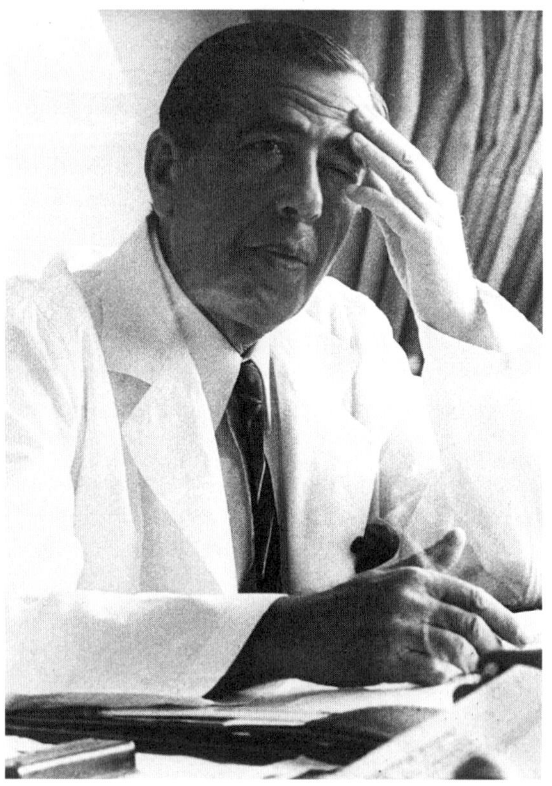

Forty-six

Wheels of justice

Spring 2001. The struggle had reached its summit. While trying to destroy each other, both sides were shedding thousands of dollars to top lawyers. I paid my Manhattan 'shark' $400 per hour, realizing that I might be left without income tomorrow. I gathered that my chances to negotiate even a silver parachute were grim without a powerful lawyer.

"Dr. Schein, how nice of you to come up." Behind his immense desk, the CEO's gigantic stature shrinks to an average size. I look around his huge office; it is much bigger than Statinsky's, a floor below, larger than Wise's, three floors down. I notice golf trophies and group pictures on all the walls.

"You are a golfer, Mr. Musk?"

"Since my thirties. The best anti-stress remedy one can find." He smiles at me. "You should start now. Never too late."

The CEO leans across the desk. "What's up? What do we need to discuss?"

"Well," I begin. "As you know, I am the problem-maker, the 'virus,' some call me." I use fingers on both hands to emphasize the quotations. "If this is the case, I thought perhaps I might be leaving. Do you remember what I said the last time you offered me a deal? You never came back to me."

"Dr. Wise tells me Dr. Gerst at the Bronx-Lebanon Hospital wants you badly. I know that Dr. Wise has highly recommended you to him."

"Oh, sure. Dr. Wise wants to get rid of me. Another reason to leave."

"What better way to get a glowing recommendation." The CEO allows himself a throaty chuckle. "I thought you and Wise were buddies. Am I wrong?"

"We were at one time." I think.

Musk sighs. "So when do you want to leave? You don't want to hang around too long. You don't want to raise your flags, waiting for the outcome, do you?"

"No. I don't need to hang around. I know that Sorkhi will eventually collapse. Remember that it was Wise and myself who sold him to the State. I was the one who reported Mantzur. You must thank me for this, Mr. Musk. I did a great favor to you and the hospital."

The CEO grimaces but then appears to ignore my comment. "When are you thinking of leaving?"

"I don't know yet. I'm still negotiating a contract. June or July, I'll let you know."

"Great. I like your openness and decision to go to a hospital that needs you. It lacks the political background of this place, so you'll be more at home there. The Methodist is special, you know. There are a few problem surgeons everywhere. One must learn to live with it. Morals and ethics have no business in hospital surgical departments. Ten years ago, when I came here, I knew a hospital like this could grow or regress. So I pushed it up. I knew that wars such as we have now would be inevitable. People such as Sorkhi and Mantzur had arrived from far away. They trained locally to become the leading local professionals. Those were the people I had to work with, to rely on."

Musk looks at the ceiling and carries on as if talking to himself. "Yes, they became the local top surgeons. I knew there would be struggles when I brought people in such as Wise or yourself." Musk bends forward again. "I know Sorkhi has problems, but he's a good man and surgeon — he removed my gallbladder, you know? Yes, he made mistakes. He should have recognized that Wise is the Chairman and should have cooperated. Sorkhi has some problems with his judgment. We could have prevented the whole mess if he'd asked Wise for advice."

He looks at me, and I see a glimpse of kindness in his blue eyes. "And you, Dr. Schein, you were also mistaken. Yes," he reiterates. "Even you made mistakes. You had a point, but there was no need to take the dirty laundry outside. You could've come to me. I wish we'd had an open communication channel between us. It is sad to see how the OPMC treats this hospital. I was told that at Sorkhi's hearings, the prosecutor made fun of his referring physicians. There are seven hundred good doctors in this hospital — why blame them for the sins of a few."

"Look," he says with finality. "You can stop working now, and we'll pay you until July." His lecture was finished. Now, it was back to business.

"Mr. Musk, do you remember what I asked for?"

He looks at his notes. "Yes, we agree to vest your pension fund fully. You'll be able to take it with you." He scribbles this down.

"I would like severance pay equivalent to at least three years' salary."

Musk raises both hands in disgust. "An employee who resigns is not entitled to a severance fee. You know that."

"I do. But I'm not just an employee. I may decide not to leave on my own. I told Dr. Wise that it would be better if he fired me. I could sue him then."

"You don't want to sue him. It could take years."

"Of course, I don't want to sue him or anybody else. But I've worked here for five years, and all was not well… considering the amount of turbulence I've saved the hospital in the future by eliminating those two quacks, don't you understand why I feel I deserve the golden handshake?"

Musk smiles. "Dr. Schein, do you think I'm an heir to the Rothschilds? This is a non-profit city hospital in Brooklyn, New York. We do not have generous sums of money! Here's what I can do for you. Leave now, and we will pay you for the next six months with benefits."

Musk is waiting for my reply. My silence unnerves him. "OK, this is the final deal," he says. "You stay with us until the day you start in the Bronx. We will continue paying you a full salary for six months after you leave. It's a lot of money, you know. We never do such things and must not advertise it like the Firestone balloon."

I nod to indicate understanding but say nothing. Musk goes on. "So we have to draft a termination agreement."

"No, I'm not being terminated, I'm resigning."

"Whatever."

"I'll have to show it to my lawyer."

"Of course." He stands up and walks me to the door. A firm handshake. I know the CEO will immediately call Sorkhi to announce the big news. "Hey Mahmud," he'll say. "I got rid of Schein for you."

I descend the few floors to our department. Wise's office is open. I hear his secretary calling: "Dr. Wise, Mr. Musk for you on the phone."

I knew that my days at the Methodist Hospital were numbered. But before letting them pay me out, I wanted to secure the nails deep into the coffin of my enemies.

* * * * *

In the mid-morning hours, Times Square appeared surprisingly calm. I walked westward to the 43rd Street and entered the vast lobby of *The New York Times*. I picked up one of the black phones near the security desk and dialed Jennifer's extension. "Dr. Schein?" she said. "You're on time, let's meet at the cafeteria, my cubicle is too small. I will clear you with security. Please take the elevator to the seventh floor."

We met in a huge cafeteria. Journalists sat around in groups engaged in lively discussions. Jennifer seemed to be in her early thirties, with expensive Italian high-heeled shoes, a modest green patterned skirt, and a matching blazer. I was sure she was a New York Jewess — definitely upper middle class.

Ms. — or was she a Mrs? — Steinhauer pulled out a tiny notebook. "OK," she said. "Let's see what you've got. The issue is unnecessary operations, correct? Mainly in elderly patients? Right?"

I headed back towards the subway. Times Square swarmed with Japanese tourists hunting for lunch. The early spring breeze was mildly cool. My mood was elated. I felt unburdened as if things were finally rolling forward — as if the house of cards I had been trapped in for years was collapsing.

* * * * *

The bulky Saturday edition of *The New York Times* was delivered before 7 a.m., landing with a heavy thud at the doorstep. Heidi picked it up and sorted its multiple sections on the kitchen table. The expected article started on the front and continued in the Metro pages. We sipped from our coffee mugs and read:

> "May 5, 2001
> License of Prominent Doctor Suspended During Inquiry
> By Jennifer Steinhauer
> The New York State Commissioner of Health has suspended the license of the President of the Medical Board of New York Methodist Hospital in Brooklyn, calling the doctor, who has a large surgery practice there, a danger to patients… Dr. Sorkhi* is the latest, and most prominent, doctor to be brought up on charges of negligence at Methodist by the Health Department in recent years… Through the years, a variety of doctors have complained to hospital administrators about Dr. Sorkhi's surgical practice, but he has never been sanctioned by the hospital… One doctor, Moshe Schein, had complained repeatedly to the Chairman of Surgery at the hospital, Dr. Wise, and was fired last March. Dr. Schein was inexplicably rehired a few weeks later…"

The article mentioned that according to numerous sources, the tensions between Dr. Sorkhi and others in the surgical department intensified four years ago, after Dr. Wise recruited Dr. Schein and that a few physicians at the Methodist Hospital believed that Dr. Sorkhi had been undone by jealous rivals. It quoted an obstetrician who said that he had known Dr. Sorkhi for many years and "If any loved one in my family gets sick, I would trust him with my heart…"

"See what your beloved gynecologist says?" I teased Heidi. That gynecologist had been changing her uterine device each year; she used to chat with his wife at the gym.

* Name changed to a fictional name.

"What could he say? What do you expect him to say? He's scared, and he's Iranian as well. Yes, a Jew, but still Iranian. Perhaps he still has some family left behind in the old country. And why do they mention your name? I thought that she promised to leave you out of it," asked Heidi.

"She doesn't cite me. The quotes are all of the others. Whatever these reporters do, they try to seem objective and balanced."

We continued reading the article, that described that while in prior years some of the hospital doctors were sactioned by the State and retained, another prominent doctor under investigation had recently retired quietly.

"This is Mantzur," I said, "the old fox is smart. He knew when to take off his surgical gloves. He understands that he has lost the war. It seems that the Padrino will never decorate the pages of *The New York Times*."

We read on, that one surgeon who had been critical of Dr. Sorkhi said the whole affair "…is really too bad because the Methodist has a great spirit…"

"Yes, great spirit indeed." I sighed.

"And what now? What will Musk, Statinsky, and Wise do?"

"They'll just wait to see how things evolve. They call it "damage control" — waiting for things to cool off, hoping there will be nothing further in the papers about it — they know that papers turn yellow and people forget."

A few months later, I logged into: https://www.health.ny.gov/professionals/doctors/conduct/ and then I typed in Sorkhi's name in the search window:

> Action: License revocation
> Effective Date: October 12, 2001
> Nature of misconduct: The Hearing Committee sustained the charges finding the physician guilty of incompetence and negligence on more than one occasion; gross negligence; providing treatment which was not warranted by the patient's condition and failing to maintain accurate records.

Then I typed in Mantzur's name:

> Action: License limited precluding the practice of medicine
> Effective Date: September 26, 2001
> Nature of misconduct: The physician did not contest the charge of negligence on more than one occasion.

So the two guys were finished. Sorkhi was advised by his lawyers not to appeal. He left New York to practice in his 'old country.' He periodically visits his family, which continue to live on Staten Island. *The New York Times* published a brief statement about the verdicts and nothing more. After watching New York hospitals and keeping doctors and administrators on their toes, Jennifer Steinhauer was transferred from the newspaper's health desk. The newspaper did not bother to replace her.

* * * * *

At night, the lights of the southern tip of Manhattan slowly retracting, the stern of the Staten Island-bound ferry is perhaps the most glorious place in New York City. I breathed in with pleasure the smell of the sea, exposing my face to the cool breeze. I felt elated. The truth is that I was happy with myself. I wouldn't tell anyone, but I was rather proud. I did it — I managed to destroy the invincible mafia of the Methodist Hospital almost alone. Why did I do it? Certainly not for personal gain. I lost time, health, position and money; my family suffered the repercussions. Didn't I do it to let justice prevail? Wasn't that my prime motivation, to do the right thing? No. That's just a cliché. Maybe it was my kamikaze reflex, the tendency to take risks. Others call it courage. I don't know.

That is what I wrote then. But today, looking back at those years at the Methodist Hospital, I do not miss it at all. I feel so lucky and relieved that those angst-ridden years are behind me. In Brooklyn, I was under constant siege by the Iranian mafia. But now I also see their side: they probably feared my overt hostility and my role as Wise's attack dog.

After I left the Methodist Hospital, Wise, free from the opposition I had destroyed for him, continued to thrive, reigning over the department he continued to expand. During the American College of Surgery annual meetings, I would stumble across Wise every year or two. Initially, we used to greet each other, perhaps shake hands, and move on. As years passed, he would pretend not to see me.

I could guess what was in his mind: "I provided shelter for this immigrant, I harbored him when he had no visa, no license, no income, I made him a full professor, and look how he paid me back, publishing that book…" (*Life Means Nothing Behind the Green Wall*, which I published after leaving the Methodist Hospital, was not complimentary to Wise). Yet, in retrospect, Wise was the most enjoyable chairman I ever had — humane, highly intelligent, capable, and of an excellent sense of humor. But he wanted me to be absolutely loyal — to unleash me against his enemies but to be able to tell me whom to spare and when to stop.

I was not suitable for this task.

Some years ago, I met, incidentally, Wise's wife near the entrance to the Hilton Hotel in San Francisco. We hugged and kissed. "Oh Moshe, why did you leave my husband?" she asked.

"Laila," I replied, "I did not leave him. It was he who dumped me."

"No, no, no, he loved you so much."

In retrospect, each fact has a few alternative versions.

One remembers that freezing winter afternoon many years ago. We were having post-lunch drinks at Wise's Great Neck mansion, looking through the panoramic windows at the frozen, misty Long Island Sound. The house described by Scott Fitzgerald in *The Great Gatsby* was just beyond a curve in the shore. I was sipping Cointreau and listening to Wise's life story.

How the little Hungarian boy, László Weisz, had survived with his parents the deportations and the massacres of Budapest's Jews. How at the age of fifteen, he arrived alone in Australia; how, despite speaking little English, he talked his way into admission to a prestigious British-type boarding school in Sydney. I imagined the short, chubby boy with a thick Hungarian accent at a posh school — the abuse he probably suffered. It was a story of a *wunderkind*: medical school in Sydney, surgical training at premier English hospitals — under the most famous professors, a fellowship in Johns Hopkins, Baltimore, finally landing in a faculty position in the prestigious Barnes-Jewish Hospital in St. Louis. With his New York meteoric career, I was already familiar. How did he do it, I often asked myself — climbing to the top, academically, professionally, simultaneously becoming immensely rich. The short answer would be: his superb emotional intelligence. The boy who arrived in Australia must have been a charmer. He continued charming anyone on his road across the world and upwards. The only person he failed to charm was Mahmud Sorkhi. To overcome this obstacle, to take down Sorkhi, he had to charm me… and he did. Temporarily.

I can only guess how Wise maneuvered his way up to the top, but I saw how he maintained his status and influence. For example, he would invite a notable guest speaker to our weekly grand rounds each week. "Make a list," he would tell me. The list consisted of the "who's who" in American surgery — chairpersons, famous surgeons, editors of major texts; he did not object when I added to the list my own friends, even those from abroad. Who wouldn't accept a free flight to New York, a stay in a five-star hotel in Manhattan, a fancy dinner, transportation in a limousine, or in Wise's sports car du jour — if the guest was really important. All expenses were covered by our departmental academic funds, to which, we, the full-time surgeons, had to contribute a percentage of our private billing. Wise was exempt from such a contribution; he took home 100 percent of his private practice income. However, he controlled the funds.

With the notable guests, we would dine in New York's best restaurants — Wise knew them all. I used to observe how Wise played the host: down to earth, modest, friendly, but never servile. He would speak softly, limiting himself to small talk and letting the guest lead the conversation. That is how he was able to pick up the phone and call all those important people across the country asking for favors. "Leslie is speaking."

During the years with Wise, I tasted New York's high life. One remembers the steaks at Linger Longer, the Italian cuisine in old world establishments that probably do not exist anymore, the eighteen-year-old single malts at rooftop bars, the residents' graduation parties at the Ritz — mandatory tuxedo, limousines. How can one forget the departmental Christmas parties on the shores of Long Island, mountains of seafood, delicious pastas, and drinks flowing like water from the open bar? Drunk surgeons and wives dancing the *Macarena* — Sorkhi and co-mafiosi leading the pack. That was all alien to me, but I was drawn into it. I cannot claim that I did not enjoy it. However, after this was over, I did not miss it.

Once I signed a resignation agreement with the CEO, Wise started avoiding me, behaving like I didn't exist. Just before leaving the Methodist, I decided to use my travel funds to attend a surgical meeting in India. I booked the flights and hotels and submitted the usual request for reimbursement. "Dr. Wise is not going to approve your request," Wise's secretary announced. I intercepted Wise in the corridor that connected our offices. "Why don't you approve my request?" I asked. The Chairman walked on, ignoring me. "It's my money," I shouted behind his back, "I contributed tens of thousands to the department's funds. You contribute nothing." Wise stopped, turned around and said: "Just go. I do not want to see you here anymore. Stay at home." I do not remember what I screamed at Wise's back when the elevator swallowed him. Only that a minute later, the CEO came rushing down from the top floor. "What's the problem?" he inquired, "Why the shouting in the corridor? India? You want to go to India. Of course. You can go anywhere, why not Japan? Do not worry. Leslie will approve the funds."

That last direct encounter with my boss left a bitter taste. Message: be nice to the people you conquer, and try leaving a favorable last impression. Dr. Leslie Wise died in 2016 at the age of eighty-five. He was a wise man.

After departing the Methodist, I wrote a book about my experience with the Iranian mafia. Its title was *Life Means Nothing Behind the Green Wall*. The author was named Professor Z. It was a roman à clef. This is when I gained experience with literary agents, editors, and publishers. I realized that the literary world, and presumably readers, are more likely to appreciate books about bad politicians or lawyers rather than about charlatan doctors, killing surgeons, or medical malpractice. It seems that people like their doctors to be heroes, not monsters. They need to trust them in daily life as well as in books. After going through numerous agents and publishers, I self-published the book in 2003. Of the two thousand printed copies, more than a thousand were left unsold in boxes in the garage. It is still available on Amazon for 31 bucks.

How can I not mention Syed? Syed Gardezi (the character Salman Chaudri in my book) was a Pakistani surgeon, the son of a general, who had repeated his training (as most international medical graduates do) at the Methodist, under the leadership of Mantzur and Sorkhi, just before Wise took over the department. Syed was in his late thirties when I arrived on the scene. He was of medium height, moderately obese, light skinned, already balding. His manner was easygoing, his voice soft, the tone jocular and friendly. He lived close to us in Staten Island, so often we would commute together to Brooklyn, in his or my car. We would talk a lot during the long drives, early morning, late evening. He was a devoted Muslim but did not broadcast his beliefs. Somehow, we became friends. At the time of Dr. Wise's arrival, Syed was a fresh attending surgeon in private practice. Cunning as he was, Syed did not join his old teachers in their holy war against Wise. Surprisingly, the young Muslim declared an alliance with the new Jewish chairman. The latter, noting Syed's popularity among the various hospital communities and staff, gradually adopted him as his 'Rasputin' — the expert on hospital politics, the psychology of the 'opposition,' a spy and a key negotiator. Some say he was a double agent. If a single person had greatly benefited from the downfall of Sorkhi and Mantzur, it was Syed, who then became the busiest private surgeon at the Methodist. Following Wise's example, Syed lost interest in me once my role in the game ended. I recall meeting him once again — I think it was in the cafeteria of the convention center in Chicago. I saw him standing in the line with an empty food tray in his hands. "Hi, Syed," I approached him, "where do you want to sit? Let's eat together and chat." "Good to see you, Moshe. Sorry, but I can't. I'm with this bunch…" he pointed to the two girls behind him, probably surgical residents at the Methodist. I nodded.

Syed died suddenly in 2012 at the age of fifty-four. Surprisingly, the top-earning surgeon at the Methodist left behind heavy debts. His wife had to sell their New Jersey mansion and move out with their kids. Where did the money go? Muslim charities? Another woman or women? There are only rumors and guesses. At least, unlike Rasputin, he died of natural causes at home.

In the summer of 2001, I looked for the last time at the Statue of Liberty through my office window and left the Methodist Hospital. I do not remember being sorry or sad. In fact, I was happy with myself and elated, looking forward to the next job. The Bronx, here I come, I thought.

* * * * *

Syed Gardezi, RIP.

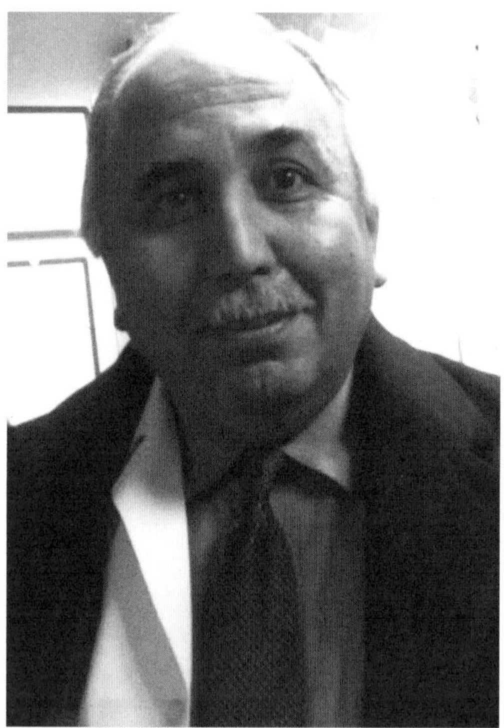

Forty-seven

The slums of the Bronx

September 11, 2001. We were eating breakfast with "Good Morning America" on TV. The sky was cloudless outside the window – a perfect early autumn Staten Island day. I emptied my coffee, grabbed my backpack, and walked towards the garage stairs when Heidi shouted from the kitchen: "Look, the Twin Towers are burning!" I turned back. We watched on the screen the smoking north tower, and a few minutes later, the airliner rammed into the south tower.

"I have to go," I said, "the hospital may be receiving casualties. Who knows how many there are."

My daily route to the Bronx-Lebanon Hospital would take me across Goethals Bridge to New Jersey, northbound on the Turnpike, over the George Washington Bridge into Manhattan, and finally into the chaotic, unbearable Cross Bronx Expressway. But that morning, I found the Goethals Bridge already closed by the police. I had to turn back, to be locked in on the island with its entire population for the few next days. At home, from the windows of the second floor, we could see the black smoke staining the otherwise blue sky over the southern tip of Manhattan. I felt numb to the ensuing pandemonium and public hysteria that affected the city and the nation; it happened only a few miles away but it felt like it could have occurred on the moon. It was a terrible tragedy and loss of life – against the perspective of history, this was like one or two trainloads transported to Auschwitz.

* * * * *

When I agreed to leave the Methodist Hospital, the only full-time position available for me in New York was at the Bronx-Lebanon Hospital. Here, the surgical Chairperson was Dr. Paul Gerst. The man, then in his mid-70s, had been running the department for thirty-seven years. He was a shrewd New York Jew who had noticed, early after moving to the Bronx from the Presbyterian Columbia University Hospital in Manhattan, where he practiced as a thoracic surgeon, that the only way to attract good-quality residents to an area infested with drugs, crime, and AIDS, was to import them from India. Thus, throughout his protracted rule, more than ninety percent of his surgical residents derived from India. Over the years, the entire faculty of the department (as well as the entire hospital) consisted of Indians who had graduated from the hospital's residency programs. The old Jew ruled 'his Indians' — whom he had selected, trained, and elevated — like a ruthless, harsh, but generous king. They, his Indians, worshiped him in return. Like sons would worship an aging, senile father. They willingly surrendered to his dictatorial rule — benefiting from his gradual decline — to gather a clinical monopoly and financial benefits for themselves. The old man had been smart enough to stop performing operations years ago, thus losing touch with modern clinical surgery. However, he insisted on running all clinical meetings, including the M&M meeting, like a Russian tsar.

The reason the old man wanted to recruit me to his homogenous department was stated to me at our first meeting. My interview with him was conducted in his disorganized, dusty, mildew-smelling room. "They are excellent surgeons," he was talking about his department's faculty. "I trained and re-retained the cream of India, but they are not interested in academia. They do not write. I need you for the residents, to teach and publish." He was sitting on a high, easy chair behind his desk. I was placed on a low, rickety chair at the room's far corner.

"And what will I be operating on?" I asked, "It appears all these guys here, physicians, oncologists, gastroenterologists, are Indians. They've known each other for many years. Why should they refer patients to me or anybody whose name does not start with Prasad or ends with Kumar?"

"Don't worry," said Dr. Gerst,"He did not seem to appreciate my sense of humor — later I found out that he had none whatsoever — "I will look after you!"

"Let me think it over," I said.

Noticing that I was not convinced, he promised: "I will open an additional general surgical service for you."

"But Dr. Gerst, I don't think…"

"Call me Paul," the old man interrupted, "you and I will be friends. Nothing of what happened to you in Brooklyn could repeat itself here. Please come and join me."

"I appreciate it very much. But please, I need to think about it."

"What was your base salary in Brooklyn? 275,000? We will start you at 325,000. In a year or two, you will make more than the others. Trust me." The old man was persistent.

I sensed the man was a harsh, ruthless, rigid autocrat, and that it would be impossible for me to tolerate his style for long. I knew that taking on this position would be like relocating from a fancy dump in Brooklyn to a rundown landfill site in the Bronx. However, the professional and financial guarantees were promising. Besides, I had no better immediate alternative — the severance agreement with the Methodist was ready to be signed. So, eventually, I accepted the offer. Hence, just after freeing myself from the Brooklyn Iranian medical 'mafia,' I got entangled with the Bronx medical Indian 'family' and an aging, paranoid boss, who eventually proved to be a relatively benign mixture of Professor Ferdinand Sauerbruch of Berlin and Joseph Stalin of you know from where.

* * * * *

The Bronx-Lebanon Hospital was wedged between the Cross-Bronx Expressway and the Grand Concourse. Its modern tower dominated the scruffy neighborhood, which was not grand anymore. The hospital's interior was shabby, and it took thirty minutes to reach the tower's upper floors in the overcrowded elevators. The hospital was founded at the end of the 19th century on the Grand Concourse; the latter modeled after the Champs-Élysées in Paris. It had served the middle classes that inhabited the solid apartment buildings lining the boulevard. But now nothing was left — not even the trees — of the old grandeur; only sealed synagogues with decaying Stars of David engraved on their walls told us that the previous inhabitants had moved to Long Island or New Jersey, and the neighborhood had become predominantly Spanish speaking — a 'little Dominican Republic.'

When I began my sojourn in the Bronx, I pledged to play it low key: be friendly, humble, and shut up. This was promoted by the dictator's welcome greeting: "Moshe, everybody knows about you. You have a bad reputation."

"Why?" I objected. "I didn't do anything wrong."

He ignored my comment. "Look, all I'm telling you is that our CEO has warned me that this hospital does not enjoy being featured in *The New York Times*. Nor would I tolerate…"

"So why did you hire me?"

"Because I figured out that I know how to control you."

To his credit, I have to admit that the older man really tried to be nice to me, so that I would warm towards him. But our styles, personalities, and *weltanschauung* were so divergent that all such attempts would prove futile. A month into my stay in his department, he invited me for a tête à tête dinner at a cozy Upper West Side French bistro. Here, with me sipping wine, he sticking to club soda, he opened up a little, telling me — prompted by my habitual curiosity — about his family tribulations and his rather sad and lonely existence as a widower. But the father-son-type atmosphere did not last long. Walking to our cars, he stopped and poked me with his thick index finger: "Moshe, I want you to remember this and never forget it – I'm the boss, I make all the decisions, I want to know about everything, and I know everything."

"Sure, sure Dr. Gerst, of course." But the coziness between us disappeared instantly, ruining my postprandial digestion.

"So when do I get my own service, like we agreed?" I asked.

"Not now, it'll have to wait. The others won't accept this." The 'others' were his Indian 'puppies' that naturally were not too keen to lose even a single hernia operation or a breast lumpectomy. The puppies had it well under the wings of their *pater familias*. In return for succumbing to his abuse during mind-numbing meetings, he granted them absolute clinical freedom and financial perks. They enjoyed the security of sizeable salaries and, at the same time, a thriving private practice. And this they tried to defend with their teeth: they knew that things might change when their guru and protector retired or was forced to leave.

Like the Iranian brethren in Brooklyn, the Indian puppies of the Bronx-Lebanon Hospital controlled the tributaries of referrals, which were coming from the gastrointestinal physicians – usually a brother-in-law, or a cousin; or from the oncologist – commonly one who had trained with them twenty-one years ago. Even when I was on emergency call, the 'money-making' cases, such as tracheotomies in Medicare patients, were shifted by the ICU Doc Patel, or Doc Kumar, to the puppies. But as my salary was reasonable, I decided to keep my mouth shut, to do what I was hired to do, and be happy with the sort of cases I had been used to getting in New York hitherto – emergency cases, mainly indigent, coming through the ER or the 'service clinic' – a bleak maze of smelly cubicles where impoverished patients were seen.

My first year in the Bronx was relatively calm. The commute took an average of an hour each way and occasionally turned into a nightmare on one of the bridges or at the tollgates to the Turnpike. *But this is New York, right? No need to complain.* Like all other surgeons' offices, my office was a converted flat in an old apartment building that now belonged to the hospital. In the summer, the ancient noisy AC hardly managed to cool the suffocating room; in winter, freezing wind blew through the cavity wall spaces. Intense aromas of Indian spices permeated the air from the apartments above us, where the residents and their extended families lived (commonly both husband and wife were residents, and the grandparents were imported from India to look after their children).

However, I was enjoying my time with the Indian residents. I found them bright, dedicated, and respectful. It was a second or even a third surgical residency for many of them, having completed residencies in India and the UK already. To the puppies, I smiled, and they smiled back; they had a reason to smile – they earned almost double of what I did. But the dictator was an ongoing irritating factor, and the natural course of events was downhill, heralded by multiple flare-ups.

At his weekly staff meetings, Dr. Gerst, a millionaire driving a 1970 Ford, clad in an ageless, eternal, fading, blue blazer, gray flannel trousers, and unpolished brown moccasins – with unkempt long white hair, constantly showering dandruff on the collar of his blazer – did not tolerate any deviation from the protocol.

And the protocol meant absolute attention to his chatter about irrelevant paramedical banalities. If one were to look away, stir in their seat, or look at a piece of paper, the dictator would be upset. The Indian puppies accepted this as a natural phenomenon: he had brought them from India to the promised land, and for this, they adored him, nourishing that kind of love-hate relationship one has with an older father. But I started to rebel, resulting in repetitive expulsions from the meeting, like the expulsion from the class of a misbehaving seven-year-old pupil: "Dr. Schein, you cannot read newspapers in my meeting, I do not want you here," the old man would roar.

At the American College of Surgery meeting in San Francisco in 2002, the aging leader hired – this was his habit each year – a posh restaurant to entertain the graduates ('our alumni') of his program, now dispersed throughout the country. We all sat around long tables, wives included (I did not bring mine), with the boss presiding over this family-like reunion. He made each of the alumni stand up and introduce themself. One after another, the distinguished graduates of the grand tyrant rose and uttered something like this: "I am Dr. Rashid Kumar (or Satish Patel). I graduated from the program in 1972 or 1982. Currently, I'm in general surgical practice in Orlando or Vegas. I'm very much into minimally invasive surgery doing hernias, Nissens, and..." Such statements were usually followed with a deep bow towards the eminent chairman: "Sir, I'm indebted to you for the excellent training. You were always an inspiration to me. Thank you very much, Sir."

It went on and on, speech after speech. My wine glass was empty. In desperation, I called a waiter to refill it. The observant leader noticed my aberrant movement and called me to order. My glass remained empty. After an hour, the appetizers arrived, immediately followed by a dish of overdone salmon. It provided an interlude of thirty minutes to sip some wine and chat with one's neighbors. But just as the entrée plates were being cleared, the dictator resumed the educational activities. Engaging specific persons in some irrelevant medical dialogue, he demanded that all fifty people around the table listen attentively and keep silent. He seemed to need absolute control of this social gathering, precisely like Stalin used to do each night at his Moscow dacha. I had had enough. I stood up and said: "Thanks, Dr. Gerst, for the excellent food and wine. But we are now in San Francisco, not at the hospital. I thought I was invited to a social function, not a structured CME activity."

I stormed out. None of the puppies around stirred in their seats or said a word. The residents gazed at their plates.

From then on, our relationship deteriorated rapidly. The dictator demanded the last word on the fate of all publications coming out of his department, including the list of authors of each manuscript. He instructed me to add surgeons (his 'boys') who had contributed nothing to the authors' list. "According to the Residency Review Committee," he said, "they must show significant academic activity; they need a few publications. Please do add Dr. Grishpatel as the second author." I refused. We stopped talking and communicated through memos.

However, not surprisingly, the main venue for confrontations was the M&M meeting, over which the old man had been fiercely presiding over the last thirty-five years. He continued doing so years after laying down (wisely) his knife.

Now, let me state that the Indian 'mafia' in the Bronx was surgically and intellectually more sophisticated than the Iranian one in Brooklyn. A few among them were solid ethical surgeons, but others were not. Like in Brooklyn, I saw old and terminal patients undergoing futile operations and younger non-terminal patients receiving death sentences for the wrong choice of operations and faulty treatment of complications.

Very rapidly, I noticed the pattern at the M&M meeting conducted by the dictator; there were a few rules: all operations are *indicated,* the terms 'non-indicated' or 'unnecessary operations' are taboo; the indication for an operation is not discussed because *apriori, all operations are necessary.* Furthermore, *all* deaths are *non-preventable* and always caused by *medical* complications or the natural course of events. So, for example, when discussing mortality in a terminal poorly nourished AIDS patient whose anastomosis had leaked after undergoing a gastrectomy, the emphasis was not on whether the operation was indicated or not but on whether the anastomosis ought to have been stapled or hand sutured. An analogy: a drunk driver runs over a pedestrian… the discussion hinges on whether he drove a Chevy or a Ford…

For almost six months, I suppressed my desire to comment. I buried my head between my hands and tried to control my blood pressure by taking deep breaths. But at one meeting, I broke down. I stood up and said: "In this unfortunate case, I found seven gross errors which led to the eventual mortality. First, the initial operation was wrong; second..."

The boss, sitting behind his desk on the podium, was thunderstruck. But he reacted rapidly: "Sit down, Dr. Schein. You can't talk here about errors. These are your colleagues. We do not commit errors."

"But this is an M&M meeting, right?"

"Sit down and be quiet. If you have anything meaningful to say, we'll listen to you. But we can't allow this meeting to become an accusation session about errors."

"Are you shutting me up, Dr. Gerst?"

"Sit down, Dr. Schein. Dr. Radinini, you are next. Please tell us how to mark the operative site to prevent operating on the wrong side."

It felt as if I was back in Brooklyn.

For the next couple of months, I avoided the M&M meeting or got my secretary to page me out whenever a 'problematic' case was to be presented. Then, a few weeks later, they presented a case of post-diagnostic laparoscopy pneumonia. Usually, they would run over such a case in one minute, finding no problems. But as I was there, I felt compelled to stop them. I had to stop them because the 'diagnostic laparoscopy' had been performed on a patient already diagnosed with multiple liver metastases deriving from a biopsy-proven rectal cancer.

"What was your indication to perform the laparoscopy?" I asked the Associate Chairman — the local self-appointed top knife. He was the most senior puppy, waiting to become the chairman once his master retired or died in his chair.

"Well, we needed to get histological confirmation. The oncologists wanted...," retorted the second-in-command unperturbedly.

"But you had a CT scan showing a Swiss cheese liver, ridden with tumors and histologically proven carcinoma of the rectum, so why torture this terminal patient with laparoscopy?"

"We have a residency program here. We have to provide the residents with laparoscopic exposure...," the deputy tried to explain.

"What? You performed a non-indicated operation in a terminal patient only to provide residents with experience?" I looked around and added: "This is not ethical."

It was too much. The dictator closed the meeting hastily. But from that day on, I stopped getting patients referred to me, even from the service clinic. The clinic doctors told me: "Dr. P. (the Associate Chairman) instructed us not to refer patients to you. It's nothing personal, but, you know, he may become our next chairman."

* * * * *

In the middle of my third year at the Bronx, the hospital's CEO announced that Dr. Gerst would step down "after a distinguished service of thirty-eight years." But the dictator, like a dying old lion, did not accept his fate. "I am going nowhere," he declared to his confused disciples — now bracing themselves for unpredictable changes — and barricaded himself in his shabby and dusty room, brooding on revenge.

The only successful item on his revenge list was aborting the transferal of my professorship from Cornell's College of Medicine to the Albert Einstein College of Medicine, with which the Bronx-Lebanon Hospital was affiliated. A month after receiving an invitation to a faculty meeting where new members were to be inaugurated, I got a laconic letter: "Your invitation has been cancelled." No explanation. But I immediately guessed who was behind it. I was left without an academic appointment and title.

Towards the end of 2003, Dr. Gerst vacated his office. One Saturday afternoon, when I was leaving the OR, I saw the old man shuffling around, carrying boxes to his car. By himself — alone. Where are his puppies now, I thought; why don't they help the poor bugger? I felt like approaching him, taking the load off his weak arms. But I knew he might spit at me — so deep was his misguided resentment.

Dr. Milton Gumbs, the hospital's vice president, a charming, patriarchal African American, a talented surgeon, was nominated as the acting director. For some reason, he was sympathetic to me; he let me take over the surgical outpatient department. Now, being able to refer cases to me (and send the minor cases to the others), I realized how they had been shunting cases away from me during those three years.

When the administrators announced the appointment of the new chairman — another aging Jew from New Jersey — I knew that the puppies were now weakened, and that my situation was improving. But by that time, I was already committed to leaving New York, its medicine, and pseudo-academia. I wanted nothing more to do with it.

* * * * *

Dr. Paul Gerst died in 2013 at the age of eighty-six. I realize my portrayal of him is rather harsh, almost a caricature. But this is how I encountered him — at the twilight of his long professional career. Perhaps, I admit, leading an organized department in the chaotic milieu of the Southern Bronx, for so many years required a control freak, a dictator. Like most of us, he must have had a different, probably appealing personality outside the hospital's walls. He talked a lot about his sons, and he used to mention how beautiful and lovely his deceased wife was. He must have missed her tremendously. RIP Dr. Gerst.

* * * * *

Paul Gerst (1927-2013).

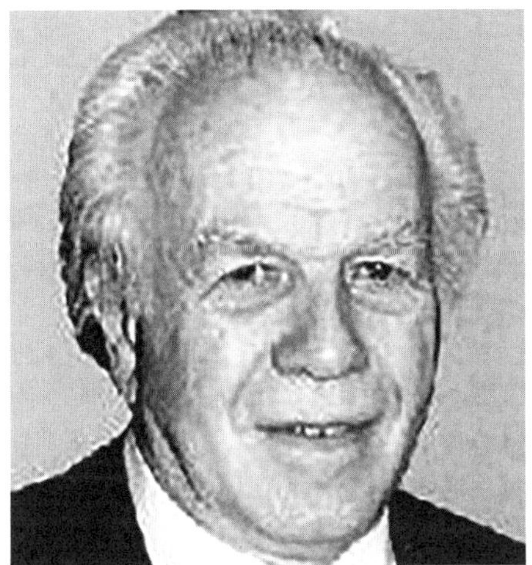

Forty-eight

So long New York

I was now chronically fed up with the New York surgical world: the unending political skirmishes, the fighting for referrals, the marginal care patients were receiving, and the chaos masked by constant lip service to how "good we are." I was tired of the pervasive corruption and sleaziness that was irritating and affecting me personally.

In New York, we had to use billing companies to process the claims for reimbursement for our private cases. At the Methodist, our team used a biller called Randy — a burly, smiling Jew in his forties. Each week, he would arrive with his much younger, attractive Puerto Rican secretary to collect our claims and to distribute the checks he had succeeded in collecting — his cut of the bounty was ten percent. At some point, the checks started to dwindle. "Your claims were rejected" or "denied" or "delayed" or had to be "re-billed" — Randy always had a long list of excuses. One day, Randy stopped coming. We learned that he had eloped with the sexy Puerto Rican to Mexico, leaving behind a wife and kids. He left with our dollars and money skimmed from doctors in other departments and hospitals. My loss was around a hundred grand — Randy's gain must have been in the millions. We were told that "the FBI is investigating," but that was the end of the story. Our group hired another biller, a soft-spoken middle-aged man, originally from Switzerland, to replace Randy. That he was Swiss made him trustworthy in my eyes, so before relocating to my new job in the Bronx, I asked him to continue to bill for me.

"Oh sure, doctor," he said, "Just mail me all your claims." I did so for half a year, waiting for checks, which never arrived. It appeared that the Swiss did not process any of my claims; it was too late to bill it again.

And I was weary of the daily life in New York. A few visits per year to the City Opera and an occasional dinner at a Zagat top-rated restaurant — hopefully, somebody else was paying — hardly compensated for the constantly congested highways and gridlocked bridges. I could not see myself spending the last twenty years of my career practicing in the Bronx or Brooklyn. Yet, the gates of the ivory towers of Manhattan were closed to me. I had nothing specific to offer them, as it had been ten years prior. Each great center was producing its own upcoming 'geniuses;' they would only import potential top-earning specialists or a chairman — by now, I knew that I was neither.

Our nest was becoming empty, so our decision was easier — we would not have moved if any of the boys were still at home. But Omri was in San Diego, pursuing a master's in musical theater, Yariv was already in one of the upstate SUNY colleges, and Dan was about to enroll in a New York college within a few months. The ground for significant change was readily approaching. Moreover, the change had to be radical — what is the point of moving to another town, suburb, or cutthroat hospital?

For years, Heidi and I were fascinated with country life. Whenever we toured or visited, be it in Europe or North America, we envied people leading what we perceived as a 'simpler' life — living in charming little chalets or cabins, near a river or a lake, among open fields, forests, and meadows. Why not us?

As it often occurs, the opportunity came suddenly, by chance, and the timing appeared perfect. It all started when Dr. Jack Cappuccino, a general surgeon from Iowa, attempted to recruit me to replace his older partner, who was then retiring. I had become acquainted with Jack through an online surgical discussion group — SURGINET — to which we had both contributed since the mid-90s. We would exchange a few personal e-mails on and off, share a drink once a year at the yearly American College of Surgeons meeting, and usually 'agree' on matters discussed online. In brief — we were good 'virtual' mates. In an avalanche of e-mails, Jack promised me the sky: an idyllic country life, a solid and lucrative job, a friendly medical community, in a little (ten thousand plus) quaint town on the western shore of the mighty Mississippi River. Above all — and this was the most convincing factor — I knew that to undertake such a radical change of practice, I would need a dedicated partner, and Jack had pledged his support and friendship. The little town was Keokuk, Iowa, located at the state's southeast corner, bordering Missouri and Illinois.

In January 2004, we flew to Keokuk for an exploratory visit of a few days. The visit was hugely successful. We immediately clicked with Jack and his charming wife. Al Z., the hospital's CEO, made a favorable impression — for the first time in my long career I had met a smiling and warmly welcoming hospital administrator. The local physicians, whom we met at a social function arranged on our behalf, seemed a friendly bunch — they were non-surgeons and thus left the recruitment details to the CEO and Jack. After all, Jack had to know with whom he wanted to work. We found Keokuk to be a little shabby. Still, the snow cover whitewashed its cosmetic sores, emphasizing the old, majestic colonial mansions standing along the cliffs overlooking the Mississippi.

Most importantly, the hospital looked modern and neat, and besides, we did not intend to live in the town but out in the countryside. On a tour with an estate agent, Heidi immediately spotted her dream house, standing alone by a semi-private lake. In the evening, Jack and I donned our Western shirts and jeans and drove to the Smurfs bar nearby at Montrose, known for its legendary burgers. We had a few beers and affirmed our friendship. Coming out of the joint, we observed the sunset on the frozen, silent Mississippi. We were allured!

In no time, I reached and signed a deal with the CEO in Keokuk, immediately followed by my resignation from the Bronx-Lebanon Hospital. We placed our Staten Island house up for sale and put an offer in on the lakeside cottage in Keokuk. Jack personally helped with anything he could, including speeding up the formalities to receive an Iowa medical license. It seemed that he was well entrenched within the medical establishment state-wide.

In June, we traveled again to Keokuk to sign the deal on the house, which now included a few more acres of the adjacent land. We were invited to stay with Jack and his wife at their riverside house on this visit. It was a large renovated mansion overlooking the great river: huge rooms, thick white carpets — outdoor shoes strictly forbidden — numerous gas fireplaces, a few studies, several sitting corners, a vast modern kitchen, a well-equipped gym in the basement, multiple guest rooms, a Mercedes SUV and a Ford pickup in the garage, a garden shed with a new John Deere and all the rest — we saw it all. It was clear that Jack was proud of what he had. "Moshe, I can't complain," he said, "I did very well for myself here in Iowa. When you come here, after a few years, you won't know what to do with the money — this is not New York!"

At a prolonged dinner — pasta with Italian sausage meatballs and several bottles of red wine — and during the cozy days spent with the Cappuccinos, I learned who Jack was. He was a few years older than me, short, slim, and in excellent physical shape. He was born in a little town in Massachusetts, where his Italian-born parents ran a grocery store — no, he didn't pick up a word of Italian. His wife, of Irish extraction, had been his high school sweetheart. He attended a medical school somewhere in Upstate New York, followed by a surgical residency in an undistinguished program in the Midwest. "My parents were poor, I went to a state college, no Ivy League for me." Jack opened his heart after uncorking the third bottle of wine, "I was too short for basketball and did not excel in other sports. Isn't this enough to develop some inferiority complexes?"

But such relatively humble beginnings contrasted with the eventual outcome: Jack practiced surgery in northern Iowa for many years, becoming a senior partner in a large practice group. A few years back he had relocated to Keokuk — "Oh, I couldn't work with the new, younger partners, I needed a change," he explained. Later, Jack listed his achievements, including his clinical professorship at Iowa State University, his leading position in a few local committees on trauma, and his frequent interviews on local TV — he made me watch a clip of such a recent event.

It was as if he was trying to tell me: "Look, I'm not just a small-town surgeon."

Discussing local hospital politics, Jack described each one of the local physicians in detail, emphasizing his relationship with the individual. There were only a few he seemed to respect or like. Jack's hobbies included collecting fountain pens and yard work. He did not admit to being an avid reader but liked watching DVDs. The Cappuccinos were not keen travelers, preferring to spend their vacations at home — they never found a reason to visit Europe. Of course, they were regular churchgoers as Catholics.

We concluded the visit sailing on the Mississippi with the CEO on his 24-foot riverboat. The early summer's day was perfect; soft light glistened on the water, the cool breeze sprayed on our faces. The cooler was well stocked with beer and wine. (Light beer and the so-called wine cooler drinks are tasteless beverages that are popular in the Midwest.) The future appeared rosy! We had no doubts whatsoever. There were no warning signs.

Such an unexpected and unusual surgical marriage of two prominent SURGINET members had been 'approved' by those who cared to vocalize their congratulations. Only Jerry, a veteran surgeon from California (one of the few who had met Jack and me personally), had raised, sarcastically, some doubts about the match and compatibility between the small-town Iowan surgeon and the Israeli Jew from New York.

* * * * *

So, what did I accomplish during the New York years besides eliminating Mantzur and Sorkhi? Some surgeons tend to pack their memoirs with minutiae, including each paper they have published, every book they have edited, and every invited lecture they have given — the exotic sightseeing and gourmet delicacies they have consumed worldwide — not to mention their romantic conquests. Being humble, I will limit myself to one paragraph.

During those ten years, I wrote and published a lot. In addition to numerous articles in peer-reviewed journals, I edited (together with Dr. Wise) a series of books, *Controversies in Surgery*. My longstanding interest in surgical infections culminated in the publication of the book *Source Control: A Guide to the Management of Surgical Infections* (together with John Marshall of Toronto). Less scientific but more satisfying was the production of *Aphorisms and Quotations for the Surgeon*, a book that continues to sell well year after year. But the book I am most proud of is *Schein's Common Sense Emergency Abdominal Surgery* (2000). This unconventional book is now in its fifth edition (2021). The various editions were co-edited with good friends — Paul Rogers, Danny Rosin, Ahmad Assalia, Mark Cheetham, and Ari Leppäniemi, and have gradually become popular among surgeons all around the world and have been translated into many languages. In some countries, it has reached the status of 'pulp non-fiction' among young surgeons. We later produced a second book along similar lines (*Schein's Common Sense Prevention and Management of Surgical Complications*, 2013) that continues to sell well. [All those books were produced and published by tfm publishing, UK.] The consequence was some degree of 'name recognition' within the international surgical community, resulting in invitations to join editorial boards of surgical journals and to deliver talks in meetings on various continents. It is somewhat unusual for such academic output to come out of a little-known community hospital. But this is where I was and from where I had to try to produce something significant.

Among those years' 'accomplishments,' one must mention the various friendships created. My rapport with the people below me was always easier and warmer than with those above. A few of the residents I helped to train have become friends, like Piotr Górecki, Adam Klipfel, Ramesh Paladugu, Narong Kulvatunyou, and others. Syed Gardezi (RIP), Jim Rucinski, Bashar Fahoum, and Satish Khaneja, all attending surgeons, were enjoyable and reliable colleagues.

But it was Pasquale, ('Lello') Lapalorcia, a surgeon of Brooklyn, who became a close friend. Lello was a thinking and capable surgeon. He was one of the few private surgeons who supported me — yes, passively and quietly but encouragingly — in my political battles. I will never forget the Italian feasts in his back garden on Sunday afternoons and the rowdy Sylvesters (New Year's Eve celebration) in his and Elizabeth's Bay Ridge house in Brooklyn. He had a warm voice and sang beautifully; people said he looked and sang like the late Italian singer Lucio Dalla. A week before our departure to Keokuk, I sat with Lello at a Greek eatery on 3rd Avenue in Brooklyn. "I envy you," he said, "I'm fed up with my practice…" I would have never suspected that this was to be our last meeting. A year later, he died suddenly. He was a character. I remember traveling with him (and his son Luigi — now a plastic surgeon in Perugia) in India. Lello carried a giant Italian thermos full of strong espresso-like coffee wherever we went. He had to have a coffee break, plus a cigarette, almost every half an hour. I remember him fondly and with love.

I vacated, yet again, my Bronx hospital office. I did not shed any tears. In fact, my foot would never step in any New York hospital again. We sold the Staten Island house at a significant profit — this was when sellers could ask for anything. One morning, a vast semitrailer arrived; the following day, the house was empty. We climbed into Heidi's Explorer with Birdi (the New York cockatiel who would scream the F word sporadically), the two cats — Goufi (born in Johannesburg) and Herbi (a New Yorker). Pablo, a German Shepherd, had been schlepped beforehand to Iowa by Omri and Yariv in my 1979 Mercedes. Pimpush, our little mongrel dachshund, who had traveled with us from South Africa, to Israel, to Switzerland, to

Milwaukee, to New York, did not come along. Before our departure, Pimpush, now nearly twenty years old, incontinent, and a little senile, disappeared. We never found her.

We traveled westwards, crossing the Hudson River. A day and a half later, we crossed the Mississippi. We felt like explorers heading to conquer the Wild West.

* * * * *

Top: Pasquale ('Lello') Lapalorcia (RIP). Bottom: farewell New York!

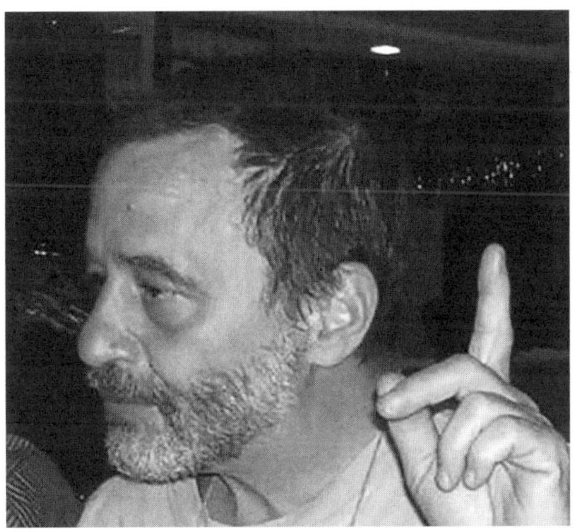

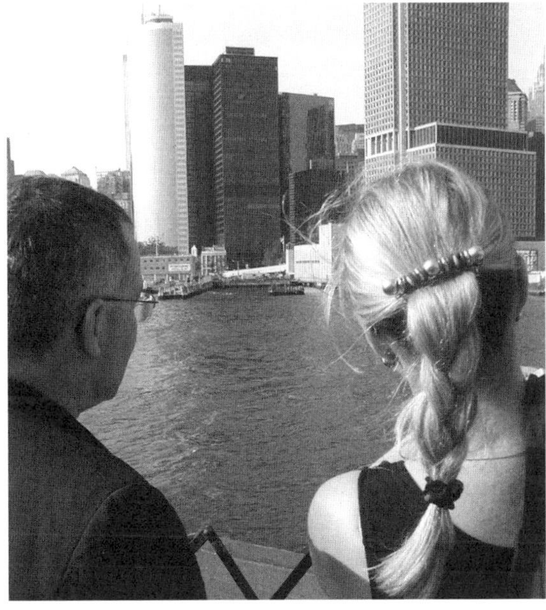

Forty-nine

My sister, Sylvia

One weekend, at the beginning of March 2004, my sister Sylvia called from Haifa: "I'm worried about you. I was thinking about your plans." She was referring to our recent decision to move to Iowa.

"No need to worry, Sylvia. The change will be good for us. We need it. We have visited the place and like it very much. What's wrong with spending the end of one's surgical career in the country?"

"I'm just afraid that you won't be satisfied in a non-academic environment, that you'll be miserable, and what will Heidi do in that little shit hole?"

"Sylvia, listen. We have considered everything and are convinced that the step we are taking is wise, so don't worry."

"But I do worry, I worry about you…"

Sylvia was found dead a week later in her apartment, lying on the Persian carpet in the living room.

* * * * *

I have hardly mentioned my sister in these pages — I did not know how and what to write about her: she was a complex and problematic person. Although not devoid of love, our relationship was unpredictable — like an emergency abdominal operation for a high-velocity gunshot wound.

"Alone. One has to learn to live alone.
To live alone. Because man dies alone.
He dies alone. But I can't be alone.
I'm afraid. And this winter frightens me.
The sea is so rowdy. And everything comes to me from the sea."

This was written by the twenty-year-old girl some thirty-six years before her death. We found her diaries and pieces of poetry in her cozy apartment on the Carmel Mountain. They were scattered here and there among thousands of history, art, travel, and cooking books, and novels. We found a few volumes of diaries among hills of clothes, expensive shoes, and perfumes — most still unused, in their original shopping bags from London, Paris, Munich, and even Haifa. One volume — the most recent — lay by her bed as if waiting to receive the last words she had planned to write. We did not discover her early diaries from her high school years. I knew about their existence; as a ten-year-old boy, I had been reading from them in secret, curious to learn about the love life of my older sister. Did she destroy them? Why?

Sylvia was just three years older than me, but the generational gap between us was wider. She had matured much earlier and had a sharper intellect than mine. Sylvia excelled in school, while I was considered 'retarded.' She had shined in Haifa's upper-crust young society — I had remained shy, awkward, and plain. Since her early teens, Sylvia had played the 'princess' role, always best dressed, extravagant, and exchanging boyfriends — who were significantly older than her — with whom, as we learned from her diaries, she was manipulative, jealous, and not wholly content.

The final entry in the last diary was dated July 5, 2003:

> "Haifa. Nothing has changed. When I think it is all finished, he arrives, and then I do not need anything else. I love him when he is with me, as I do not love anyone. I worry about him as if he was a small boy. Sometimes, in bed, I do not know when my body begins and his ends. I love his body like no man I had loved before. I'm going out of my mind if he doesn't call for a few weeks. I don't trust him… and now he doesn't reply to his cell phone, and I don't know what to do. God! There is no minute without a worry. How can one live like this? But when we are together, it is wonderful! In the last few weeks, I was depressed to death. He didn't call. I felt completely dead. At least he provides me — and he's the only one — with a taste for life."

Thus ended her last diary entry, the one which was lying on the carpet by her bed in its red leather binding. The bed was not covered — was she intending to go to bed the night of her death?

What happened? In the morning, when her housekeeper entered the apartment, she found Sylvia placed face down on the carpet in a small pool of clotted blood in the little space between her easy chair and the coffee table, which was topped with heavy glass, loaded with students' manuscripts awaiting corrections. The ashtray was full of half-smoked slim Vogue cigarettes — she used to chain smoke them but never to the end. A half-empty glass of white wine stood nearby. She had been last seen by a neighbor, late evening, on the staircase, dressed in chic evening attire. She had exchanged a few pleasantries with the neighbor. From where was she returning so elegantly dressed? We never found out. And what had happened after she climbed to the third floor, unlocked her apartment's heavy door, and entered the living room? First, she must have removed her fashionable high heels, removed her black plush satin jacket and leather handbag, and hung it on a nearby chair. Next, she poured herself a glass of white wine — not an expensive Golan or Galil wine, but something cheaper, made by the Carmel winery. We found the almost empty bottle in the kitchen. Had she been consuming drugs? There was no evidence for this except some valium lying around.

Next, she surely lit a cigarette and sat in her favorite easy chair, her legs in dark silk stockings, folded under as usual. Did she start reviewing her students' manuscripts, or did she watch TV? Did she look at one of the magazines or novels scattered around? What happened next?

There were conflicting testimonials from Sylvia's acquaintances on her prevailing mood during the few months before her death. Some claimed to have noticed her in a reasonable frame of mind: she had been planning overseas trips, writing articles, and finishing writing books. Only two days before that fateful day, she had been spotted power-walking in designer sports attire along Panorama Street. Most friends maintained that Sylvia had been delighted after finally receiving her long-awaited professorship from the University of Haifa — she loved the sound of "Professor Schein." Others argued differently: that the disappearance of Hardy had devastated her.

Hardy was her last major love in a long list of major, minor, and sporadic loves. In one entry of her diary (October 10, 2001), she had listed them in two columns:

"Finally, I decided to list all of them. Of course, I cannot remember everyone, let alone their names. For some, I will only list the nicknames I have given them:

Izi Shtadlan	Henri
Mr. Cinema	G. Winter
Mr. Shira	Jacque
Shlomo	Avineri
The son of Mrs. Beit Belgia	P
Womotzik	Adolf the German
England A	S
England B	Ari
The American with the cooking book	Shaul
Hans Abhard Myer	Tedy
Advocate Y	Avi
Guri	The French A
Yosi Ben Bassat	Natan
Doron Mendels	Gad
Hayim Goren	A
Avi Reches	Gisi
The philosopher from Haifa University	Zeev M
Moshe Adler	Zeev Kessler
Roman the Polak	Karol
The neighbor	The French B
X from political studies	Mrs. Woks' son

The insurance agent
The flower shop owner
The mafioso"

Some of the listed above I had known personally, a few I had heard of, and others were a total surprise to me. Many of them feature or are mentioned in her diaries, the diaries that served as a window into the life of a sister – the inner life of a sister that, now I realize, I knew so little about. Or did not care to know?

After graduating from high school and serving in the army, the 'princess' – who had already declined marriage proposals from serious candidates (Tedy, Zeev M) – embarked on a North American tour with Henri. He was a rich Canadian Jewish boy she met on the beach in Haifa. It turned into a 'big love,' leaving her heart broken when Henri's mother vetoed her son's decision to marry the "spoiled Israeli girl." Her next station had been in Jerusalem as a junior student at the Hebrew University. Here, the externally mature but internally confused girl romanced mostly with married lecturers or famous professors: one (A) impregnated her, paid for her abortion, and immigrated with his wife to the USA. Another was Professor Shlomo Avineri – a leading academician and politician. Sometime later, she fell under the spell of the charismatic and internationally renowned expert of medieval history, Professor Joshua Prawer (P).

Prawer, more than thirty years older, became her mentor and guardian; she his mistress. "That old Jew will ruin her life," my father predicted before his death, moaning about his daughter's affair with the notable professor. My dad's prophecy turned out to be correct. The symbiotic relationship between the two would endure for many years, during which my sister could have married and had a family.

With Prawer's connections, Sylvia had gone to the University of Cambridge, England (see lovers "England A" and "England B" in the list above), where she obtained her PhD. Obviously, the old Professor Prawer had been visiting her frequently in England. When she returned to Israel, the married Prawer, not wanting her too close to him in Jerusalem, helped to place her at the University of Haifa. Here, she was recognized as a competent lecturer and a prolific researcher, gaining an international reputation as a medieval scholar. However, being known as Prawer's protégé had been politically harmful, and consequently, her professorship was repeatedly postponed. During the 1980s, she enjoyed a steady and prolonged relationship with an older man named Shimon (S). It had a stabilizing effect on her – there were no entries in the diaries during those years. The diary resumed after S's premature death of lung cancer: "S served me like a drug, like a cognac, wine, and cigarettes. He was very effective… the first man in whom I had an absolute trust…"

Following Shimon's death, the diaries document years of depression and instability, exacerbated by our mother's terminal disease, with which

Sylvia coped poorly. As before, Sylvia attempted to cure her inner maladies by drinking wine and leading a luxurious lifestyle beyond her relatively modest academic salary. In parallel, there was a relentless search for that elusive love. And when there was no love, there was sex. While most women in their fifties complain about decreasing sexual appetites, the situation was reversed with Sylvia, as her diaries show.

Who was Hardy, whose name crowded the last few diaries, the one whom Sylvia's friends mentioned as "her great love?" Sylvia kept her personal life and affairs well compartmentalized — sharing only bits and pieces with selected people. She tended to be secretive — also about Hardy. It appears that she met Hardy in the late 1990s in Haifa. He was Dutch-German, three years younger than Sylvia, married, and a father to two daughters. Some said that he had been working for the International Red Cross and later was involved in some obscure international commerce. One girlfriend spotted Sylvia and Hardy together in Haifa a few months before Sylvia's death. Another claimed to hear from Sylvia about Hardy's recent financial troubles. Sylvia's neighbor (the "neighbor" from the list) told me that Sylvia had asked him for a loan of 20,000 US dollars "to pay off a loan" — did that money go to Hardy? (I eventually had to repay the neighbor with Sylvia's new Toyota Corolla.) Did Sylvia also try to procure cash for Hardy from a member of Haifa's underworld (the "mafioso" in the list)?

There was another reason why Hardy seemed to be responsible for Sylvia's recent financial troubles: she used to fly around Europe — Barcelona, Zurich, Munich, Paris, only to spend a night or two with him — hotels, food, and drinks paid by her. Was Hardy involved with other similar 'Sylvias' in various corners of the world, loving them for a few days, a few times a year? We will never know: there was no trace of Hardy in Sylvia's documents or laptop — not even a phone number or e-mail address — only long entries in her diaries raving about his sexual performance. Did he disappear with her money?

In 2006, two years after Sylvia's death (where was he until then?) Hardy e-mailed Haifa University; the e-mail was forwarded to me: "Dear Sir, when returning from an exhausting two-year mission abroad for my country a couple of months ago, I was told that Sylvia isn't with us anymore. A major shock to me, as I have been a close friend to her for many years, although not seeing her that often."

I exchanged a few e-mails with Hardy; he wrote back, "Yes, Sylvia, she played a major role. I owe her an unforgettable time in my life…" but never really disclosing much more. Who was or is he? What was the meaning of the "two-year mission for my county?"

So why and how did Sylvia die? Was it suicide? Very unlikely — why would she dress up and go out? And she had so many plans, and there was no physical evidence. Was she murdered? The investigation by the police was hasty, and an autopsy was not performed. However, it wouldn't have taken much physical force to place a hand over the mouth of this petite woman and stop her breathing. Was it the so-called "mafioso" who did it, intentionally or by accident — when asking her to return his money? Did he push her, and she fell and hit her head on the edge of the coffee table? Or was it just an accident? Did she try to stand up from her easy chair, slip on the carpet, and hit the table? One cannot rule out a natural cause of death: a cardiac event cannot be completely ruled out in a fifty-six-year-old woman who was a heavy smoker and receiving hormonal replacement therapy. Yes, it cannot be ruled out, but it is unlikely.

* * * * *

On a windy early spring day, we buried Sylvia in the 'new' Haifa's cemetery (the 'old' one, where our parents were resting, had run out of space) on a rocky hill overlooking the Carmel Mountain. An Arab village was plastered to the other side of the hill. Goats were roaming at the cemetery's perimeter. According to the local tradition, the burial attendants unveiled Sylvia's face, which had been covered with a white shroud, for me to identify. I saw the face of my pretty sister, now blue and bloated — dead. "Here, take it," said a bearded attendant, snatching a tiny, golden medallion still hanging on her neck. (The expensive jewelry she always wore was robbed during the transfer of her body from her apartment to the morgue.) I stared at her face, trying to absorb her last image, but the attendants re-shrouded it instantly. It is a pity that the last image of our dying or dead dear ones is prevailing.

Sylvia and I could not be considered close siblings; she was often distant, aloof, arrogant, and very moody — the smile turning into a tantrum in an instant. This always kept me on guard — remote and reserved. Most probably, she had been jealous of me — mainly of my children, whereas she, so desperately wanting them, having none — also, perhaps, jealous of my stable marriage and late financial stability. Nevertheless, there was mutual affection and warmth between us, and we talked on the phone a few times per month. However, the few well-written and shocking volumes of diaries exposed to me the real sister — the woman tormented by demons with which she was relentlessly struggling to cope. That despite her beleaguered self — crying and drinking for long nights — she could rise in the morning, get dressed, put on the face of a successful academician, and stand in front of a large class of students is admirable to me.

Whatever the actual cause of death was, chronic loneliness and a painful craving for love must have been contributory factors. Fifteen months before her death, Sylvia had written in her diary:

> "And I walk in Panorama Street and see all these couples snuggled together.

All ages. And the women are sometimes fat, neglected, ugly.

And I ask myself, what is the use of all of this?

Where am I, and where are they? They have a piece of man that cares and loves.

And me — alone. Always alone."

Sylvia has left behind a large body of historical research, including two full-length books, *Fideles Crucis: Papacy, the West and the Recovery of the Holy Land, 1274-1314* (1991) and *Gateway to the Heavenly City: Crusader Jerusalem and the Catholic West (1099-1187)* (2004). Her diaries, if adequately edited, could be her best work. But the best work of authors often never sees the light…

I miss Sylvia often. Losing a sibling is like a piece of your own flesh has been torn from your body. Every 4-5 years, each time I visit Israel, I stop at Sylvia's lonely grave. I always find a bunch of flowers lying on it. And I wonder: who has left those flowers? Someone from the lovers' list? Or from another who appeared after the list was concluded?

* * * * *

My sister Sylvia (1947-2004), at ages five, twenty-one and fifty-four, speaking at the University of Haifa.

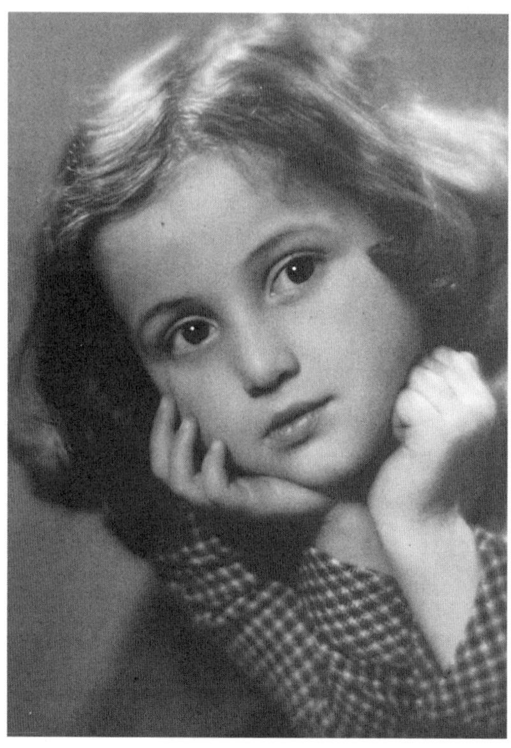

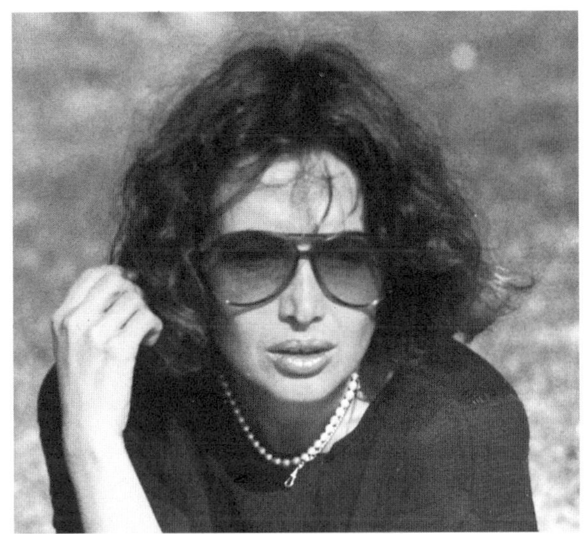

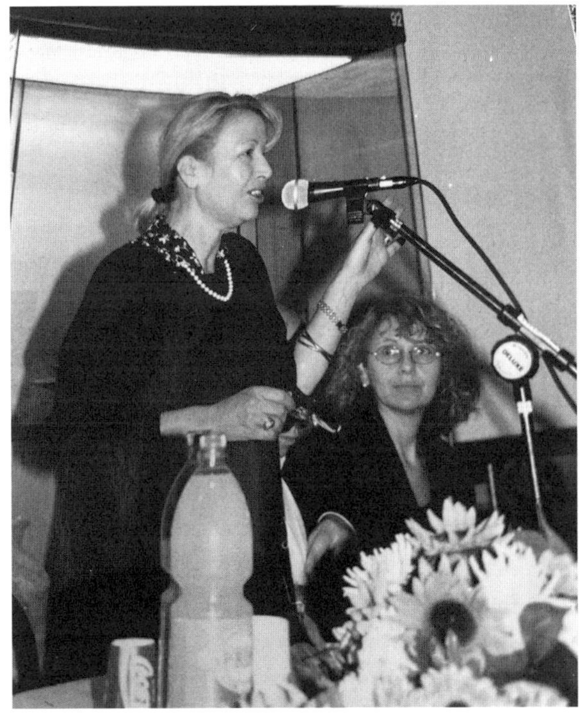

Fifty

On the western shore of the Mississippi

2004. We crossed the Mississippi from Illinois into Iowa on a warm, late August evening. We had arrived in Keokuk. We stopped at Jack Cappuccino's house, where we were treated to a dinner of penne with meatballs — the same dish we had had during our previous visit – and some red wine. This would be the last time we saw the Cappuccinos' house from the inside.

Our new lakeside, cedar-sided house was empty – our things would arrive a few days later. We retrieved Pablo, the German Shepherd, from the dog kennel, unpacked the cats and Birdie, and laid down on the thick carpets for the night. Through the open windows, light wind brought in the perfumes of the decaying vegetation. We could hear the loud lament of the bullfrogs from the lake. Ah, finally, we were in the country.

After arriving in Keokuk, I posted a series of "Dispatches from Keokuk" online on SURGINET. I hoped it would serve as a framework for a book: if others can write about "A Year in Provence" – why not "A Year in Keokuk?" Eventually, I wrote "A Year in Keokuk" but, as usual, could not find an interested publisher or agent. The following narrative cites bits and pieces from the original "dispatches" and the notes I took at that time. This is what I wrote in one of the early dispatches:

> "Late September. The summer is still here, hot days and cool nights, like in any inland desert. Depending on the direction from which it blows, the wind arrives with different smells: from the south, it carries a sweet aroma, like chocolate-chip cookies, from the corn syrup factory on the outskirts of town; from the west, a mile away, beyond Highway 61, it occasionally puffs a scent of burned rubber and scorched iron emitted from a giant railway wheels factory in the industrial zone. Unfortunately, in this country, it is difficult to escape entirely from man-made rackets and pollution. A few yellow leaves gather on the grass and float on the lakes, heralding the impending autumn – the nights are already cooler, and hordes of migrating birds are seen flying. The corn is being collected in the ocean of cornfields, stretching from horizon to horizon; autumn festivals are celebrated in the tiny hamlets scattered around us. As the night falls, it brings a loud concert of clamor from the lakes and the woodland,

an admixture of noises from insects and wild animals that we cannot yet decipher. Every few hours, throughout the night, we hear rumbling laments of trains loaded with coal or corn crawling up and down the Mississippi. And in the basement, the frantic activity of some mice…"

For Heidi and I, this move was meant to fulfill what we had dreamed and talked about for years: leaving the crowded city, the urbane life, for a simpler and healthier existence in the country. This was our great mid-life transformation opportunity — we were very excited and optimistic. I was so excited and optimistic that I wrote this for the local daily, *Gate City*. It appeared in mid-October:

"**Doctor finds Keokuk move a pleasant experience**

"With New York a 1000 miles behind us and Keokuk just a few miles ahead — cornfields rolling on both sides of the road — I calculated that Keokuk is going to be my 32nd mailing address. Poland, Israel, Italy, South Africa, Switzerland, UK, New York — towns, suburbs, streets, neighbors; blurred images in my brain. But Keokuk will be our first rural address ever — a reversed mirror image of New York City where we lived for the past ten years. Would we cope with such a drastic change?

"I also reckoned that Keokuk Area Hospital would be my 17th hospital since graduating from medical school twenty-four years ago — the first rural hospital that also is non-university affiliated and 'non-teaching.' Would I be able to function in such an environment without residents doing the 'scut' jobs for me? After years of immersion within multi-ethnic New York, working among doctors and patients who had emigrated from numerous countries, how would it feel to deal with a homogeneous population of Midwesterners?

"However, the anxieties, which evolved around our 'enigma of arrival,' dispersed very rapidly for everywhere and all around us, we encounter signs and declarations of warm welcome and friendly attitudes… In the hospital: modern, clean, well-equipped and spacious, I note that each and every patient is treated as if he or she were a VIP in New York — with patience and respect. Not the hurried large city attitude where 'time is money' and 'bring the next patient, please.' Walking around the corridors and getting wide smiles and a 'good morning' from nurses, technicians, secretaries and cleaners is a pleasant surprise…

"So, the first few months in Keokuk proved to us a most pleasurable experience; the fact that the daily commute to work takes now ten minutes instead of the 120 minutes in New York obviously enhances the euphoria of changing places. Will our report on 'A Year in Keokuk' be as positive as this one? Time will tell and let us hope so."

Some twenty years later, when I read this article, it seems somewhat naïve and over the top — probably the result of exaggerated optimism. However, I still believe that it was genuine. True, I may have been looking at the fresh Keokuk experience through euphoric lenses. Still, even today, after all that happened, I maintain a favorable opinion of Keokuk and its people. And indeed, that modest article was welcomed and hung on the walls of the cafeteria, the hospital's floors, and the operating room. Everybody thanked and congratulated me — except Jack Cappuccino, who shrugged his shoulders, threw his head back, and uttered a contemptuous "eh" — a tic I was already getting used to. For after six weeks into our Keokuk adventure, I could sense that my fresh association with Jack was not progressing smoothly. I had observed the early signs — the minor, soft signs — that would typically predict a crisis in the fresh marriage.

* * * * *

After a week of unpacking, I started learning how to function as a country surgeon. I followed Jack wherever he went. I scrubbed with him on elective and emergency cases. It did not take long to notice that he did not enjoy my assistance and presence. Perhaps the following case contributed to his fast-growing, initially latent, resentment.

Jack admitted a small boy whom he had diagnosed with acute appendicitis. The abdominal X-ray also showed significant dilatation of the small intestine (this was before the era of the 'routine' abdominal CT scan in the ER). We scrubbed together. Jack performed a keyhole incision; he removed the appendix and sucked out some darkish abdominal fluid, which to me looked abnormal. Jack was ready to close the tiny incision. "Jack, wait," I exclaimed, "this appendix looks normal. It does not explain the intestinal dilatation on the X-ray, nor does it explain the dark fluid. Don't you want to look at the bowel?"

I noticed the sweat forming on Jack's forehead. He wanted to close up. He did not appreciate me telling him what to do — in front of the OR staff. "OK, OK," Jack murmured impatiently; he enlarged the incision and eviscerated the intestine, finding a typical intussusception of small bowel into the cecum — a segment of small bowel was dead — black! Obviously, closing up without dealing with the problem would have killed this boy.

Jack said nothing. He started fervently removing the dead bowel. Jack then sutured together the edges of the small bowel to the large one. Next, he pushed the eviscerated bowel back into the abdomen. "Now, let's close up," Jack said. But when he started to close the peritoneum, I noticed that the intestine was turning dark.

"Jack, the mesentery is twisted, cutting off the blood supply. Let me untwist it," I said, trying to pull out the intestine. He pushed my hand away. He then tried to manipulate the bowel within the abdomen. I knew it was hopeless — one has to enlarge the incision, eviscerate the whole bowel, untwist the mesentery, and put it back in the correct order.

But Jack had already decided. "I'm closing… this patient needs to go to pediatric surgery."

So he closed the abdomen over the dusky intestine, went to the phone, called the University of Iowa Hospitals, organized the chopper, and in thirty minutes, the boy flew out. Eventually, his abdomen was re-opened, and the bowel untwisted — he survived.

Subsequently, Jack never mentioned this case to me, and I never said anything to him about it either. But he probably resented demonstrating his faulty judgment; that the OR team had witnessed how things evolved must have made matters worse.

I wrote in my notes:

> Friday was busy: I scrubbed with Jack for multiple cases. He's very good with routines such as laparoscopic cholecystectomy, where he does it the same as he did 700 times — never changing any step. He's a typical one-person team — not used to being assisted by another surgeon and used to doing each step alone. Clearly, he is a good guy who works in isolation and does what he does very carefully; occasionally he's a little hesitant. He enjoys being the 'lone ranger' among the nurses in the OR. I should leave him alone — not force my presence on him.
>
> On my first week in town, an oversized parcel with copies of the second edition of a surgical book of mine arrived at our office. One of the secretaries opened it: "Hey doctor, *you* wrote this book?" Just then, Jack entered the office. "Doc, did you see Dr. Schein's new book?" I watched Jack's face — it froze; he nodded, said nothing, turned around, and left the room. No word. So, I thought, a few weeks ago, he had been "so proud" to recruit a guy with "a fantastic CV and many books," but a week later, when the poor guy arrived, is he already feeling threatened?

About a month or two after my arrival, Jack and I had our first significant dispute. A young girl was referred to me for a cholecystectomy because of biliary 'dyskinesia' (allegedly, causing biliary pain due to poor emptying of the gallbladder). However, I thought she was suffering from chest wall pain. I told her that no operation was necessary and that the procedure for dyskinesia and its diagnosis with a radioisotope scan were, at best, controversial. Jack, who admitted that half of the gallbladders he removed did not contain stones, and were thus diagnosed as dyskinesia, was far from convinced. He e-mailed me:

> "Here are a couple of personal observations, which, at least locally, I know to be true. When in Rome, do as the Romans do (as long as it is not dangerous). You are in Keokuk, Iowa, Midwest, USA, not in Frankfurt or London. What happens elsewhere may not be relevant at all here. Around here, we believe in biliary dyskinesia, and we operate on it..."

I was upset. I did not appreciate the early pressure applied on me to perform procedures that, to me at least, appeared not to be indicated. I replied:

"So what did you envision, Jack? Schein is coming to Keokuk and must start to do everything that a local general practitioner expects him to do?"

I contacted the ex-chairperson of surgery at Iowa City (the local ivory tower) and asked her opinion. She replied:

"No, we don't do cholecystectomies on these people. Having said that, I don't know what the practice is in the surrounding communities. It is possible these are being done all around us. Whatever the prevailing practice, it seems you have an opportunity to educate..."

I told Jack: "See, you tell me when in Rome do as the Romans do, but even a few miles away in the ivory tower, they do not believe in what you do, and they are Romans."

From my notes:

> I met Dr. Willy in the hospital yesterday morning. Tall, fat, wears scrub pants tied around his waist with a string. Post-liver transplant (booze?). He had emigrated from Germany to South America as a young man (parents Nazis?) — now around sixty years old. He is the Director of Family Practice, the one who had referred the young waitress with biliary dyskinesia to me — the one I had declined to operate on. I mentioned the case to him. He tried to be friendly but stated, "She had a Murphy's sign." There was no point in arguing with him. Obviously, he thinks that he knows when to operate and that I ought to do whatever he asks me to do — as Jack does.
>
> Apparently, he and Jack are buddies, drinking lattes at the mall a few times a week. I do not trust the man — something seems fishy about him.
>
> We, Jack and I, seem to have some adjustments to make. As a newcomer, I have to adjust more. However, Jack, who is used to flying

solo for so many years, has to understand that he has a partner with his load of past experiences and ideas — he has to learn to live with this.

The following month, I did my first major case: a colonic resection for a diverticular stricture in a morbidly obese patient. Of course, I asked Jack to assist. I had planned a hand-sutured colorectal anastomosis, but when he said, "Let me insert a stapler," I politely agreed, watching him perform the colorectal anastomosis.

The patient eventually leaked from the anastomosis when Jack was on vacation. She returned with an abdomen full of feces. I took down the anastomosis, did a colostomy, left her abdomen open, and then shipped her to the ivory tower in Iowa City. She survived. The patient returned home from Iowa City with a massive abdominal wall defect and a high-output small bowel fistula.

I decided to go and see her at home. She lived in a dilapidated house half a mile off the main street. The surrounding houses and shacks were in even worse shape. Rusty cars and other junk blocked most driveways. The front yards were neglected. I climbed the few stairs leading to the porch and rang the bell. The husband opened the door. I do not remember how he looked, only that he said nothing. I followed him through a stuffy parlor, through an old-fashioned kitchen, into the patient's tiny bedroom. She was lying on her bed, her abdominal wound connected to a loud suction machine. The dressings were saturated with contents of the leaking small bowel. I unblocked the suction tubes and re-dressed her wound.

From that day, I would visit her regularly, helping her husband with wound care and providing advice. They seemed to accept the home visits of the operating surgeon as normal or obvious. Perhaps they understood my guilty conscience. My visits were functional; they never asked me anything, and no refreshments were offered. At the same time, I did not feel any hostility or recrimination. Occasionally, they accepted without a word a twenty-dollar bill to buy gas for the ride to a follow-up visit with the doctors in Iowa City. She later returned to Iowa City to have her fistula closed and colostomy reversed. Then I lost touch with her. Nevertheless, the home visits stayed in my mind.

Obviously, this represented a major surgical disaster. When Jack returned to town, he would not admit any responsibility for this catastrophe. He asserted that my operative report — describing the site of the leak in the rectum just below the anastomosis, where he had inserted the stapler, and most probably created a hole in the rectum — was "dishonest." This would turn out to be the sentinel event — this is when Jack decided, "Schein is an incompetent surgeon."

There were more soft signs. Jack had been out of town when I saw one of his postoperative patients with pus draining from his wound. I opened the wound and wrote in the chart: "drainage of an infected wound." On his next visit, the patient consulted Jack, but then Jack left town again, and the patient had to see me. Now, I could read what Jack had written in the chart: "The wound looks clean. I do not see any evidence of the alleged wound infection." So, I thought his partner drained pus, and he says the infection was "alleged."

An entry from my notes, early November:

> Jack: very surprising. E-mail personality — warm, welcoming, "We'll be friends, we'll be sharing partners, assist each other, support each other…," and here he is remote. Socially, there is NOTHING. We invited them for dinner twice, but nothing on their side; we invited them again, and he declined to come. Two months, and he has never asked my opinion about anything and never asked me to scrub in with him unless I offered myself. People tell me that "Jack is very competitive," and he may be. After many years alone in private practice — it is impossible to change one's skin.

One Friday afternoon, I entered his office.

"Jack, what's wrong with you? You hardly talk to me."

He looked away, "I'm not in a good mood. This is how I am. I can have bad weeks."

A week later: "Jack, how do you feel? Is your mood better?"

"Not really."

"Why don't you try a small dose of Prozac?" I said, "I'm not kidding."

To Heidi, I said: "I suspect that I'm the cause of his depression. Perhaps he cannot stand me. He feels trapped with a partner he doesn't want. I think that there is something in me that seems unbearable to him. I bet he already decided a week or two after we arrived that it was a mistake. I wonder why? My look? My accent? The different surgical background I brought with me? That I do things differently? It must be a combination of all of these factors."

* * * * *

I was not overly busy during the first months in Keokuk. While Jack saw about twenty patients on an average office day, I consulted only on four or five. Whereas his operating days were fully booked, mine were half empty. Only later, I would fully understand why I did not get more patients.

I found myself with free time on my hands. And free time, as any hillbilly or redneck is aware of, means fishing! So I took to fishing with all my soul.

I was told by the locals that our small lake had been under-fished for many years and that it was swarming with all sorts of fish. I bought a fishing rod, hooks, lures, sinkers, and bait. I found a rusty johnboat sunken below a broken dock — the previous owner of our house left it behind. I emptied it of sand, muck, decaying vegetation, and a water snake. However, I did not know how to fish — I had never fished before — I had to find a teacher. I found Scott, one of our OR technicians, to teach me the basics of fishing. He was tall, robust, and blonde — a Minnesotan of Norwegian stock with a mild and warm personality. Further lessons in the advanced fishery came from Bob, the head pharmacist in the hospital, and David, one of the internists. My fishing buddies were my only friends in the hospital; the fishing they taught me proved to be the main pleasure and a longlasting benefit of the year in Keokuk.

A dam divided our lake into two parts, interconnected by a large-bore pipe. The upper lake was well stocked with beautiful large crappies — I would catch a few dozen of them on a good day. The largemouth bass, however, favored the lower lake. I would return home in the afternoon, grab a rod, and walk down the lawn to the waterline. A few minutes later, I would walk up to the house with a few fat, good-sized bass — ready for dinner!

On the Mississippi River, I fished for bigger fish. On freezing winter days, I would climb the river ramp by the corn processing plant Roquette, a third of a mile downriver from River Lock 19. Here, a huge duct was discarding hot, sweat-smelling, foamy fluid — a byproduct of processed corn — into the river. The water at this site was not frozen, and the odor and warm temperature attracted the carp. The Mississippi carp were line-breaking monsters. Huge! I used to snag them with large triple hooks. Their filets were delicious. In summer, the famous Mississippi catfish were there. I became pleasantly obsessed with fishing. It helped to maintain my sanity during that ever-increasingly stressful year.

The house had been vacant for two years, awaiting a buyer. Its exterior needed some fine-tuning. We found Stan, a master handyman — who also became a good friend. Stan replaced the cedar sidings and repaired the expansive wooden front deck. The roof had to be redone, and an outdoor jacuzzi had to be installed in the front garden.

* * * * *

Top: the house in Keokuk, Iowa (2004). Bottom: our private lake.

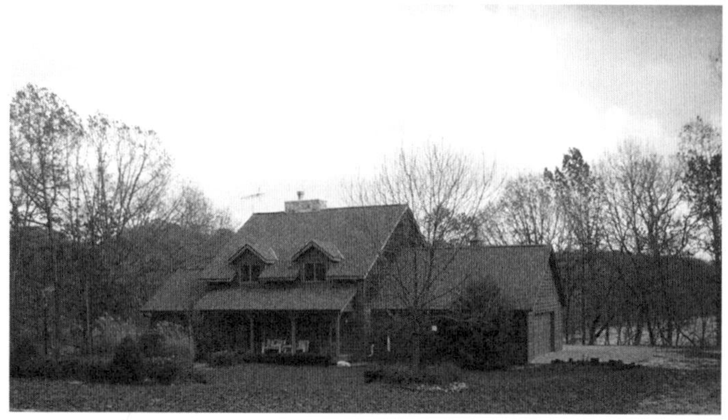

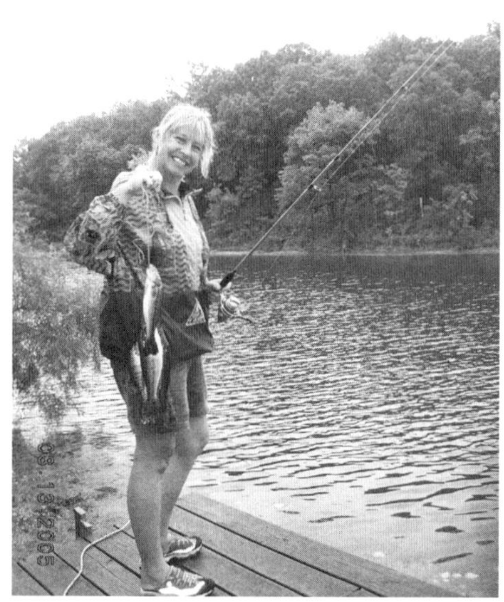

Fifty-one

The making of a rural surgeon

A white Thanksgiving. According to the old locals, there had not been a white Thanksgiving since the 60s. The snowflakes changed the world — painting the ugly, scarred emptiness of late autumn in white. Now, we would walk down from the porch onto the virgin snow, follow the footsteps of the deer, down the slope over the ramp that divided the two lakes, then uphill on the other side of the ramp, where, at sunset, the deer used to gather. We would turn eastbound, follow a dirt road, through a hole in barbed wire onto vast white fields, past a few farmhouses and the railway tracks; in an hour or so, we would reach the great Mississippi.

Our house was cozy and warm. I bought a chainsaw. Our little forest had tons of dead trees, so we were not short of hard, dry wood to feed the fireplace in the living room. The mile-long dirt road accessing the house, which was, according to the season, muddy, flooded, frozen, or covered with snow, called for an appropriate vehicle. I bought myself a 4x4 F-150 Ford pickup. I thought this would enhance my new image of a country boy — a country surgeon.

* * * * *

Meanwhile, I had to develop an optimal modus operandi to coexist with Jack — or in parallel to him. I sensed that the key to my success and survival (yes, already then I guessed that Jack would want to get rid of me) was to rapidly learn the trade of the rural surgeon — to satisfy the needs of the patients and, more importantly, the referring physicians.

Most surgeons function within a specific type of practice during their entire professional career. If they decide to move around, they prefer to move to a familiar environment. Hence, academic surgeons tend to relocate from one university hospital to another. If they decide to go 'private,' they would do it within the walls of the ivory towers or community teaching hospitals. On the other hand, with a few exceptions, rural surgeons shift to the country early after completing their training. They might move from one tiny town to another, perhaps from a larger rural setup to a smaller one. However, changing to a surgical rural practice after twenty-four years in an academic or teaching environment, one is suddenly exposed to new realities, which mandates a radical readjustment of practice. Here are a few points, not in any particular order of importance:

There is no one around to clean the shit after you. It takes a few weeks or months to realize that everything depends on you, however minor it might be! No interns, residents, or physician assistants to solve even minute, silly problems. Do you want to sleep well? Then think about the tiny details before going home, for they (nurses) will wake you up for *anything*. Forget about being a big shot, putting in the last stitch, and leaving the operating room — if you forget to tape the chest tube to the drainage system, then twelve hours later, at 3 o'clock in the morning, you will be driving through the ice to treat the collapsed lung.

You are first in the line of fire. Initially, when the ER, nurses, or patients had been calling — usually about minor problems — my reflective thought was, *What the fuck do they want? — why don't they call the resident on call?* Then I grasped that nobody was there to solve the problem except me and that I had forgotten how to manage minor complaints such as postoperative nausea, having for years left all the minor issues to the juniors.

There is no immediate feedback. This was perhaps the critical issue for me. Working with doctors, even younger than yourself, you always have somebody to confer with. When you decide to operate, or during the operation, you speak to your juniors all the time — you explain and teach, which helps your thinking process. They ask questions and (hopefully) challenge you: Why do you want to operate? Shouldn't we wait? Why don't you do what the other surgeon did last week? You explain — you think, and it keeps you alert. Should you become crazy and decide to do something stupid, the chief resident would ask: What are you doing? Of course, many nurses are smart; many understand what you are doing and what should be done. But they would rarely confront you directly. Instead, they will do it later on behind your back. You can speak and explain, but the feedback from the nurses and scrub techs would usually be supportive and positive. I was missing the real-time input, the discussion, and the previously irritating "Why are you doing this?"

Assistants. Your assistants in the OR, the nurses and scrub techs, are passive. They know when to remove the clamp when you tie the ligature; they can 'fry' the tissue with the diathermy between the jaws of your dissecting clamp. However, they rarely have the guts or impetus to take the initiative — they reposition their hands or shift a retractor from site to site only when told to do so. Operating with partners or (sound) residents is different: they take initiative, move their hands spontaneously, and do things — sometimes too much. The acute change from *active* assistants to *passive* nurse assistants can be painful. You realize you cannot wait for the assistants to read your mind: you must stop, reposition the retractor, and say, "Would you please..." Old country surgeons are accustomed to doing it all alone, so much so that they do not tolerate being assisted by active colleagues. They would rather scrub in with the good old OR girls, who are always agreeable and supportive — always laughing at their jokes.

Operating from the right side of the table. As an academic surgeon, I had started all operations, whatever their magnitude, from the right side of the table. The operations were performed by residents, with me assisting from the opposite side. But here, I had to get used to operating from the 'other side' — like a British driver suddenly dislocated to the streets of Manhattan, to the other, 'wrong' side of the road. Anatomy often looks different from the other side — one must adjust the operative technique accordingly.

You do a little of everything. In a small town with a limited patient catchment area, one cannot develop a high volume of interest in a specific field. Instead, one has to do a *little of everything*. Therefore, one should preferably arrive at such a practice with significant experience because the existing volume cannot support a learning curve in uncommon maladies. This limited volume is why rural surgeons tend to stick to their old guns doing 'the same'; it limits the impetus, or courage, to change.

You cannot take chances. Even a single major complication in a small town may harm your reputation. Anything that goes wrong in a small hospital is considered to happen *because* of you — your alleged or real 'inexperience,' or the limited local facilities. On the other hand, when the complication occurs at the university's ivory tower, patients consider it an act of God, developing *despite* the best efforts of the great doctors. Doing twelve emergency colon resections per year in a large center, you can select ten for primary anastomosis and accept one leak. But in the country, if you do three such procedures yearly, you will opt for a colostomy, which precludes leakage. Nobody will ask why you did a colostomy, but if the patient leaks and dies, they will ask, "Why not a colostomy?" Although the one-stage procedure is based on good evidence, in the country, good evidence often stops at the library's doors. In general, complications in a big center tend to be diluted — in the country, they are concentrated and thus more notable.

You have to know the limits of the system. It is not only that there are things that you do not know to do or believe that others can do better. Here, in a small town, there are also things you can do but should not do because the system cannot support you. Suddenly gone are the days when you leave the OR and hit the bed while others work on your patient in intensive care, trying to keep him alive. Now, it is your job to stay up and look at the multiple details of supportive care day and night. However, caring for sick patients is sometimes not doable, and you have to ship them away. You realize that transferring the critically ill patient *before* the operation is preferable rather than *after* it. Learning when not to tackle a case, and where to refer it, is as essential to your success and reputation as your operative skills.

The CT is your friend. It's funny how rapidly I had changed my attitude to good old CT scanning. Just a few months prior, I had given hell to residents for ordering CTs indiscriminately, laughing at the physicians and ER doctors for overusing imaging. But in the country, I rapidly found that the CT is my best friend. The negative CTs — showing that there is no problem, ordered more readily and liberally than pizzas — helped me to sleep well. "No appendicitis, no free air, no free fluid, no obstruction — send him to my office tomorrow." Forget about the literature and evidence — who cares that overall, routine CT scanning has no advantage? The only 'evidence' a country surgeon wants is to play it safely, solve problems instantly, maintain a good quality of life, and satisfy referring doctors and patients.

Everybody knows each other. In a rural town, each patient you see is somehow related to somebody you know, you need, or you will soon meet or need. Rumors, alleged or confirmed, of your arrogance, impatience, and negative attitude spread rapidly and are unforgiving — destroying your reputation. You have to be 'nice' always, positive, and at eye level with the local population.

Hide your impressive CV. If you arrive at the small town with a list of academic accomplishments, hide it! That you have published hundreds of articles and written a few books is not interesting to your patients. All they want to know is that you are a caring doc and can safely remove their appendix. As to your new colleagues, it is doubtful that they have ever written anything or engaged in academia — for many of them, it means nothing. To some, academic medicine is considered a derogative term. "If you are such a great academician, what are you doing here?" some may ask, suspecting there must have been some reason for leaving everything behind and migrating to the remote country — a scandal or malpractice.

Be modest. As a surgeon in rural America, you belong to the top 1% of the community. Your salary could be almost tenfold of the county's average. Locals know it. One must not show off, annoying the population with a flashy lifestyle. You want to avoid dressing up like a Manhattan surgeon or driving a new Mercedes Benz. If you do, no one will say a word, but it will not make you popular — everybody knows you, and you are always watched.

In Keokuk, I learned and internalized some of the above lessons rapidly. Many more came to me later, helping me establish myself as a country surgeon. Keokuk provided the basic training.

* * * * *

One day, I discovered that a patient I had scheduled for a hernia repair underwent the operation in Jack's hands.

"Oh he did not like your bedside manners," Jack explained without blinking when I confronted him. Most patients referred to our office from family practice were landing on Jack's schedule. However, I knew they were usually referred to "general surgery" without mentioning a specific surgeon's name. To my inquiry, our soft-spoken receptionist shrugged her shoulders, pretending she did not understand, but what did I expect her to say? And Jack just looked at me and said, "The patients want to be seen by me. You are developing a bad reputation."

What bad reputation? I was wondering, is it true that patients dislike me? For twenty-five years, I had never had a patient complain against me, so why now suddenly? Is my non-Midwestern body language irritating them? Or is Jack trying to show me that I am not suitable for the job and the place, thus manipulating the referrals? Indeed, one late evening, Jana, a recovery room nurse, approached me and whispered, "I have to tell you this: be careful. Your partner is badmouthing you. He hasn't a single positive thing to say about you."

The second week of November was my weekend on call when the situation exploded. On Friday morning, Jack handed a patient over to me with intestinal obstruction, instructing, "Treat her conservatively until Monday." He wanted to leave, but I insisted we examine the patient together.

A large volume of brown, thick, feculent fluid was draining from the patient's nasogastric tube. "This is a bad prognostic sign," I said to Jack, "It's improbable that she's going to open up without an operation." Jack shrugged his shoulders and left. Obviously, he had some urgent plans for the weekend. At rounds on Sunday, I noted that the patient was deteriorating — she needed an urgent operation, I was convinced. I called Jack's house. His wife replied that Jack was fixing something on the roof, "he'll call you later." I waited a few hours and called his house again. Jack sounded aggravated, like *why are you bothering me? I told you that I'll decide on Monday*. He hung up on me, sped to the hospital, and rushed the patient in for an operation. On Monday, in the office, we argued hotly about that case, and we agreed to bring our differences in front of the CEO.

I documented this in my notes:

> December 16. We met this afternoon in the CEO's office. It lasted over two hours and was painful and depressing. The CEO opened with a brief statement: how he likes and respects both of us; that the conflict between us seems to have gone into the open, at least within the hospital, but not as yet into the community, and we have to find a

solution and contain the damage. "Let us talk without going down to the level of he said or she said," the CEO concluded. However, a virulent and chaotic exchange between Jack and me followed. The CEO, a benign and polite middle-aged Midwesterner — who had hitherto been extremely warm and welcoming to me — was sitting there, suffering and holding his head between his two hands.

"May I start?" I asked the CEO. I pointed out that it seemed that Jack had started to dislike me very soon after I arrived at Keokuk; I described the arguments concerning the various patients and the scarcity of surgical work and referrals — "Is Jack actively diverting patients away from me?" I concluded. I turned towards Jack: "Look, you brought me here. I left a job behind, sold a house, and moved here, so what now? You have recruited me. You have to find the solutions!"

Jack replied. He spoke calmly in measured sentences, avoiding eye contact: "I knew Moshe for about eight years. We met on the net and had some social interaction during surgical conferences. I wanted him to join me. Unfortunately, what I learned about Moshe over the last few months is not what I was expecting or hoping for."

"Be specific, Jack. Provide examples?" I hissed.

"Well, to start with Moshe, I do not appreciate how you manage patients. Your bedside manners are inappropriate."

"What?!" I jumped up

"Let him speak," the CEO interjected.

"I am not satisfied with how you operate," Jack continued in the same controlled fashion," you don't seem to have any respect for the tissues."

"Examples! Provide examples — do not bullshit." There is nothing more hurtful to a surgeon than being told that his operative technique is faulty. Jack's comments penetrated my flesh like stab wounds.

"I assisted you on that colon case. I saw how you'd closed her abdomen. It was awful to watch." He was referring to the colon resection that had leaked.

"Please, Jack, do not teach me how to close bellies. I close my abdomens as is written in textbooks, and I don't have any problems with the results of my closure. I do not recall having an abdominal dehiscence or evisceration. Now, if your method is different — it is your problem, not mine."

"Moshe, you wanted examples, and I give you examples, and I will give you more. Patients and doctors don't appreciate the way you function. Therefore, I do not want to be associated with you anymore. You must leave town or relocate to a separate practice."

I looked at the CEO. He appeared pale and distressed — apparently, he did not expect the meeting to evolve this way.

"Jack, you are bullshitting again. Who is not happy with me? Provide names. Don't bullshit." I was angry. I knew that Jack had problems with me but did not suspect how deep his loathing of me was.

"First, look at the gallbladder you didn't want to remove. The patient was furious, and so was Willy." Willy was the patient's physician — an old buddy of Jack.

"But Jack, there was no indication to operate. The fact that you do hundreds of unnecessary operations does not mean I have to do the same."

"Don't interrupt. Let me talk. The truth is that patients, as well as doctors, are not satisfied with you. The patient with ascites whom you had drained in the ER complained about your rough attitude, my patient with the biliary fistula you saw when I was away told me how painful the procedure you performed in the office on him, and a young hernia patient whom you'd booked for an operation, changed his mind and came to see me — he told me that you are not trustworthy."

I turned to the CEO: "You are walking around the hospital and speaking with OR nurses, floor nurses, doctors, right? Did anyone ever complain about the attitude of the new surgeon? Nurses were present in the ER or the office when I had that alleged poor attitude with those patients, right? Were there any formal complaints about me from any patient?"

"No, there were no complaints about you. Nothing of this sort has ever reached my ears," said the CEO stoically.

I continued. "I go out of my way to be nice to everyone, but this seems insufficient. Perhaps in this little town, I am too foreign to them? One of my worries about coming here was whether I would be accepted. Jack, you have practiced here for almost ten years. Everybody knows you; you have operated on everybody's father and grandmother. So, I assume that when that hernia guy went home after consulting me, his friends asked who his surgeon would be. The guy with an accent he probably replied. He's new, they may have said. Don't let the new guy touch you. Go to Dr. Jack; he did my father's hernia. And you, Jack, you encourage such an attitude, delighted to get all the referrals now, leaving me with nothing to do. How would it feel if I sent you to another country, where people talk another language, into a new system, where you are ignored — everybody's going to the local established surgeon?"

"I knew it, I knew it," Jack half giggled, "sooner or later, you'll start accusing us of being xenophobic, haters of foreigners. Before you suggest that we are anti-Semites, do not forget that my son is married to a Jewish girl in Chicago. The point is that I'm a much better surgeon than you are — I know it! Patients and doctors know it as well! You are using the fact that you are foreign and Jewish as a crutch."

I looked at the CEO. He seemed lost in our senseless argument, waiting for us to finish venting our anger. To Jack, I replied, "Your head is inflated like a balloon — your superiority complex as a surgeon is ridiculous. What matters are the results. There are many ways to do things, but you, isolated in a small town in Iowa for so many years, think your way is the highway. And you know what? You have a significant number of complications. I see them from time to time, including some serious errors in judgment. Do you wish me to provide you with a list?"

"I've been in practice for thirty-five years, and I was never sued!" Jack declared bombastically.

"As you well know, the number of lawsuits does not necessarily reflect the quality of care. And anyway, we didn't come here to talk about how good you are and how bad I am but to find solutions."

"Absolutely!" The CEO woke up, "Let us be constructive. Now, after you both have vented your emotions, please calm down and come to the point."

I realized that my only chance to survive would be to be pragmatic and positive; this would be what the CEO would appreciate. I said, "Jack wants me to leave town or resign from the Surgical Specialists of Keokuk, but I'm not going to do either. I can't. I plan to stay here, hopefully even after Jack retires. Basically, on a personal level, I like Jack" — I lied, of course, for at this moment all I wished was to kick his ass — "and I think I'll be able to continue our partnership on any level he wants. But we must accommodate each other. He must stop transmitting his negative feelings. A few days ago, a nurse came to me. She said that he's badmouthing me — this has to cease."

"Who is she? I need to know?" inserted Jack

During the discussion, voices were raised, and virulent sarcasm prevailed. But gradually, under the calm guidance of the ever-friendly CEO, our anger melted. I continued appeasing the CEO by telling Jack: "Look, I respect you as a surgeon. I go around town saying how excellent you are..."

"Moshe you know that I like you too, as a person," eventually Jack grunted.

"So Jack, let us try harder to coexist, but if you wish to divide our practice or use a separate letterhead, it is OK with me."

"No, Moshe, we'll keep everything as it is. I have to admit that until now, I haven't been encouraging referrals to you."

The CEO stretched in his chair, wiped his sweaty red face, and said, "Well, I'm happy that you guys got some catharsis, and it helped you restore your senses. Of course, the administration would like your partnership to continue. Separation of practices would cost us and would need a lot of explaining to do. Jack, you are a trusted and respected community member, which gives you an advantage over Moshe. And Moshe, we are delighted to have you in town. Gentlemen, from now on, please, any dispute between you, however minor it is, please conduct it through me, let me negotiate it. And now let us shake hands."

We shook hands, exited the room, and Jack dragged me to see a 'problem' patient, who turned out to be just an interesting case. I politely joined him.

After the meeting, I was thinking: so what now? Naturally, I was hurt. Over the years, nobody had accused me of being an incompetent surgeon. But I had to try to understand Jack's attitude, for this is how he was — pathologically competitive. He had to be the better surgeon, so those around him had to be incompetent. If I could, if it would have been a viable option in professional and financial terms, I would have left town. What was the point of taking abuse from that man? But going away would have hurt our interests. We had to survive here for at least a few years. I had to swallow my pride, continue, and do my best.

The alleged complaints of patients and lack of referrals were more problematic. I was investing much effort in being nice to patients: I sat down at their face level, conducting the encounter in a non-hurried and relaxed fashion, and never ended any interview without asking, "do you have any more questions?" I tried to insert humor and cheerfulness into the encounters when and if appropriate, and I tried to be friendly to those who seemed primitive or ignorant. However, I needed more than this; a few of them did not feel comfortable with me. After so many years in public hospitals — South Africa, Israel, Brooklyn, Bronx — my body language may have become too rough, too abrupt for the Midwesterners, with their highly mild manners and outgoingness. I could work on my Iowan social skills, but it would take time until the community considered me an equal alternative to Jack. I saw a long way ahead of me — frustration, isolation, and struggle.

I met Jack in the office the following day. He was polite and sounded philosophical, telling me how stressed he was about the whole affair, about the severe headache he had developed after last night's meeting. I even noticed a tear or two in the corner of his eyes. I was getting used to the abrupt changes of mood — piety and compassion followed by ruthless contempt, extreme humbleness intermingled with utter conceit. On that teary morning, he again mentioned a few of his complexes, including his humble origin and stature: "I'm short, too short, always the shorter kid around..." Jack was half an inch taller than I and commonly declared this critical fact to the OR nurses. It was hard to estimate how much, if at all, his wife was contributing to his psychological makeup. She had been his red-haired, Irish, high school sweetheart. Unfortunately, she did not age as gracefully as he did. Instead, she transmuted into a stout lady with thinning hair. Although they were portraying a happily married couple, I could sense the tension between them.

There was a deep bridge between Jack and I, a gap in mentality, character, past experiences, *weltanschauung*, and much more. Our relationship was doomed, but that morning, we both agreed to give it another chance.

* * * * *

The enduring tensions at work and the uncertainties about the future could not detract from the pleasures we took from country life. Never before had we experienced the four seasons so distinctly and acutely — so radically different from each other. The autumn was red and fiery, with vast amounts of dead leaves flying around, followed by a cruel, icy, and windy winter — lakes frozen, blocks of ice floating and blocking the Mississippi. Then spring would come, like a Mediterranean spring: gentle, fragrant buds and flowers, sparked by sunshine, warmth, and water, growing at top speed. And finally, the summer arrived — almost tropical — scorching and oppressively sultry.

And the numerous storms: rain storms, hail storms, frozen rain storms, tropical storms, snow storms — flooding our lakes, ripping up the dirt road, the lightning directly destroying an ancient giant oak tree. The nature around us was majestic: deer walking the woods, rabbits jumping in the brush, raccoons climbing the fences of the chicken coup, beavers damming the nearby brook, giant turtles crawling at the side of the lakes, and the lakes themselves, as I have already mentioned, were a fisherman's paradise — two hundred yards from our porch.

The lakes provided, from early spring until late autumn, a loud nocturnal orchestra dominated by the baritone of bullfrogs. In winter, the nights were so silent that we could hear the blood flowing in our ears — that is when the turbines in the nearby railway wheel factory were not groaning and grinding.

It is all that I did: work, fish, read and write, and walk around the property. Heidi instructed aerobic classes at the YMCA, worked a few days a week at an antiques mall, and looked after the garden and chickens. We did not socialize much except the occasional dinner with Stan, our handyman, and Howie, the estate agent who had sold us the house. We did not attend church, play golf, or own a yacht. Thus, we were not members of the golf or yacht club, respectively — to which the "who is who" in town had to belong. This mostly self-induced isolation possibly contributed to my eventual downfall. To survive and prevail in a small town like Keokuk, one needed a certain political support base from the community.

* * * * *

Thanksgiving 2004.

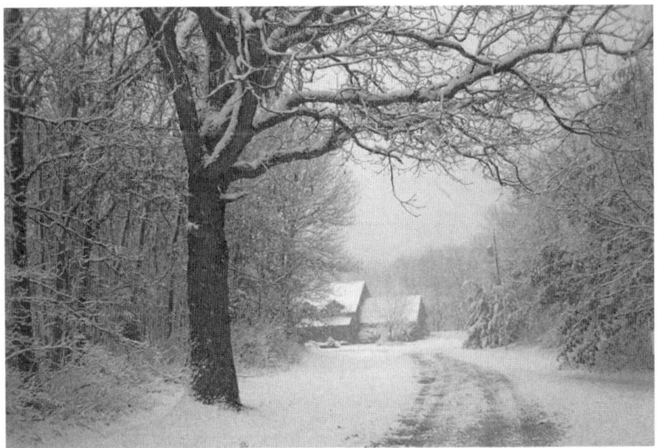

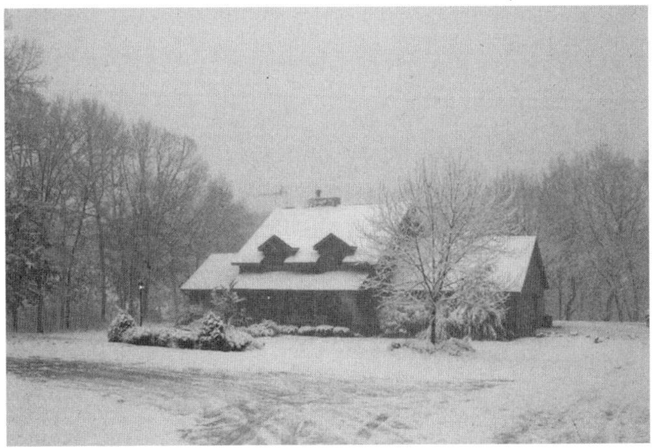

Fifty-two

It could have been a good year

A tense and awkward cease-fire between Jack and I persisted during the winter of 2005. We continued sharing calls, covering each other, but with minimal interaction. I sensed that he was 'observing' me, waiting for the opportunity to strike. The casket of dynamite was ready, but the match to ignite the fuse was missing.

From my notes:

> A big fight! Yesterday, when I returned from the OR to my office, I found a handwritten note signed by Jack on my table. It read: "I noticed you had scheduled a colonoscopy for 2/23. You have done a few others since December. My recollection of our last meeting with the CEO was that you would not perform colonoscopies any longer. Let me know if you have a different opinion. Jack."
>
> I replied by e-mail: "Jack, yes, I have done a few colonoscopies since then, and I recall having called you once or twice when I had some uncertainties, and you were kind enough to come in. You kindly offered to teach me colonoscopy, which had not been a part of my practice in the big city. To be independent, I must do many of these procedures under your supervision or with you on 'standby.' Whether you want to supervise and assist me is in your hands. There are two colonoscopies scheduled for tomorrow. I will be glad if you continue supporting me; if not, you are most welcome to scope these patients tomorrow. I will see you tomorrow morning at the trauma meeting, and you can tell me then what you've decided. Take care, Moshe."
>
> Today at 7 a.m., Jack and I met at the trauma meeting. We nodded politely to each other. After the meeting, we walked together towards the OR. In the corridor, I asked, "So what did you decide, Jack?"
>
> "We've got an agreement that you won't do colonoscopies," he persisted.
>
> "Never! We never had such an agreement," I insisted.
>
> I was standing against the wall with Jack close to me. I could smell the early morning double cappuccino on his breath. "You're lying, you're not honest, you always lie, like in that operative report of the colectomy case," he said, bringing his face — distorted with anger and hostility — closer and closer to mine. It was then that I reflexively placed my forehead onto the bridge of his nose. He withdrew a few steps,

massaging his bruised nose with his hand. He succeeded in restraining himself and did not strike back at me. I looked left and right: no one had witnessed this. *Good!*

"You assaulted me!" Jack hissed — or was he crying? — "I'm going to the CEO."

"I assaulted nobody; you brought your face into mine. OK, let's go up to the CEO," I said, following Jack up the stairs.

We stormed into the CEO's office, finding him having his early morning coffee and reading the *Des Moines Register*. Jack, still nursing his nose in his right hand, exclaimed, "He assaulted me. He head-butted me!"

"He lies," I retorted. And so it went on again, like two toddlers in a kindergarten. Jack turned to the CEO and said: "Don't you remember that he agreed not to perform colonoscopies?"

The CEO sighed: "Sorry, Jack, but I do not remember that such an agreement had been discussed."

Jack pointed his finger at the CEO: "If this is how you support me after eight years… and I thought you were my friend… I am resigning." In mid-sentence, he turned around and stormed out of the office.

"Jack, Jack, stop, stop, come back," the frustrated CEO stood up, shouting at the open door. But Jack was gone.

"Leave him. Let him go. He needs a psychiatric evaluation," I said with contempt. I then went to the OR to perform the two colonoscopies, for which David, one of the internists, agreed to back me up.

On the same day, late afternoon, I saw Jack loading books and pictures onto his F-150, parked outside the Surgical Specialists of Keokuk building. Later on, I noted that the door to his office was unlocked — our office doors were lockless, but some weeks prior, Jack had installed one on his door. *Paranoia?* His room was bare and empty. Where did he go?

* * * * *

From that day, Jack decided to separate himself unilaterally from our practice. He continued seeing patients in our building but did not 'reside' there.

He acted on a few fronts: demanding the CEO to formally separate our practice and evict me to another hospital-owned location; laying a complaint against me before the Executive Committee of the Medical Staff for the alleged assault; and spreading rumors about my questionable surgical skills — including an alleged excessive rate of postoperative wound infections. He could not make a formal complaint to the quality assurance bodies because he had no evidence whatsoever to support such claims.

On my part, I asked the CEO to hire an outside surgical expert to assess the quality of surgical care I had provided hitherto and my surgical skills. I demanded that such a person be brought from out of state — not one of Jack's acquaintances from Iowa City. I also requested the CEO to poll the patients I had treated to refute Jack's reproach about my deficient relations with patients. Such a poll was organized, and the CEO reported an "excellent" level of patient satisfaction. A 'surgical leader' willing to review my practice was located in Boston and scheduled to arrive in May.

The CEO, after prolonged consultations, issued a document entitled "Administrative Decisions," which called for complete separation of practices, with me vacating the office and moving to another building to allow for Jack's return. I agreed but pleaded to delay my move pending the assessment of the Bostonian reviewer.

The Executive Committee of the Medical Staff convened to discuss Jack's allegation about my physical assault on him. I denied everything. There were no witnesses to the event, but the Committee perceived that something must have happened because Jack's nose had been observed to be traumatized. Nevertheless, the committee members — familiar with Jack's overt and covert crusade against me, a few of them not recognized as his admirers — appeared sympathetic to my case.

On April 29, 2005, I was called before them to hear the verdict that was voiced by the Chairman, Dr. Philips, the Chief of Radiology, who, over the previous months, had become my confidant and non-formal adviser: "Moshe, we understand that the first months in Keokuk have been very stressful and frustrating for you. We do realize that any specific speech or action under consideration needs to be evaluated in its context. It is certainly clear to the members of the Executive Committee that the circumstances that confronted you were contributory. Nevertheless, the Committee has found that your behavior was verbally abusive and involved inappropriate physical contact."

"But there were no witnesses to that encounter," I objected.

"Yes, we understand that your personal space was invaded, and you reacted," interjected Art, another radiologist, the only African American on the staff. Philips ignored him and continued: "While understanding the specific circumstances, we have to warn you that any future incident of shouting, threatening, profanity, physical contact, or any disruptive speech… will meet with the consequences as outlined in the Medical Staff Bylaws, section IV, including options for limitation, suspension or termination of privileges."

A few days later, the CEO summoned me: "You do not have to vacate your office; you're staying where you are. Jack has just resigned from the hospital's full-time staff. He is moving to a small hospital across the river." I sensed that the CEO was happy for me.

"So from now on, I'm the only surgeon in Keokuk?"

"Until we find you a partner, you will be the only full-time surgeon on the staff. Don't worry; we'll get you a locum whenever you wish to rest or go out of town."

The CEO must have read the deep relief in my face. He added: "However, Jack will maintain operative privileges in our hospital."

"I understand," I replied. "Jack has planned it well: a lucrative full-time day job across the river, private operations in our hospital, and no night calls. So he'll continue drawing on our referral base?"

"Moshe, we'll do everything to support you. And by the way, I've rescinded today the visit of that Boston surgeon. The Executive Committee maintains that now that Jack has left, this would be a waste of money. After all, we believe that the allegations concerning your performance were not serious."

* * * * *

After twenty-five years in practice, I was starting to lose my surgical confidence. Before Keokuk, I was confident that I knew what to do, how to do it, when not to do things, and when to refer to people who can do it better. I knew that often, I knew more than others did, and people would ask me what to do. Now, the situation had changed. In Keokuk, I realized that it did not matter what I had done in the past, what I knew, what I had written, or what had been written in literature. What mattered now was what Jack would say about me. And no one was around — for we were the only two surgeons — to arbitrate, defend me, and say, "Hey, this guy's all right."

While a certain degree of uncertainty is inherent in anything we do as surgeons, and taking risks is what we are accustomed to doing, now I sensed an increasing anxiety when being uncertain. Whereas in the past, I accepted that uncertainty is part of the 'game,' now I tortured myself on what previously were easy decisions. During operations, I would search for a single red blood cell, like a junior resident. After the operation, I would excessively worry about the outcome: will the anastomosis hold? — like I had worried after my first independent anastomosis many years ago. On some patients, I would round five times a day — not that it was necessary — but to relieve my anxieties. I was like a chef, who only a few months ago taught in a French cooking school — who used to scold young cooks for overcooking the béarnaise sauce — now standing in front of a lowly pot of chicken soup, not sure whether to add salt or pepper and how much. I was convinced that if the soup was too salty or too bland, Jack would use it against me.

Often, during these months, awaiting the next blow from Jack, I thought that what was happening to me, which seemed surreal, was what had happened to my enemies at the New York Methodist Hospital in Brooklyn. What I felt now — the isolation, threat, decreasing confidence — was, paradoxically, what Sorkhi and Mantzur must have felt when we drove them out of the hospital and took away their licenses. I asked myself, is this karma?

One morning, Dr. Delgado stopped me in the corridor between the cafeteria and the library: "Dr. Schein, how are you? Can you spare me a few minutes? I've got to tell you something." He grasped my left elbow, dragging me to the deserted doctors' lounge. As we sat down, he exposed a broad set of bright teeth, grinned, and, looking directly into my eyes, said: "Fuck them!"

"Fuck who?" It was my first contact with Dr. Delgado since I had arrived in town, except for one brief "hi" when Jack had introduced him to me.

"Fuck them, fuck everybody, just smile like I do, see?" another white grin, "and say fuck you. I know the story, trust me, I've been here almost thirty years, they tried to do it to me, but I'm still here, good life, good money. They say that you enjoy fishing, eh? So go and fish and don't care about what Jack is doing and about referrals. Just have fun, smile, and fuck them. We've met in the OR on your first day, remember? I could've warned you then, but it was too early, you wouldn't have understood, now you do, hah?"

"Dr. Delgado, when exactly did you arrive in this town?" I tried to intercept his monologue. All I knew about him was that he, a slightly built man in his mid-sixties, was a semi-retired general surgeon with an office across the river, who occasionally used our OR. From the scrub nurses' remarks, I gathered that he was 'nice,' did mainly colonoscopies and minor operations, and operated well.

"Oh, I came over many years ago. I'm oriental, you see, from the Philippines. Have you met any Filipinos in New York? I worked hard and was taking calls, but they never offered me a salary or a contract — like yours. The surgeon who'd worked here before Jack was excellent; we worked well together but he left. Want to hear more about Jack? Go up to northern Iowa and ask."

"Ask what? What would they say?"

"Just go and ask. Jack used to call me a 'hack' as well — did I care? You are lonely? You need somebody to help you at night, you know, to support your feet, like this" (he went on his knees and touched my ankle)… "just call me anytime. You want to get more confident in colonosopies, come and do it with me, any time, we orientals are open, we carry our hearts in our hands."

"But Dr. Delgado, I met many nice people here, positive, supportive."

A look of disdain. "Supportive? All they do is smile like this." Another grin. "When they walk away," now he was pacing across the room to demonstrate the point, "they think to themselves *fuck him*; do you understand?" He stopped pacing and stooped over a chair, showing me his behind; with his index finger he pointed to his butt: "See, they want to fuck you in here, don't let them!"

* * * * *

The end of May brought the best days of that year. The rain was over, the sky blue, and a gentle wind was stirring the young foliage on the trees, rippling the brown waters of the lakes. The smell of wild herbs and freshly cut grass brought to mind alpine meadows in summer. Only the ringing of cowbells was missing. It was a perfect spring; never before had we been immersed in the country for so long. We enjoyed every minute.

After my archenemy left the practice, I felt reassured and more confident. At the same time, I warned myself not to be euphoric and forced on myself a certain, healthy dose of paranoia; Jack still lives in town, he keeps his privileges in the hospital; Rachel, the OR director, is still his friend — watch your back Schein! Smile, do your job, and hope that as soon as you find a new partner, they won't try to get rid of you — a known tactic of "let him find his replacement."

And indeed, after a decade of surgical reign, Jack had left behind a few well-entrenched devotees. Chief among them was nurse Rachel, a solidly built, plain-looking middle-aged woman. It was well known that Rachel and Jack attended the same Catholic church and ate Sunday breakfast together — with their respective spouses — at the Hy-Vee food store; when Jack and his wife were out of town, Rachel would look after their house and walk their incontinent dog.

Local 'historians' could tell that before becoming the OR director, Rachel had been Jack's office nurse, and there was, *allegedly*, something more significant between the two. Rachel was good at her job: strict and organized, she led a well-functioning OR. From the start, Rachel's attitude towards me had reflected Jack's. The honeymoon had been short-lasting; then, concurrent with Jack's crusade, she had become cold and remote but still professional. But as soon as Jack resigned, she became overtly hostile and finally started boycotting me. "Good morning, Rachel," I would say when entering the OR. She would look away. While initially she would scrub on my cases or assign one of the more senior assistant nurses, now she kept her silent distance and dispatched the younger, newer staff to my OR. Occasionally, however, because of a shortage of OR staff, Rachel had to take night calls; this compelled her into direct contact with me.

On one such night, she had to assist me in a laparotomy of a grossly obese patient: she did it 'automatically' and did not utter a word. She did not move her hands unless I told her to relocate them, and then she let them re-freeze in their new position. It was like operating with a human mechanical retractor, a metal retractor but one with an active thought process, one which despises you and wishes a disaster on your procedure. After I complained to the CEO that I found it challenging to operate with Rachel, she did not scrub with me anymore; instead, she would stand against the wall, sulking, blaming me with a pair of hostile eyes for the resignation of her surgical hero. I tried to ignore her, but the atmosphere in the OR was not the same — no jokes, no laughter, very tense. Her hawk eyes were watchful: how fast is he? How much blood did he lose? Oh, is he going to open this laparoscopic case? Jack wouldn't convert!

Sometimes, on leaving the OR, I would observe Jack — he would visit occasionally — and Rachel immersed in an intimate conversation in her little office. I knew that I was under constant scrutiny by them: anything and everything I did, which may appear questionable to them, was probably recorded.

Was I paranoid? Yes. I had to practice surgery as if I was an alleged juvenile sex offender working in a kindergarten.

However, the summer of 2005 was kind to me. I worked hard, and it seemed, at least to me, that my position as Keokuk's main surgeon was stabilizing. It appeared that my ex-partner's plan to attract most of Keokuk's patients was unsuccessful. Since he was unavailable for emergency calls, all surgical emergencies went to me. This allowed me to prove myself to skeptical physicians, who until then had remained on the fence but leaned towards Jack. Also, the group of three internists — the jewel of Keokuk's medicine — decided to refer solely to me, which solidified my position. And the 'goddess of surgeons' stayed on my side so that the outcome of whatever I did, however difficult and complex, was favorable. Reassured about my long-term prospects in Keokuk, we had a swimming pool constructed on the lawn between the house and the lake to find refuge from the sweltering prairie days.

In September, we celebrated our first year in Keokuk. A month later, at the conclusion of the monthly meeting of the medical staff, the Chairman, the radiologist Bill Philips, unexpectedly said: "I hope you'll all join me in a few words of appreciation for Dr. Schein, who was left alone to carry our surgical load and is doing such a good job…" Everyone clapped his or her hands. I produced a severe face, nodded my thanks to the Chairman, and then mockingly looked towards the CEO and said: "I don't need applause, but I demand a new Cadillac in return for my efforts." Laughter: the loud but polite chuckle professional Americans allow themselves in such circumstances, to alleviate the constant interpersonal tension and distrust, deceitfully confirming that yes, after all, we are all such good friends.

It could have been a good year…

* * * * *

Keokuk, Iowa, in the Summer of 2005 when the boys (from left to right: Omri, Yariv, Dan) came to visit; Pavlo, RIP, sitting on the left.

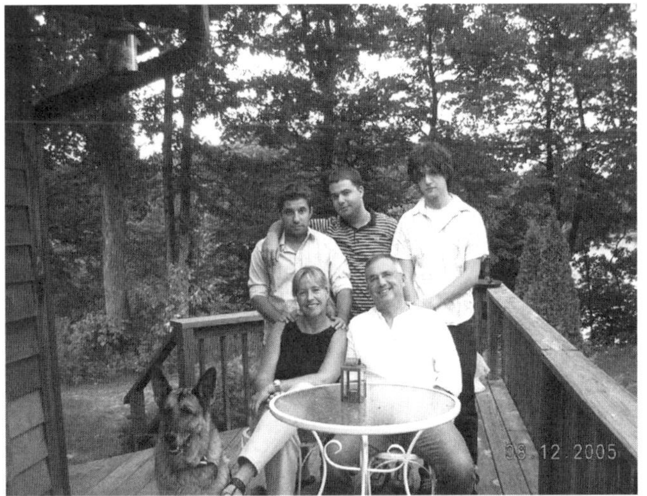

Fifty-three

Indira of Keokuk

Early October 2005. The situation suddenly started deteriorating. As is often the case, I did not realize then that I was sliding down a slippery slope. As expected, Jack and Rachel orchestrated the evolving events, but the personality who provided the motive to unleash the onslaught against me was Dr. Ravikumar — our anesthesiologist. To myself, I called her "Indira" since she looked like Indira Gandhi: petite, slim, dark-skinned. Outside the OR, she was always clad in a traditional sari, wearing elaborate Indian gold jewelry. After training in India and Pittsburgh, she arrived in Keokuk almost thirty years ago, becoming the sole local anesthesiologist.

Indira was married to an Indian-born psychiatrist; together, they represented a 'royal,' rural couple — an Indian-styled mansion on the river, a private airplane, a collection of Rolls-Royces, Bentleys, and Mercedes, stocks in many local businesses, ownership of agricultural land, and influential seats on some of the city and county civic boards.

Indira ruled her small anesthesia department (she employed two nurse anesthetists) and the OR like a queen. At the same time, she was hard-working, readily available, and a careful, albeit old-fashioned, anesthesiologist.

My relationship with her had been 'correct' during the first year — almost cordial. Often between cases, she would tell me about herself and her family — repeatedly emphasizing her "superb training in Pittsburgh," where she "could have stayed on as a professor." Typically, however, she never asked me any questions. She did not seem to like Jack, with whom she had a few unpleasant encounters over the years, but never took sides in my ongoing conflict with him.

Once, I remember, she approached me at the sink where I was scrubbing for an operation: "Moshe, do you have any social life here? Do you meet people?"

"Yes, a couple or two, we have an occasional dinner with them."

"They don't like us foreigners, you know. We have invited local people to our place over and over again. They never reciprocate. People need company, we need to meet and eat together." I made a mental note: *we must invite them for dinner*. It would never materialize.

From my notes:

> 1 October 2005. In the morning, I had an unpleasant confrontation with Dr. Ravikumar, our lady anesthesiologist. Larry is a middle-aged alcoholic from across the river who, for a few months, has been begging me to repair his large and unsightly abdominal incisional hernia.

"You are high risk for such an operation. You have cirrhosis. Why don't you have the operation at the University Hospital?" I kept telling him. However, because he is not insured, the University Hospital would not accept him for an elective operation. "OK, I will operate on you if you stop drinking for three months," I told him eventually, "But I won't touch you if I smell even a drop on you." So Larry stopped drinking, and his liver function normalized. I referred him to David, my internist buddy, who agreed that a hernia repair would be reasonably safe. I sent him to the hospital's financial office, where arrangements to pay in installments for the operation had been worked out.

The operation was scheduled for this morning at 8 a.m.; however, at 7.45 a.m., when I walked into the OR, I was surprised to find Dr. Ravikumar standing at the reception desk, clad in her red sari, instead of attending to my patient. She said: "Dr. Schein, your patient is not a candidate for an operation. He has cirrhosis, you know. Let him have his hernia repaired at the University Hospital. It's perilous to do him here." She did not pause for a breath but continued: "and he can't pay us." I was furious: why did she cancel my patient five minutes before the operation? But arguing with her would not help: "Your patient is drunk. He smells of alcohol!" said the Indian woman.

I stormed out of the OR and complained to the CEO in writing:

"…Of course, anesthesia has the right to discuss and question the fitness of patients and the indications for operations, but for elective cases, this should not take place minutes before the planned operation in an already starved and stressed patient. Patients are seen and assessed a few days before the operation at ambulatory surgery — this is when anesthesia should screen them. What they did with this patient was inappropriate, dysfunctional, and unethical. I contend that they have to apologize to the patient for calling him 'drunk' and canceling his surgery for non-medical reasons…"

5 October 2005. Dr. Ravikumar did not return my greetings. *Oh well. Who cares?!*

This afternoon, when I reviewed a CT with Bill Philips, he said: "Moshe, I have to tell you this: you cannot be confrontational. Letters to the CEO are counterproductive. Dr. Ravikumar is scared of you. Other doctors told me this as well. Everybody knows about your Brooklyn story. They know that you blew the whistle on some docs."

Well, it seems that Jack's propaganda is effective… But is my friend Philips a friend or a plant? I had a tackle with the anesthesiologist despite my utmost efforts to appear peaceful and benign. Notwithstanding my pledge to change — I'm still irritated when patients are mistreated.

November 7, 2005. The CEO called me this morning: "Moshe, a woman has just left my office. She'd dropped in to tell me that… this is her version… that the new surgeon, that must be you, hah, 'gave her the finger.' According to her, it'd happened yesterday at the intersection of Main and 9th Street. To make matters more interesting, the woman is none other than the wife of John Smith — you may know him; he's the President of the hospital's Board of Trustees. So I thanked her for informing me about the incident and promised to investigate her complaint. Moshe, I can't believe that you showed her the finger. Tell me what happened?"

It took me a moment to correlate this with yesterday's minor incident. I had left the hospital at lunchtime, driving slowly toward Main Street. I didn't follow my usual route but turned into Blondeau Street. Immersed in thoughts, I missed a stop sign. When crossing the intersection, I noticed a car turning in from the left, with its driver waving her fist at me. I smiled and waved back, turning the palm of my hand up, like, "I'm sorry." When I arrived at the intersection with Main Street, the other driver pulled her car along mine and continued waving her fist.

I opened the window and shouted, "I am sorry." Realizing she couldn't hear, I stepped out of the car; I wanted to approach her and explain. By then, the traffic lights changed to green, and she sped off. I shrugged to myself and forgot the incident.

The CEO listened to my version and said: "Sure. I knew it had to be some misunderstanding. But please write her a nice letter, explain and apologize. Welcome to the joys of small-town America…"

That's all I needed to have a problem with the President of the Board of Trustees. I met him once after operating on the infected hand of his daughter — she seemed to me a drug addict, and I suspected that the cause of the infection had been a human bite, but I said nothing. John Smith appeared to be a friendly and reasonable gentleman. But they say his wife is as crazy as the daughter, and now she's after me. Why? Why should she have interpreted a friendly hand wave as the 'F sign'?

November 14, 2005: Monday. What a day!

Just after 8 a.m., I brought a patient (Mrs. A.M., who had been involved in a car accident) from the ER to the OR for an emergency laparotomy for intra-abdominal bleeding.

In the OR corridor, I spotted my ex-partner, Jack, concluding one of his frequent morning social visits to nurse Rachel. I overheard him questioning the indication for the operation ("Why doesn't he ship her out?"). I thus predicted that Rachel would be dispatched to the room to observe — *what is Schein up to?*

During the brief laparotomy, I found a significant amount of free blood originating from the shattered spleen. I removed the spleen. The patient had multiple associated injuries that we could not evaluate appropriately before the operation; therefore, my intention was not to extubate her after the operation but to take her immediately for a CT of the head and chest. At that stage, before the CT, I had not decided as yet in my mind whether I wanted to keep her or airlift her out. So, after I closed the abdomen, beginning to suture a deep laceration in the patient's arm, I said to Indira: "Please do not plan to remove her endotracheal tube. Keep her sedated until I decide."

"She's waking up," interrupted the anesthesiologist, "I can't keep the tube in, she's in bronchospasm, better to let her breathe on her own." Before I started to object... the tube was already out. The patient was transferred to the recovery room.

Ten minutes later, when I emerged from the changing room, where I had dictated the operative note, I found Indira and a bunch of nurses crowding around the patient's bed. I saw a positive pressure mask — one of Indira's old-fashioned rituals — fitted over the patient's mouth. "What's up?" I asked.

"She's not breathing too well. She's still bronchospastic. We'll try this mask and give some bronchodilators," Indira explained. I looked at the monitor's screen: O_2 saturation of 85 percent, *shit*. I felt the patient's pulse: 140 and feeble. "Can we get a portable X-ray, please, now!" I said.

"She's still spastic," repeated Indira.

"Look at her left chest. See how it swells up," said a recovery room nurse. She was right! I touched the chest and felt the crunchy air under the skin: *surgical emphysema!* She was blowing a tension pneumothorax!

I felt for the femoral pulse, but there was none: *she's dying on us*. "Give me a chest tube," I shouted, "reintubate her now."

The chest tube went into the left thorax with a loud *pssssssssss* as the pressurized air was hissing out. We took a portable chest X-ray. While I was fixing the chest tube to the skin, Bill Philips rushed in with the chest X-ray film in his hand: "Moshe, the other lung is totally collapsed."

Within thirty seconds, I had another chest tube in, draining the right thorax as well. The patient stabilized and started to improve. Now I was able to gather my thoughts: *she had survived a few minutes without functioning lungs!* Only a minute or two separated her from death. I also understood now what it was that had almost 'killed' this patient: it was my good old friend Indira. Obviously, the left pneumothorax had already developed during the operation, resulting from associated lung injury that had not been apparent before the anesthesia (not seen on the chest X-ray in the ER). Instead of looking for and treating the cause of the emerging respiratory difficulties, Indira had blamed it all on bronchospasm. Instead of ordering a chest X-ray, she removed the tracheal tube. When the patient continued to deteriorate, she used that positive ventilation mask, which pumped air under pressure into the other lung, injuring it as well.

With the two lungs recovering, the patient was improving rapidly. Still, I decided to ship her away anyway: she'd need to be ventilated, and it was better to do it in a proper intensive care unit. While the chopper crew was 'packing' the patient for the airlift, I told Indira: "You see, this started during the operation. You should not have removed the endotracheal tube."

This episode impressed the bystanders. Many people were present in the recovery room, watching me save that patient's life. But Indira was not impressed — she continued talking about that imaginary bronchospasm. In her mind, she did the right thing.

It took only another week, when fate brought me another encounter, this time a 'terminal' encounter with Indira.

From my notes:

Saturday, November 19. Another drama with Indira yesterday. Friday late afternoon, after a long day — I'd done a few emergencies already — Dr. L., our obstetrician, summoned me to see a woman in her 23rd week of pregnancy who had presented with acute cholecystitis. Together with the obstetrician, we agreed that the best approach would be to proceed with an operation to remove the gallbladder. In the OR, after placing the patient under general anesthesia, Indira approached me at the scrubbing sink. She said: "What you are doing is dangerous for the baby... no one would perform a laparoscopic cholecystectomy during pregnancy."

"Who says it is dangerous? You?"

"Well, in Pittsburgh, no one would operate on a pregnant patient," Indira was mumbling.

"Nonsense," I exclaimed, "perhaps you have to update yourself after all those years. Take some CME!"

Of course, we both were irritated and shouted at each other. Nurse Rachel arrived and joined the discussion... I closed the OR door in her face using my foot and told her to leave the room. She replied: "I can't. I must see that the patient is doing OK while you two are arguing." "Just leave," I told her, "you make me nervous... and let me operate." I forced myself to calm down and took out the gallbladder. Today, the patient is well and going home. She is not aware of what a fierce argument her management had evoked.

Now, let's see the outcome of this. It is the third consecutive confrontation with Indira. She's good for routine cases, but her judgment is often faulty. But she's the Indira of Keokuk, the ruler of the Indian aristocracy with a wide-reaching influence. We'll see...

A week later, the CEO would tell me, "Moshe, the snowball is rolling..." Clearly, the snowball had started to roll on that Friday, or perhaps much earlier: that is when Jack had decided that he did not want me in Keokuk.

* * * * *

Fifty-four

The lynching

It was late afternoon on the Monday following the last scuffle with Dr. Indira. I was sitting in my underpants, dictating an operative report, when my friend Dr. Philips, radiologist and Chairman of the Medical Board, entered the OR changing room. He seemed agitated. I guessed instantly it had to do with last Friday's events.

"Moshe, you must appear before the Executive Committee of the Medical Staff tomorrow at 7 a.m. There are serious allegations against you by the Department of Anesthesia and the head OR nurse."

"Nonsense, Bill. Bullshit, yes, bullshit – this is my response. Look, I'm tired. I've been on call constantly for thirty days, had a rough weekend, and just finished a difficult laparotomy. Please let me dictate and leave me alone."

"Moshe, sorry, you'll present yourself tomorrow sharp at 7 a.m. We'll listen to your version of what happened."

"Bill, I knew that they would complain about me. I could have complained about them too, but what's the use? When I do complain, nobody listens. You know that it's all part of Jack's vendetta..."

"We'll discuss it tomorrow morning. See you then." He walked towards the door, but I stopped him, unable to suppress my rage and disgust: "No, Bill, I won't be there. I'm tired of playing to their tune. I'm not going to jump and reply to any frivolous accusation. That game is over for me. I'm tired and need to rest and think. I won't be there tomorrow morning."

"As you wish. But be aware that anesthesia has declared that, as of now, they won't provide anesthesia to your patients."

The following day, during morning rounds, Bill Philips paged me: "The meeting is postponed to 1.30 p.m. Will you appear? If not, we'll discuss it without hearing your version. It's your only chance."

"OK, I'll be there."

* * * * *

Again, we sit along the same long oak table. It was only six months since I was last sitting here, defending myself against Jack's allegations that I had assaulted him with a head-butt. What was their verdict? Was I reprimanded? Will they warn me to behave myself? So much has happened since and before. How can I remember the details of all the political troubles following me like tireless ghosts? Why don't they leave me alone?

As usual, the members of the Executive Committee of the Medical Staff enter the room one after the other, a few minutes late. I look around. Bill Philips, the radiologist, is the Chair. A WASP, originally hailing from the south, he has been — or so I think — sympathetic to my cause all along. To his right, I see Art's heavy bulk; he is our second radiologist, an African American hailing from Chicago. I like him: ever friendly — the only black doctor in town ought to support the case of the only Jew, right? On the left side of the table sits the 'Prince,' Dr. D: tall and gaunt — perhaps the only physician around who always wears a necktie — he is considered the leading physician in town. He did his graduate studies at Princeton and never fails to mention this to you. As the only physician born locally, he has become the established healer to Keokuk's VIPs. At his side sits Dr. H., a lanky Iowan, a pilot in his free time, and a partner to the Prince. On my right hand, I see Dr. Don Brown digging into a paper plate of chicken wings; he is our orthopedic surgeon and the rotating Chief of Surgery. Originally from Iowa City, he arrived in town only a year before me; he is of average height, chubby, with round eyeglasses on a pleasant face, contorted in an everlasting Midwestern grin. I perceive him as one who would never take sides overtly but take them covertly when it served his interests, while always maintaining that sunny Iowan oh-how-happy-we-are-loving-each-another attitude. *He's a potential enemy,* I make a mental note to myself; he spends too much time in Rachel's OR office.

Philips shuffles his papers and opens the meeting in his pompous, albeit civil, drawl. I do not listen. I know that politically correct garbage by heart: serious allegations, our role with regard to the medical staff… protect doctors from abuse… eradicate inappropriate behavior, blah, blah, blah. Instead, my mind is formulating immediate strategies; how should I respond? I sip from my cup of coffee and play with the thick volume of Medical Staff Bylaws, which I brought with me.

"Dr. Schein," concludes Philips, "would you please share with us your version of the events and respond to the allegations made against you by the anesthesiologist Dr. Ravikumar and Mrs. Rachel Kelly, the head OR nurse."

"Could I please see the specific allegations? According to the bylaws," I open the white volume, taking time to find the specific section, "here, section 6, second paragraph, I quote: 'A request for an investigation or action must be in writing, submitted to the Executive Committee of the Medical Staff.' Could I please see what's in their letters of complaint?"

"Well, the letters are being produced, but let me tell you what they accuse you of…" Bill consults one of his papers, "they use the words 'Dr.

Schein behaved in a loud and threatening fashion in the presence of witnesses.'"

"Yes, I understand. But before making any statement, I need to see their letters. Do you want me to reply to accusations that may affect my fate in this hospital without being able to see them?"

"Um. Look, Moshe, this session is *investigative*; we ask, and you reply. When and if the issue moves to the next *judiciary* stage, you'll have the right to view documents and bring your legal consultant. We need to move on. Please talk to us."

"Yes, just tell us what happened," says Dr. H. The others nod in agreement.

Don't surrender, do not yield. Obstinacy may pay off. I reply: "I need time to think and formulate my reply. I'm tired and stressed. I didn't sleep last night. I would prefer to reply in writing. You'll have my written version by tomorrow morning. I don't want to discuss the current allegation in isolation without bringing up the whole background. To me, it's all one story — an ongoing witch hunt, call it a lynching if you want — initiated against me by my ex-partner Jack and his buddies."

Silence. The Prince is the first to reply, serious as ever: "Be assured that we are aware of the specific background you allude to. But the hospital is now facing an urgent dilemma. We have to deal with it promptly. Therefore, we'll have to proceed with this investigation with or without your input."

"What's so urgent? Why can't you wait until tomorrow?" I persist.

"Dr. Ravikumar, after what took place last Friday, isn't ready to administer anesthesia to your patients. Mr. Terry, her nurse anesthetist, wouldn't work with you as well, and as you are our only surgeon, this is a serious matter."

Bastards. Let me spit it out then. I stand up. "I want to start with the background against which this episode is taking place…" I tell them about Jack's campaign again, his friendship with nurse Kelly, and her hostility towards me.

"Moshe," Bill Philips stops me, "let's focus on Dr. Ravikumar. Nurse Kelly's allegation is a side issue. Please carry on." Philips, who is seriously committed to transcendental meditation, has perfect manners.

"OK," I empty my cup: "Until last September, my relationship with Dr. Ravikumar seemed smooth. At least on my side, there was always an attitude of gentle and friendly respect. On the morning of that day — was it the 19th? — however, Dr. Ravikumar decided to cancel the scheduled elective hernia operation of a patient from Nauvoo…"

"Dr. Schein. I've discussed this case with you before. You were rude to her, arguing in the corridor," says Philips.

"Come on, Bill. It's your interpretation of events."

Philips looks at his watch, "We know the background. Why don't you come straight to the events of last Friday? A few of us have to go back to work."

"Sure, Bill, but please let me mention what occurred last Monday, just a few days before the key incident, OK?"

"Do you mean the trauma case? It has nothing to do with Friday's events. Please come to the point."

"But…"

"Look, Moshe, we are running out of time," said the tall internist H., who, as a part-time job, owned a few blocks of flats for rental. "This is only a preliminary meeting. You'll have another opportunity to address us if you wish. Now, please let us focus on last Friday. What happened?"

I sense that they are in control, and I am in their hands — all my resolutions to be obstinate, to dictate the pace of events, have now evaporated.

"OK. I'll tell you what happened on Friday," and I tell them about the pregnant patient with gallstones and how she arrived at the OR.

"So now I'm standing, scrubbing my hands like this," I imitate the procedure with my hands, "and then Dr. Ravikumar arrives at the sink, you know, to rinse her laryngoscope. She leans towards me and tells me that what I'm doing is dangerous, that one doesn't operate on pregnant ladies." Silence. They are listening attentively. "Then I asked her, why? Didn't she ever see people performing cholecystectomies in pregnant patients? She replied emotionally, her face near mine, that no, never, it is not done, it's dangerous to the child. So now I'm becoming upset… here I am busy scrubbing for the operation for which she has already agreed to anesthetize the patient, and she's telling me that what I do is dangerous. So I asked why didn't she discuss her anxieties before putting the patient to sleep. But Dr. Ravikumar doesn't listen and insists that it's dangerous… for the child… that she did obstetrics at Pittsburgh University, and never, ever saw anyone operating during pregnancy."

Now I walk towards the conference room's door with my hands raised. "So imagine that this is the open OR door. Now I'm moving towards the room holding my wet hands upwards, and on my left side, I see nurse Kelly, her face white; I know that she's arrived to see how I am abusing her old friend Ravikumar."

I do not tell them how ugly, contorted, and hateful was the nurse's face. Suddenly, I had had enough — why should I tell them anything? I'm exhausted. I return to my chair and whimper: "I can't go on… I'm too emotional…" I put my head between my hands — my emotion is real and fake at the same time — I know that some Americans appreciate naked emotion and a few tears.

Nobody says a word; they all look at me, waiting.

"I won't go on, I can't," I repeat.

Silence. I pour myself a glass of water.

Fuck them, should I leave?

Then I stand up and continue: "OK, let me finish the story. So here is my patient and her fetus, under anesthesia, induced by this anesthesiologist, who now claims that what I'm going to do is dangerous."

Again, I approach the door. "So my hands are wet and sterile, so obviously I can't touch Dr. Ravikumar, nor nurse Kelly, and therefore I can't threaten them whatsoever. I now walk through the open door into the OR, where Joan, who is nurse Kelly's daughter, and Mr. Becket, a scrub tech, are present. I don't remember who else was there, and as I walk into the room, I tell Dr. Ravikumar that she thinks what I'm doing is dangerous because she's outdated, that she needs to take a CME vacation, to educate herself. Then, when inside the room, I use my foot to shut the door behind nurse Kelly who is left outside. Of course, I can't use my sterile hands to do so. How often have I complained to the CEO that I don't wish to have nurse Kelly's interference during my operations? And now I wanted to calm down, restore my peace of mind needed to perform the operation."

"You used your foot to close the door in nurse Kelly's face, right?" Dr. Philips interrupts me.

"Yes, of course, I told you that my hands were sterile."

"How much force did you use to close the door?" asks the Prince.

"As much as needed to close the door."

"So you kicked the door, slammed it in her face, eh?"

"I used my foot, and you can term it however you wish." *What a moron!* "But then nurse Kelly opens the door and enters the room. I approach her, my hands now covered with a green towel I received from Mr. Becket to dry them, and I calmly say: 'Would you please leave the room, I can't operate like this, you make me nervous.' She says something like, 'I won't leave as long as you two are fighting.' I say: 'Just leave, the fight is over, now we have to operate.'"

Silence. I continue: "So now nurse Kelly leaves the room. We do the operation. No word is spoken. The patient wakes up and goes home the next day. After the operation I call the obstetrician and tell him about the episode. He comments laconically that Dr. Ravikumar had talked to him before the operation and had no problems whatsoever. I think that's all." I sit down.

"Moshe, do you have anything else to add, perhaps you forgot to say something?" asks the ever-polite Dr. H.

"Yes, Tom, I should add that my ex-partner is well known for throwing tantrums in the OR, abusing nurses, and making them cry. Did anyone complain about him?"

"Moshe, enough, hold on," interrupts Philips, "you'll have an opportunity to continue. Thank you for coming."

"Thanks guys." I leave the room.

* * * * *

Agitated and starved, I entered the adjacent doctors' lounge to find Dr. Delgado clearing the last doughnut from the tray. He flushed his toothpasty smile at me, like a bright sun shining in the background of his brown face: "So Moshe, they fucked you already?"

"How d'ya know?"

"The rule here is that everybody knows about everything within five minutes, and everybody pretends they know nothing. What they do is smile, smile. Hey, didn't I warn you?"

"Yes, you did… but, you know, this is minor. I have survived heavier fire before; they speak, show you how important they are, and only play at being judges or umpires…"

But Delgado was not listening. His smile did not leave his face when he turned around and showed me his butt, as he had done before, and pointed to his anus. "Is your ass stretched enough, Moshe? I hope it is because they are going to fuck you big time. Did you ever believe that your ex-partner would let you take over Keokuk's surgery? Besides, you have underestimated Dr. Ravikumar, don't you know that she and her husband own half of the property in town? Never underestimate the Brahmins, whether they are fuckin' white or Indians. What did I tell you? I told you to smile and keep your ass tight. And what did you do — you relaxed the anal sphincters. You have boys in college, eh? Like me? We have to continue to provide for them. I wish you good luck." He pressed my hand and left the room, still smiling widely with snow white teeth.

Half an hour later, just as I entered my office, a secretary informed me that Dr. Philips had just called. "They want you immediately back in the conference room." I rushed across the street, through the back gate of the hospital, and re-entered the meeting room. They were still sitting, like when I had left them earlier.

"Thanks for coming back," said Dr. Philips, "please sit down." I did. Philips continued with all the gravitas he had gathered as a head boy in his private school in Georgia and later as a president of some obscure college fraternity: "The Executive Committee of the Medical Staff has discussed at length the serious allegation against you and decided to temporarily revoke your operative privileges in this hospital, pending an investigation. According to the bylaws, we must report any revocation of temporary or permanent privileges to the National Practitioner Data Bank. To avoid this, at this stage, you may voluntarily ask for a vacation as of today."

I was stunned. *Those boys are moving fast!* I looked around the table and said: "You do surprise me, guys. Did all of you vote to suspend me? No one was against?"

"We didn't vote," replied Dr. H., "This is a preliminary hearing. We had to solve an acute situation before the Thanksgiving weekend. We'll continue next week. Anesthesia won't work with you, so the problem is now solved as you won't operate and won't be on call."

"And who will provide care for surgical emergencies in my absence?"

"No problem, the ER will be instructed to ship them elsewhere," said Philips laconically.

"Look, guys, I don't mind a short vacation, but I must tell you I'm surprised. I did nothing wrong."

"Moshe, the Executive Committee of the Medical Staff will conduct a careful hearing next week after Thanksgiving. We'll call witnesses. You'll have a chance to speak again. Until then, enjoy the holidays, everyone. This meeting is adjourned."

* * * * *

That afternoon, I dropped in at the CEO's office. He had always been friendly and supportive. I knew, however, that he was wedged between the Trustees, above, and the medical staff, below — his existence depended on his ability to satisfy both, which was impossible. Behind his courteous and smooth Mid-American façade, I had noticed seeds of fairness and remnants of a rebellious personality — in his free time, he was writing playscripts — partially suppressed by many years of managerial occupation.

As I walked through his open door, he turned around from his computer and shook my hand. He didn't say, as usual, "What's up?" — he knew already.

"I'm suspended, you know?" I uttered.

The CEO looked at me and said nothing.

"What now? Who will take over my patients?"

"From what I understand, you can continue seeing your in-house and office patients. But no operating and no ER calls. Now you can enjoy your red wine." A faint smile.

"What are my chances?"

I noticed him tensing up, forcing himself to look at my eyes: "Moshe, it seems to me that the snowball is rolling…"

As I left his office, I saw the President of the Board of Trustees waiting to see the CEO. I nodded and smiled at him, but he did not notice me. *What is he doing here?* It was his crazy wife who had that delusion about me showing her the finger. *Is he here to discuss me, or am I paranoid?*

The snowball is rolling. What does it mean? Rolling in which direction? On my way out, I stopped at radiology, where I found Bill Philips mumbling ten words per second into his microphone, dictating yet another radiology report. Each day, I had come to this room to review images with him, and we would talk about restaurants, politics, and gossip. He and his wife had dined at our home, but we were yet to be invited by them — "after we move to our new house."

I asked: "Bill, what exactly would the next stage be? Should I get a lawyer? Will I be able to call on witnesses? Can I be present during the proceeding?"

"I advise you to study the bylaws, hmm. I'm sure you already did. The next phase will be investigatory. We'll ask questions, and we may take action. No, you don't have the right to call in your witnesses, and you can't be present — this is all confidential. However, depending on the outcome, you can ask for a judiciary hearing, which is more like a court proceeding, with your lawyer, a court recorder, the whole spiel." Bill had trained in Boston and liked to show off his Yiddish. "I hope you have full trust in the members of the Executive Committee. They are all your friends, and you can exclude any of us if you think there may be some conflict of interest."

"Thanks, Bill. I trust you all. However, I'm not sure about Brown — he's too cozy with Rachel Kelly."

"No problem. What about Dr. L.? He is a respected and long-term member of the staff."

"Sure. I've no problem with him; actually, that pregnant lady with the gallstones was his patient. But Bill, why not stop the bullshit? Can't you negotiate a ceasefire with Dr. Ravikumar? You know I'm not as difficult as she tries to portray me. Ask the nurses in the OR how nice I am with them."

"Hmm, are you sure that they will come out to defend you? Don't forget their loyalty to Kelly and Dr. Ravikumar. Again, the Executive Committee doesn't care much about Kelly — we must address Dr. Ravikumar's complaints. And she's scared of you. I'd warned you about this before. She's concerned about your Internet activity, your surgical discussion group."

"Look, Bill, how can she know? If I write something, it is to a limited Internet list or private friends."

"And what about Jack? Isn't he feeding her concerns?"

"Jack resigned from the Internet list almost a year ago."

"How can you be so sure?" The radiologist looked at me mockingly.

Later that night, I picked up the novel, *The Plot Against America*. But my mind was jittery and not prone to Roth's endless sentences — it was occupied with another plot — the plot against Schein, authored by Jack, his alleged lover, and a sari-clad, middle-aged Indian woman.

* * * * *

The snow arrived after Thanksgiving and buried Keokuk in white. A deep chill followed. The lakes froze over instantly, and young deer loitered about, probing for food under the snow. Our chickens huddled in their chicken coup, their egg production halved. Now, with my operating and ER privileges on "voluntary leave," I enjoyed the sudden leisure, awaiting, with no excessive anxiety, the outcome of the preliminary investigation by the Executive Committee of the Medical Staff. I judged my chances to survive this episode as sixty percent — surely the committee members would not get rid of their only surgeon… who's doing such a good job. But on the other hand, deep in my heart, I worried. *Didn't the CEO say something about the snowball?*

After Thanksgiving, I arrived at the conference room at 7.30 a.m. as requested. In the corridor, I saw nurse Rachel Kelly; I guessed she had already been interrogated. I opened the door and peeped in. I saw the diminutive but fleshy figure of Dr. Ravikumar, surrounded by all the tall men of the committee — engaged in what appeared to be a cozy discourse. *Bad sign — she's not being interrogated; she's one of them.* Bill Philips noticed me: "Moshe, please wait in the library. We'll call you in a few minutes."

I was summoned in at 8.30 a.m. There followed the usual mini-speech by Philips about my rights; then, "Could you please describe again the events of Friday, November 18?"

"Sure." I stood up and played it again. Having performed it already alive and in writing, I knew it by heart.

Philips: "Would you like to say anything else"?

"Yes. That my body language may differ from what you are used to here… I speak using and raising my hands, and my voice may be an octave louder. If any of you watch Italian movies, you can see that people speak and move their hands differently… and somebody could define it as threatening."

"But do you realize your style may not conform to local standards?" asked Philips.

"Yes, perhaps, but we all have different DNA. Some are tall, some fat… and some move their hands when they talk."

"Thank you, Dr. Schein. Please make yourself available in about thirty minutes." said Philips.

When they summoned me back, I smiled at them, but not even Art smiled back. They were somber, frozen-faced, like in a funeral. "Thank you for coming back. Please take a seat."

I did. I was trying to control the gathering anger. "Dr. D., would you please summarize the Committee's decision?" said Philips.

The Prince shuffled his papers. His long, pale, thin face looked at me at that moment like the face of an inquisitor, albeit a puritan-protestant one. A month ago, I had been invited to his house to watch a ball game — Iowa

City against who knows — I understand nothing about American football and thus had excused myself. I saw Dr. H's benign face, now grim, carefully studying the polished surface of the table, restlessly moving his long legs. On my left, Neville — the ever-cheerful Neville, ever eager to share his expertise on restaurants, cars, and wine — gloomily studied his fingertips. Dr. L, the obstetrician, looked ahead staring into space — his task was to sit here — a replacement for Brown, the orthopedist to whose presence I had objected.

"Moshe," started the Prince formally, "Moshe. I was your friend, and you know it. You were my surgeon, my only surgeon. I believe that all present in this room were your friends." The others nodded their heads gravely and murmured their approval. "But this is too much… you abused Dr. Ravikumar, who is a petite and soft-spoken woman. We've known her for many years… we see she could not have started the argument with you."

"But…"

"Let me continue: we had warned you six months ago after your encounter with Dr. Cappuccino. Let me quote from the letter this Committee had written to you: 'Any future incident of shouting, threatening, profanity, physical contact, or any disruptive speech… will meet with the consequences as outlined in the Medical Staff Bylaws. Included would be options for limitation, suspension or termination of privileges.'" The Prince paused and looked at me sternly, like a headmaster at Eaton.

"Well, what's new? You allow them to provoke me, and then you take their side. Jack has been screaming in the OR for many years… did you ever discipline him?" I said with disgust.

"Many people fear you in this hospital," retorted the Prince.

"Who are they? They, they," I sneered contemptuously," Who are the many people? Stop hiding behind empty words and show me some evidence?"

"Look at you. This is exactly your style… interrupting and disrespectful."

"But if I am accused, I should know who fears me and why?"

"Not at this stage… many people are afraid of you. We warned you, we can't let you work here." Now, even the cool Sir Osler of Keokuk lost his composure, "and you've shared information with patients… which may subject doctors to litigation."

"What?!"

"Yes, after the hernia affair, you spoke with the patient and blamed the cancellation directly on Dr. Ravikumar."

"For God's sake, whom should I have blamed? Myself? God Almighty? She canceled him — not me... not you, and the patient was upset. I would be, too. On which side do you work, eh?"

The Prince ignored me and continued: "...thus we decided to revoke your privileges in this hospital. We advise you to resign now — if you resign, nothing will be reported to the National Practitioner Data Bank. Alternatively, of course, as you know from the bylaws, you have the right to appeal. I should emphasize that, naturally, if you decide to appeal, this would be reportable. You have three days to decide."

This was not what I'd expected. A warning? Yes. You're a bad boy. Apologize and be nice to Dr. Ravikumar, yes. But not a summary execution à la Soviet *troikas* during the great purge of the late 1930s. I was stunned and enraged. My mind was grinding like a crushing computer: so what now?

I have to resign. If I continue fighting, they'll report me, which means there is no chance of another employment. Until when?

And meanwhile? How will I pay for the boys' schools? What will Heidi say? I looked around the table at each one of my henchmen. I knew that the person responsible for my fall was not among them. As I left the room without a word, I recognized that my ex-partner Jack had finally won!

On the way home, I saw ice forming on the snow-covered gravel road. I parked in the garage and walked into the kitchen, where Heidi was busy slicing vegetables.

"Already home?"

"Yep. I have been fired."

I remember saying so when the kids would ask me, "Dad, why are you home early?" I would reply: "I was fired. From now on, we'll eat only bread." They never thought it was funny.

* * * * *

Fifty-five

Adios Iowa

After a day or two, the cloud of acute depression started to lift off. Instead, a nagging anger emerged: *fuckers!* Just two weeks ago, I was their surgical hero. A few days later, they were obeying orders to kill me. It was fast: chop chop, chop. Don't let him breathe. Brutal!

I started to obsessively analyze the steps leading up to my lynching. I found out that the methodology used was well described on the Internet. Apparently, I realized, the phenomenon of lynching colleague-physicians, exploiting for this purpose peer review mechanisms – the exact mechanisms that had been originally developed to improve quality of care – is not uncommon across the country. So how does it work – or specifically how did it work in my case?

Step 1: Spread rumors about the new surgeon: incompetent, poor bedside manners. Blame your complications on him.

Step 2: Harass and humiliate the new surgeon as much as possible; try to force him into open confrontations. Then, complain that he's aggressive.

Step 3. Engage the community: at the bank, grocery shop, country club, coffee joint, especially the community leaders; let them always know that "he is an ongoing problem."

Step 4: Work on his referring base: "His wound infection rate is excessive, and he's poorly trained – what do you expect from someone trained abroad?"

Step 5: Make the doctors scared of him: "He's active on the Internet, he discusses your cases, he had reported doctors to the State in New York, he writes books… probably busy writing something about you."

Step 6: Exhaust him – let him work hard, tire him, isolate him, and stress him.

Step 7: Use your allies to irritate and provoke him; wait for an opportunity…

Step 8: Use your allies to ambush him.

Step 9: Immediately gang up against him…

Step 10: Lynch!

Step 11: The lynching should be formally conducted according to the hospital's Medical Staff Bylaws, with all discussions and discussants being immune from future litigation as all peer review procedures are.

The victim is caught like a fish, hanging and quaking on the hook. And the fish has very few options. Once he loses the hospital's clinical privileges, his contract and income automatically expire. He could hire a lawyer and start a legal battle against the committee that had disciplined him. But such legal actions tend to last years, and usually fail as the courts prefer not to interfere with the inner mechanisms of the medical peer review process — *let the docs kill each other as long as it stops them from killing us!* Besides, such prolonged legal wars are very costly, especially to someone who has lost his job and is unlikely to find another soon — for as long as one is engaged in legal procedures against a prior employer, few prospective employers would consider him. So the most reasonable option, the one chosen by most lynched doctors, the one I opted for, is to resign promptly, negotiate a severance agreement with the hospital (rarely successful), and look for another job — thanking heaven for not being recorded in the national database, hoping for at least neutral references when the future employers contact the last one with the usual questions of "How was he? Why did he leave?"

I continued asking myself why it had happened to me. The individual doctors who eventually lynched me were not Jack's friends; actually, they were those who preferred to work with me. So what motivated them to change face so swiftly and move against me? I received a few e-mails from surgical friends that may help to provide a plausible explanation.

A Canadian surgeon wrote: "…when living in a small town, make sure your beautiful wife wears only a good Republican cloth coat, nothing splashy except if you take a few days in the city to cool your jets. Definitely watch out for cops, no speeding, if you have had just one drink, your wife must drive. You have no idea how many people think Jack saved their kid from a certain death from appendicitis and would dearly love to pay him back; even having to stop to take the breathalyzer will stigmatize you. 'You know that fucking *kike* got caught for drink driving the other night. The lucky prick was just under the 0.08.'"

Yes — the car. Showing the finger to the wife of the President of the Board of Trustees did not endear me to him. He probably thought: "That *kike* showed the finger to my wife; this against the background of questionable competence and a chronic discord with Jack. And now he's attacking our anesthetist, who has been our neighbor for twenty-five years, and her husband's a good friend of mine. The *kike* has to go." So, the order for the kangaroo court by the Executive Committee of the Medical Staff may have come from above.

Another surgeon wrote to me from the North East: "I do not underestimate that good old middle American anti-Semitism is playing out in this whole process. In my experience, this is never far under the surface..." An interesting comment, especially when coming from a gentile.

Another American surgeon wrote: "I once worked in a small town and I know how insular, xenophobic, and insecure the doctors can be, how limited their political views, how narrow their perspectives, and how difficult it is for them to accept anything or anyone outside the ordinary. This is a psychological self-protective adaptation that secures the established self-satisfied mediocrity from outside criticism."

A retired academic American surgical guru wrote: "The lesson to be learned, I guess, is always to be on the lookout for anyone who might harm you and move to neutralize them first. In the Keokuk case, that would have been the members of the hospital's Board, as well as the nurses. Even if you couldn't entirely neutralize the old girlfriend, testimony from other senior nurses to counteract her comments might have been helpful. Everything, of course, is clearer in retrospect."

Another 'foreign' American surgeon commented: "...we are foreigners and do not know the 'rules of engagement' here. You can smile all the time and be unassuming, but then they nail you for an alleged anything. One lesson is that with the absolute first signs of hostility, you must go and complain of a hostile work environment; regardless of whether it is found to be true or not, you are immune from being fired because this would be considered a retaliatory firing. This is just one example of the things we don't know, and the local people grew up with from childhood."

But there must be, I think — there always is — another side to the story. Whatever was Jack's psychopathology, that he had turned against me so rapidly and with such vehemence, must have some grounds — I had to have irritated him to a significant extent. George Orwell wrote: "Autobiography is only to be trusted when it reveals something disgraceful. A man who gives a good account of himself is probably lying since any life, when reviewed from the inside, is simply a series of defeats." So what was so disgraceful about me that may have irritated others? A body language that often transmits arrogance or *chutzpah*, a nonchalant smirk, impatience, small irritating comments, endemic political incorrectness, and unsolicited advice or criticism — such behavioral traits are not uncommon among my generation of Israelis.

Unfortunately, we cannot penetrate Jack's head to learn more: was I 'too foreign' to him, too personal and colloquial — in a way so natural to us Middle Easterners but repelling to some American professionals? Henry Roth, an octogenarian New York Jew, wrote in his memoir *A*

Diving Rock on the Hudson: "...he was an everlasting Falasha, their dominant society that he detested for its banality and that detested him, he was sure, with equal intensity for his alien views, elitism, his alien response to their mass-produced, disposable values..." "He" was the author himself, recovering from his famous writer's block of more than fifty years. Didn't they, I pondered — those who did away with me — manage to detect my alien views? Didn't I sit in the OR nursing station, between operations, reading *The New York Times* on the Internet? Did I stop to consider that this might have irritated them — reading in public the mouthpiece of the liberal educated elites? And what about the nights at the Yacht Club or during operations, whenever they would ask, "Doc, did you watch the ball game yesterday?" I would reply that I am not interested in watching a bunch of overgrown people running after a small ball. Didn't I consider that for most of them, watching ballgames or anything to do with local baseball or football represents an entire religion?

No, they did not demand of me to be one of them, to follow their ways, but that, like Roth wrote, "his alien response to their mass-produced, disposable values" must have irritated at least a few of them. And yes, we should have tried schmoozing with Keokuk's aristocracy rather than avoiding them; we should have not come to Keokuk with some romantic agenda of exploring how a sole New York Jew would fit into rural southern Iowa, just on the edge of the Bible Belt — perhaps we should have tried merging in naturally. We should have laid low, played it out low-key, as advised by Dr. Delgado, as the Indian doctors do, and this is the key to their American success: they continue being 'Indian' at home — but at work, they do their job, smile and shut up.

But another voice told me: stop blaming yourself. You did what you could. You were doomed when Jack — a formidable and resourceful adversary — turned against you. You did not know this, but your end had been written on the wall — everybody knew it except you. Now, move out of here.

* * * * *

Being fired for the first time in one's life at the age of fifty-five is an excellent reason to develop depression. But I had no time for it. With three sons in college, a mortgage, and all the rest, I had to find other employment. The 'deal' arranged with the hospital was unconventional: in return for six months' salary, I would resign because of "personal motives." Both sides should avoid "derogatory or defamatory" statements and further litigation. Nothing that took place would be reportable to any state or federal authority; in fact, the whole story did not exist, or did it? It did not because any record of the actions taken by the Executive Committee of the Medical Staff — if ever recorded — had already been shredded — the 'lynching' had never happened.

I was lucky! Others are lynched and kicked out without even a cent of payout. I have to contribute such a smooth divorce to the benevolent CEO: I believe that he was genuinely sorry about my saga and also, obviously, wanted to avoid any unpleasant repercussions for his organization.

Alas, one pitfall concerning my retrenchment agreement with the hospital was that I did not ask for 'tail' malpractice coverage, which should cover any future litigation stemming from my practice in Keokuk. I knew nothing about it, and the hospital did not volunteer without me asking for it. So, a year later, when a Keokuk patient sued me (it was a frivolous claim, and I won the case in court), defending the case cost me thirty grand.

My next task was to find a new job. Now that we had tasted country life — even if only on the 'tip of the fork' — we did not want to return to a big city or suburbia. What we had in mind was something even more remote, more pastoral. Some place further up north, as far as possible from the Bible Belt, and what it represented.

The skirmishes with Jack tainted my education as a rural surgeon, but I had enjoyed playing the new role and wanted to continue. Looking at myself through the eyes of a potential employer, I did not see an overly attractive candidate: fifty-five years old, a foreign medical graduate, no USA specialty training, an unconventional CV — too academic and unusually frequent job changes. Who would want to hire me, I asked myself…

However, ultimately, we were invited for a series of interviews in those few States where I was licensed. After visiting at least ten rural locations in Upstate New York, northern Iowa, and Wisconsin, the best match appeared to be with an employer in Northern Wisconsin — starting May 2006.

* * * * *

Towards the end of April 2006, we left Keokuk. The spring had already arrived. A fragrant breeze was blowing from our lakes, where the fish were spawning by now. We locked the empty house — we had renovated it only a year ago. We drained and covered the six-month-old swimming pool. We would manage to sell that house only a year later, with a significant loss. With the help of Stan (our handyman and friend), we placed the chicken coup, including the chickens, on his trailer; the three cats, born in Johannesburg, New York and Keokuk, respectively, Pablo the dog, and Birdie the bird, were distributed among the cars. (One chicken would die of exhaustion during transport; Romi, the youngest cat, would be eaten by an owl a few months later.) I left the old Johnboat to a 'redneck' neighbor.

As our small caravan climbed the dirt road towards Highway 61, we turned back and photographed on our retinas the cedar wood house, the freshness of the foliage, the lush garden, and the gleaming lake — all illuminated by the sloping morning rays of the sun — we knew that we would never see our dream house again. Or would we…

Driving north, with the Mississippi to the right and corn fields to the left, this paragraph from *Curlew: Home* by Tom Montag came to my mind: "We (Iowans) welcome the weary traveler; we are glad to see his money; and, soon enough, we are happy to send him on his way. Perhaps we do not trust those coming through; there is some unease, some discomfort, and we exercise caution, carefully watching the strangers among us."

Perhaps this is a good way to say goodbye to our Iowan chapter, which had been fleeting but stormy, enjoyable but painful.

But hold on a sec: what was Jack up to all those years? I would walk past Jack during the American College of Surgeons annual meeting every year or so. Once, I spotted him emptying his bladder at the restroom of San Francisco Airport. We would recognize each other but not even share a head nod. After I left, Jack continued seeing patients and operating in Illinois and Keokuk. The Keokuk Hospital hired another full-time general surgeon every year or two; it seemed that as long as Jack was still practicing in town, no competitor could survive. I hear that he has finally retired close to his mid-70s.

I have had not a few struggles and enemies — real or assumed — during my life. All were forgotten and forgiven over the years. All except Jack. His Jekyll and Hyde unpredictably dual nature — outwardly holy, soft, and sweet; sometimes shockingly obnoxious, vindictive, and primitively cruel — made him a dreadful enemy. Some deep wounds cannot be pardoned.

Al, the benevolent CEO, became ill and retired years ago. Then, the hospital was bought by a large 'system' and changed its name. Eventually, in September 2022, the Keokuk Hospital closed down. This is the fate of some rural hospitals where money rules the healthcare system.

* * * * *

Leaving southern Iowa in the morning.

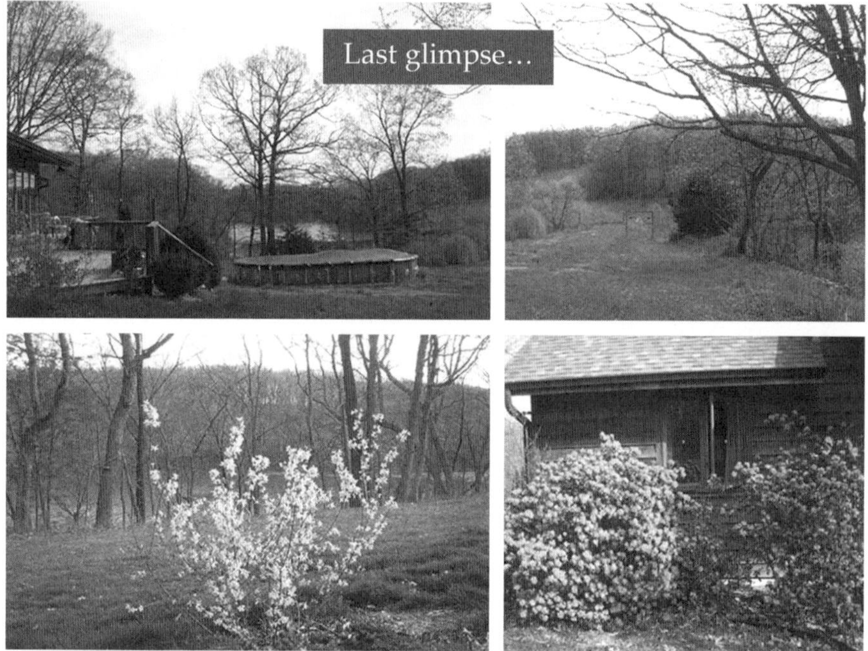

Fifty-six

Coming to northern Wisconsin

A year after we had settled in Ladysmith, Rusk County, Wisconsin, I wrote:

If this memoir were to continue, it would continue like this: Late April 2006. The temperature dropped gradually on the road from southern Iowa to northern Wisconsin. It was late spring when we had left Keokuk in the morning. Nine hours and 450 miles later, the trees were bare in Rusk County, and the grass was patchy with old snow. We settled in a solid log house, nestled on a ridge overlooking the Thornapple River, a mile above where it empties into the more expansive Chippewa River. Around us: the Blue Hills, forests of pine, oak, hickory, and birch trees; rivers, flowages, ponds, and lakes; dairy farms and logging plants; hunting and fishing, canoeing, and cross-country skiing. A few weeks later, the spring arrived, and the foliage on the trees, the vegetation along the river — now teeming with spawning sturgeon — obscured the river from vision. From the covered north-facing porch, the view remained unhindered: the prairie extending into the horizon, with red sunsets — the scent of cow and horse manure drifting from the farms. Next came the summer: warm but dry, with the dust washed away by sudden, violent rainstorms; there is little use for air-conditioning in these parts. The summer was short-lasting — perhaps three and a half months. The autumn that hastened to arrive presented itself with majestic colors. Finally, the winter was brutal — the big freeze lasting at least five months. It felt like coming to paradise!

At that point, I placed the memoir on ice. I stopped writing on it until eighteen years later.

* * * * *

My local friends laugh when I describe northern Wisconsin as "a paradise." Even though a perfect paradise does not exist, finally, after many stormy years, we settled into a stable and healthy existence. It still feels like a paradise, even after twenty years; years that passed across like a violent summer storm on the northern prairies — swift, unexpected, eventful, exciting, followed by intervals of relaxing calm.

I remember our first visit for a job interview at the Clinic in Ladysmith. It was deep winter, January 2006. We drove up from Keokuk, crossing I-94 and continuing northwards through miles and miles of snowy-frozen forests. We passed through lonely — one gas station, one bar — hamlets. We saw desolate farmhouses — the red barns like mushrooms in the white fields. "It looks like Siberia," I told Heidi. "Where is this Ladysmith?" We checked in at the local American Inn. We smelled chlorine drifting from the indoor swimming pool on the first floor, where local kids were splashing on that Sunday afternoon, watched by their parents, who were setting out boxes of pizza, soft drinks, and beer for the après-swim party.

Some ten miles north of town, we found Cedar Lodge — a lonesome bar grill. Two or three couples were drinking at the bar, and heavyset people in working clothes were eating inside. All were wearing baseball hats while munching their food. The burger was excellent, as it always has been in that joint in the many years to follow. The wine was less so, with a rudimentary selection — this being a beer and cocktails country. We drove back to the hotel through the night. There were no cars, no lights, and the town was deserted. When we went to sleep, I said, "I don't know. This isn't very promising. It looks like a hole somewhere in Kamchatka."

Heidi replied, "I like it. I have a good feeling. So many trees. Unlike the empty cornfields of Iowa. Good night."

The following day, I put on my suit and tie, below a heavy Carhartt coat, and walked on the freshly plowed road to the Clinic just across from the motel. It was the last time I would wear a tie in northern Wisconsin. The local clinic was one of the subdivisions belonging to the 'big' Clinic — a hundred-year-old healthcare system with over fifty locations in northern, central, and western Wisconsin. The Clinic's one-story modern-looking building lay alongside the four-story old red brick structure — the County Hospital. The hospital with its administrative and nursing staff belonged to the County — not to the Clinic — but its medical staff were all employed by the Clinic — 'on loan' to the hospital.

The interview proceeded as usual. You meet everybody for 15-30-minute sessions: the local clinic administrator, the center chairman doctor, and most physicians. A series of friendly little chats: they do not ask you much; they expect that the Clinic has vetted your credentials before inviting you for the interview. You suspect they have skimmed over your CV, which lay on their desks. A few may ask about your family or "do you fish or hunt?" Or, "Do you like the outdoors?" Pondering in their minds: is he suitable for country life?

Next comes the traditional interview lunch: they sit at the long conference room table. The 'providers' who are interested and not busy join individually. A free lunch is always welcome. Each loads a disposable plate with food on the side table: sandwiches, salad, and cakes ordered from some local eatery. They grab a soda in their other hand and join you at the table. There is some minimal small talk, never anything serious. Rarely, would they ask you any questions concerning surgery or medicine. Probably, they are thinking *we will never see this guy again*. So many interviews. People come and go. Why bother?

After lunch, I am escorted to the hospital to meet with Mr. Shaw, the hospital's administrator, a big smiley man in his sixties who seems a straight shooter. He explains the cooperation model between the Clinic and the hospital: "You are employed and paid by the Clinic, but we depend on you to manage your patients in our hospital. We pay the Clinic for your services." Over the next few years, I would find Mr. Shaw a solid administrator, a humble, down-to-earth man of the old generation. His demeanor and his shabby office echoed Midwestern modesty — the opposite of the female administrator who would replace him six years later. Next, I am led on a hospital tour — a typical smallish 'critical access' rural hospital. I visit the operating room: only two operating rooms, a recovery room, and a cozy little surgeon's changing room. It's even smaller than the one in Keokuk, I think. I meet a few smiling nurses — Pat, Cindy, and Nancy. We exchange a few pleasantries and smiles.

Any such job interview involves a formal dinner with selected medical staff representatives, including their significant others. It takes place in a favorite local eatery. It is part of the courting process: look at how nice we are! What about you and your wife — are you nice as well? Would you guys fit in? Of course, the impression on both sides is subjective: we have seen charming assholes and vice versa.

So here Heidi and I and four other couples sit at a barn-like restaurant, munching lovely burgers and drinking beer or wine. Through the large windows, one can see the moon reflected in the frozen lake, and the loud voice and hearty laughter of Dr. Joseph Bachir echoes from one wooden wall to the other. Joseph is the surgeon whose job I am now being interviewed for. He is sixty-five years old and wishes to retire. I have already realized that he is the one who selected me for the interview. Later, I would understand that he influenced the Clinic to hire me. Joseph, short, stocky, handsome, with a swarthy face, an intense nose, talks excellent English with a heavy Arabic accent. His life and professional story is even a little more complex than mine: a Christian Syrian who studied medicine in Moscow — it was when the Soviets were offering free education to individuals from the 'third world.' Next, he went to the UK and trained in surgery in England and Scotland. Unable to secure a consultant position in the UK, he emigrated to the USA. Eventually, in the early 1980s, he landed in Ladysmith as the first qualified surgeon in town. Before he had arrived, as it was common in rural USA, surgery was performed by the local general practitioners. Over the years, Joseph became a famous citizen of Ladysmith: not only *the/our surgeon* but also an outspoken member of the Clinic and the school board chairman. Patients appreciated his skills, his warm human touch, and his gregarious, if forceful, personality, wrapped with a loud sense of humor. Even today, almost twenty years after Joseph left, old patients mistake me for being Dr. Bachir. "You sound like him, he was such a good surgeon, a lovely man," they say. In my mind, there is no greater compliment to a retired surgeon than being remembered by patients!

A town tour, including housing options, is part of any such job interview. Thus, the following day, an estate agent took us on a drive around Ladysmith and Rusk County.

"What kind of home do you have in mind?" he asked.

"In the open country, not in town, preferably something like a small farm," we responded.

With the country covered in snow and ice, everything looked the same — it was impossible to appreciate the lay of the land and surroundings. But the large, solid log home, nestling above a frozen river, surrounded by snow-covered trees and white fields, seemed attractive. "No real farms for sale?" asked Heidi as we returned to the agents' SUV in deep snow. He insisted that this was the best country house currently up for sale. Later, we would learn that this log house belonged to him and had stood empty for almost two years. A new doctor comes to town — this is his chance to sell…

In the afternoon, as I was warming myself in the hotel's jacuzzi, I got a call on my mobile phone. It was Joe, the center's medical director. "Moshe, we want to offer you the job." He mentioned the proposed yearly income — a hundred thousand more than I had made in Keokuk. Immersed in the hot water, the offer made me feel even warmer. Perhaps, after all these years, we may reach the promised land. "Thanks, Joe. I appreciate your offer very much. We have a few more interviews scheduled over the next month or so. We will decide and let you know. OK?"

That night we were invited for dinner at Dr. Bachir's lakeside house. We drove through the moonlit white forests, crossing frozen rivers and vast fields glittering blue white on both sides of the road. The wooden house was immense. A few fires were burning in the stoves. A large single malt whiskey was offered, followed by tasty Middle Eastern food… It was cozy, and we felt at home. Arabs and Israelis have so much in common. It was an opportunity to ask about Dr. Armando Garcia, the other local general surgeon I had not met yet.

Joseph said: "Armando spends each February in Acapulco with his kids and numerous grandchildren. He'll be back next week. If you accept this job, you'll share calls with him. That is until he leaves. His contract will end in a year or so."

"Tell me more about him," I asked.

"He's a Filipino, even older than me. The guy trained somewhere in New York, did a colorectal fellowship and was the colorectal guru at our clinic's flagship hospital for many years. I used to refer my major rectal cases to him, you know, the very low rectal cancers and so on... a truly superb rectal surgeon. A great technician..."

"So what is he doing now in Ladysmith?" I interrupted.

"Ah, a few years ago, he had a heart attack. Yes, during an operation. It scared him. He decided to retire. Then, he immediately got bored. The man loves to operate. So, a year ago, when I started planning my retirement, I thought, why shouldn't I bring Armando in to work with me during the transition period until they find a full-time replacement? You know, replacing a small-town surgeon can take years. Armando loved the idea, and they gave him a three-year special contract."

"So, assuming I take this job, he'll be my partner for another year or so. How is he as a partner?"

Joseph took a large sip of whiskey. "Frankly, we don't speak much. He does his job, and I do mine. He used to be friendlier over the phone when I used to refer cases to him. You will find out. I must admit only this: he loves to take out colons and rectums. Sometimes, it seems that the mere presence of a colon is for him an indication to remove it." Another prolonged laugh.

The next day, we drove southbound on Highway 61 to Iowa. We had the feeling that we would be back.

We went for a few more interviews in rural south Wisconsin, north Iowa and Upstate New York. But nothing proved as attractive as what the Clinic offered in Ladysmith. We were fascinated with the Northwoods. Perhaps, we hoped, this 'marriage' would be successful this time.

* * * * *

Spring 2006: first month on the Thornapple River, Rusk County, Wisconsin.

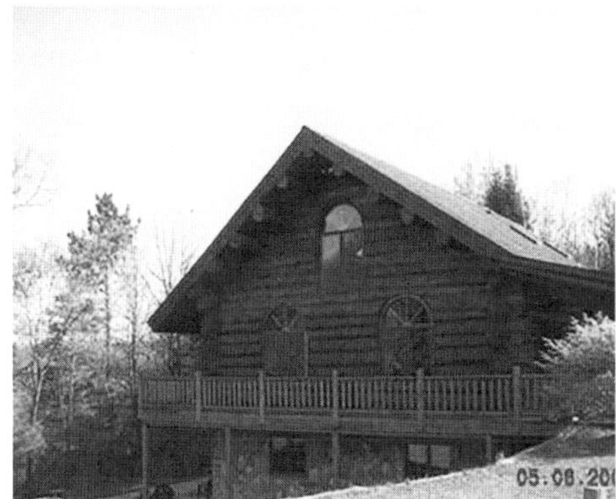

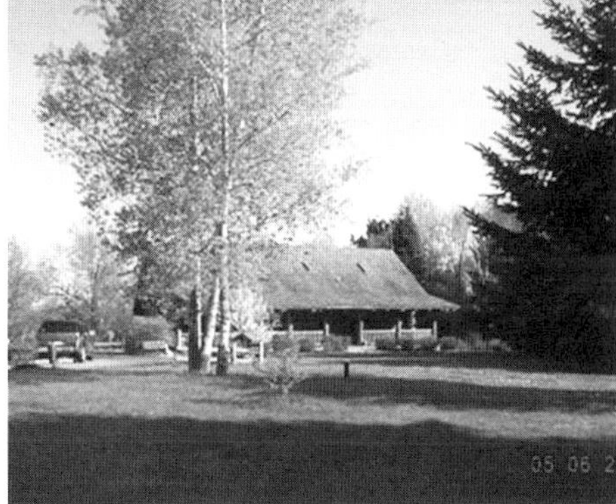

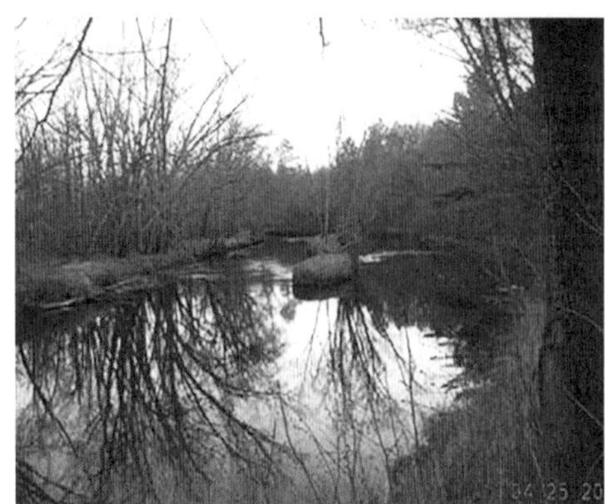
04 25 20

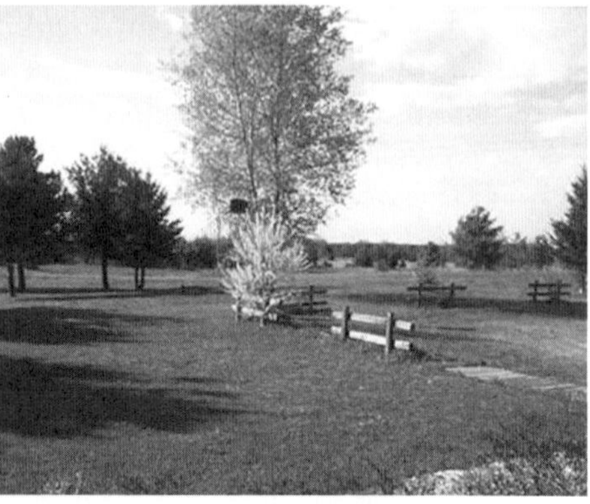

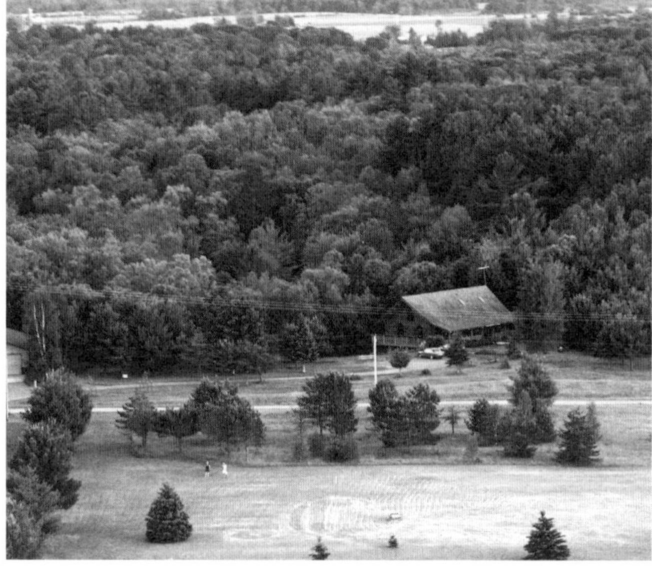

Fifty-seven

Ladysmith, Wisconsin — the early years

Twenty years. In hindsight – the best years! How do you summon up long years of practice? Without a diary, we depend on our faulty memory, which tends to recall not the smooth, uneventful, happy sailing but the big storms that shake the boat and endanger the passengers.

I will divide the Wisconsin years into three parts: the *early years* of the voyage, generally pleasant, albeit shaken by a few little storms. Next came the *years of Princess Charlotte* – who navigated the boat from a hurricane to a typhoon, eventually aborting it in disarray. Finally – the *final years* of sailing – down into the mystic…

The Clinic thrived in those days. It had a large group of experienced family practice physicians and internists. We had a busy obstetrics service run by family practice docs, supported by us general surgeons who did the C-sections.

It was a new skill that I had to learn from scratch. Hitherto, C-sections fell into the domain of trained gynecologists wherever I worked. To acquire the needed aptitudes, the Clinic obliged me to perform ten C-sections with a gynecologist in a neighboring town. Whenever the gynecologist had an elective planned case, I would jump into the truck, drive down, and scrub in with him. Anyone who has ever taught residents to operate knows you must let them do the procedure step by step – under your careful tutoring. Letting them watch you is not enough. But for many community surgeons, teaching colleagues is an alien concept. *Who has the time and patience? Let him come and see how I do it. I'm busy.*

So, I would scrub in and assist the gynecologist, who hardly spoke. After ten cases, I was 'credentialed' to do it independently. To a general surgeon with experience in major abdominal and vascular surgery, a C-section seems 'easy;' some call it an "obstetric I+D" (incision and drainage) – like draining an abscess, in this case not draining pus but extracting a baby. However, soon I realized that a C-section in the middle of the night, on a morbidly obese abdomen (so common around these parts!), assisted by a single scrub technician, is not exactly a walk in the park. Luckily, I had Bob Nogler to scrub in with me on many nights. Bob, a family practice doc, had been engaged in obstetrics for many years, including C-sections. He is the one who taught me what the other gynecologist did not: how to extract the newborn, how to grasp his head, how to rotate the shoulder…

As always, I learned from my own mistakes. I remember one of my early solo cases: a colossal woman, with a scrub nurse who was not the most skilled of assistants. The thick abdominal wall falls repeatedly over the uterus. The baby apparently is in distress — so I am told. I see nothing — operating in a black hole. *Just extract the baby,* I tell myself. *Get it out.* I open the peritoneum with scissors, vertically as always. Suddenly, I see the balloon of the Foley catheter looking at me. *Shit — I've breached the urinary bladder.* I open the uterus, shell out the baby, and suture the uterus; finally, I meticulously repair the bladder. Everything is all right. The patient recovers smoothly. The next morning, everybody knows: Schein had opened the bladder — the 'exciting' news broadcast by the same nurse who doesn't know how to retract properly. So, this is how I learned that the pregnant uterus can push even a well-drained bladder upwards, just beneath the peritoneum, where it must be opened to expose the uterus. From now on, I opened the peritoneum as high as possible. It is something that I did not see mentioned in any book. Gaining confidence, I started enjoying the little drama involved with these procedures, but occasionally, the drama became excessive.

A few years later, one night, I rushed in for an emergency C-section: "You must come immediately, fetal distress, bradycardia, meconium, probably the cord is around the neck…" When I arrived, the patient was already lying on the OR table, screaming. The young husband was holding her hand. The nurses were frantically opening the sterile sets and arranging the instruments. Another nurse was pressing a fetal stethoscope against the bulging tummy. "I can't hear anything," she said.

I looked at the certified registered nurse anesthetist (CRNA): "Spinal in?"

"Yes, I tried, but I'm not sure it's working yet…"

"Give her a general, now, let's go, we have to move…"

"Get me lidocaine two percent," I told the nurses, splashing some betadine on the abdomen. I injected the local anesthetic.

I placed a midline incision into the lower abdomen, opened the peritoneum, sliced the lower segment of the uterus, and fished out a blue baby that did not seem to be breathing. I unknotted the cord that had strangulated his neck and handed him to the pediatrician. She managed to revive the baby…

Delivering the baby took a minute or two. I noticed that the CRNA was still busy preparing for general anesthesia. Now, I took my time and injected more lidocaine under the skin and fascia. Still, when I attempted to eviscerate the uterus, the patient screamed and moved her hands towards the sterile operative field.

"Hold her hands, tie them down," I screamed, "Why isn't she sleeping yet, for God's sake?"

Suddenly and violently, the patient tried to sit up. The drapes and instruments slid down from the table.

"Hold her down," I shouted, looking at her husband standing there passively, "do you want her to die!" It took a few minutes for the general anesthesia to be induced. I eviscerated the uterus, sutured it up, and closed the abdomen. Both mother and baby did well.

Two days later, a tall, hefty woman, like an oak tree, stands at my office door. She comes in and sits on the only other chair available. I look at her: a coarse face, a cheap red business suit, and chunky low heel shoes on huge feet. In her fifties? Who is she to storm into my room? "Yes," I say, "how can I help you?"

In slow motion, the woman takes a notepad and a pen from her pocket, ready to take notes. "I'm Debbie," she says, "the new Vice President for Nursing."

"Oh really. I heard about you. Welcome…"

I offer her my hand but withdraw it half way when it is not reciprocated. Wow, I think, now head nurses of any small hospital are calling themselves vice presidents.

The woman has no time for small talk or civilities; she goes straight for the jugular: "Doc, there is a complaint against you. The day before yesterday, during a C-section procedure, you screamed at a patient and her husband. What can you tell me about it?" With her pen ready, hovering on her silly little notebook, she stares at me with her poker face.

I am speechless. What a cheek! I feel the blood rushing in my head, coloring my face with anger. *Control yourself.* "Would you please leave my room immediately!" I say and show her the door.

"OK, doc, you will be hearing from us."

That was my introduction to the 'sphinx,' so I started calling that bulky, rough, expressionless woman.

But the 'sphinx' and the CEO who recruited her arrived only later — they belong to the following chapter.

* * * * *

Dr. Armando Garcia — my so-called 'partner,' the second general surgeon at our local clinic — was by natural selection the senior surgeon among us two. Not only had he already been in Ladysmith for a few years, but he was a well-known colorectal surgeon around northern Wisconsin. Therefore, he inherited Dr. Bachir's spacious office and procedure room while I was allocated to a cubicle and a procedure room half the size.

I met with Dr. Garcia immediately after his return from Acapulco. When I entered his office to introduce myself, I saw a slim, short man — no more than 5′2″ — with thinning white hair and features suggesting South Asian

DNA mixed with that of some Spanish ancestors. The smooth face made him look younger than his chronological age of seventy. His demeanor was mild, polite but official; he spoke very softly. He wore a blue suit, a white shirt, and a tie – no other doctor in our clinic dressed so formally. Our chat was brief. I asked about his background, training, career, and current practice. He asked nothing except one question just when I was leaving his room: "By the way, how come you are a Fellow of the American College of Surgeons? You didn't train in the US. You are not board-certified, right?" I understood immediately: he wanted me to realize that he – who had arrived from the Philippines many years ago, trained in New York, and therefore was board-certified – belongs to a different, elevated, better class of surgeons.

The pattern of my interaction with Dr. Garcia was established on my first weekend on call. Each Friday of his 'free' weekend, immediately after lunch, Dr. Garcia would walk down the corridor, passing the open door of my cubicle rapidly; he would then exit the Clinic through the back door, hop into his chunky Cadillac and drive down to Marshtown, to spend the weekend with his wife at their main home. During the week, and on his weekend call, he stayed in a little condominium overlooking the river, a 4-minute walk from the Clinic – a route he had only driven.

That Friday was my first weekend call. Dr. Garcia stopped momentarily in front of my door. He said, "There's one patient for you to see in the ICU. She is three days after a colectomy for diverticulitis. She's doing well. Just babysit her for me until Monday. Bye." The handover was completed.

The next day, I rounded on his patient. She was recovering uneventfully having passed gas and bowel movements. I removed her nasogastric tube and started her on a liquid diet. She seemed ready to go home on Sunday, but I decided to keep her another day – let Garcia enjoy his handcraft and discharge her on Monday. I advanced her diet.

Late Monday morning, Dr. Garcia stormed into my cubicle. I noted his agitation immediately. He hissed at me (he never shouted): "Why did you remove the NG tube? She's vomiting. She's distended. Where have you been trained? Never do it again on my patients!"

I was aghast. Garcia proceeded down the corridor before I managed to utter a proper retort. I sensed a feeling of déjà vu – two weeks into my new job, and here I have, perhaps, another partner like Jack of Keokuk. The nightmare from which I had just managed to escape…

Atypically, for my nature, I decided to swallow my pride. *Let him be the 'big dog.' I will do my job… and we will see the outcome.* I made a point of treating Garcia respectfully, as one would treat an older, more senior partner. I would force myself to ask him for a second opinion, even when it was unnecessary. I accepted the fact that he was busier than I was. I suppressed my resentment, watching how some referrals were diverted to him — even on the days I was on call. I realized that with his charming ways — manly focused on the ladies — he was popular among the supporting staff, the nurses, and the girls at the appointment-scheduling desk.

I even made a point to assist him with his colorectal operations. He was not too happy about it. Some surgeons, like him, prefer to operate with dedicated assistants who are not qualified surgeons — assistants who do not ask questions or criticize and do not understand whether the operation is indicated — whether the punishment fits the crime. I would appear in the OR just before the operation started and volunteer as the first assistant. I would say: "Dr. Garcia, this is such a complex case. No wonder it was referred to you from out of town. Obviously, you are the man to tackle it… I would love to assist and learn from you…" He would concur with a head nod or a grunt. How could he refuse me in front of the entire OR team?

Some old surgeons gradually lose their technical skills but preserve their mental acuity and solid judgment — the opposite is true for others. My growing impression was that Garcia belonged to the latter entity. I found him a superb technical colorectal surgeon. Watching his tiny hands elegantly remove colons and rectums, it was obvious that he had been repeating the same steps for many years.

Once, he boasted to me: "I did more than a thousand sigmoid colectomies for diverticulitis." After observing how laissez-faire his indications for these procedures were, I believed these numbers.

Another Garcia-related story left an imprint on my mind. It was another Friday midday, perhaps a year later. Garcia was on his way home for the long weekend. He stopped at my open door: "Moshe, I have a patient in the ICU. I removed her sigmoid on Monday. She isn't doing well. You know, bad pneumonia, she's septic. I left her to the internist. I don't think that you'll have anything to do with her. Bad prognosis." He shrugged his shoulders and shuffled down the corridor.

Five minutes after Garcia's Cadillac left the parking lot, I was already examining his 'pneumonia' case in the ICU. I took the patient immediately for a laparotomy and dismantled her grossly leaking colorectal anastomosis. I was thinking: what is wrong with Garcia? Is he one of those people who condemn their patients to death because they do not want to bother with the complication or, more likely, do not want to be associated with such a life-threatening complication? Is Garcia another version of Dr. Mantzur, my old 'friend' from the New York Methodist Hospital?

After receiving the colostomy, the leaking patient improved rapidly. Come Monday, Dr. Garcia was back. His head reappeared at my door: "Moshe, thanks for looking after the ICU woman. You should now take her over. OK?"

"Of course, Dr. Garcia. As you wish."

Like Drs. Mantzur and Sorkhi, I was thinking, once they screw the patient, they do not want anything to do with them. Let others deal with the problems and the families. *The faster we forget — the better.*

The above was not an isolated case — it followed a pattern with Garcia. This time, however, I decided to act differently. No more acts of professional suicide like in Brooklyn. No more open critique like in the Bronx. Anyway, I did not have a choice. Doctors hired by the Clinic sign a two-year contract as "associates." Only after two years, if approved by their peers and the management, are they voted as "shareholders" — a sort of tenure ('hard to get rid of') status. Those who were denied a permanent job would have to go elsewhere. Besides, there was nowhere to complain: our small hospital, where Garcia's sins were committed, did not then belong to the Clinic. Its quality assurance bodies existed on paper only. As to the Clinic, Garcia had been their hotshot surgeon for thirty years.

Meanwhile, the mild, smiley Garcia attempted to undermine me in his quiet and subtle fashion. I believe he intended to prevent me from getting the permanent status so that he could stay on at the end of his special contract, which was to expire within two years. It was clear that there was no room for two surgeons at our small center in the long term. Formally and superficially, we continued to be 'partners,' but practically, I was on my own. I looked after my patients day and night, rounding on them weekends and nights — even when he was on call. I avoided operating before going out of town.

I did not want to leave my patients under Garcia's care. I did not trust him.

* * * * *

It happened on Friday afternoon during the autumn hunting season. A big man in his thirties was brought in to the ER after being mauled by a bear. He had been sitting on a tree stand when a bear cub climbed up to him, followed by his mother. Luckily, the hunter tied himself to the tree so the mother could not drag and finish him off. Bear claws are a lethal weapon, so the man had sustained numerous deep, long, and rugged wounds to his entire body. He lost some blood, but there was no evidence of any internal injuries. I took him to the OR, cleaned and debrided the wounds, dressed them, and said: "I'll reoperate on him in seventy-two hours."

Jessica, our CRNA — in her late thirties, a pleasant and not bad-looking Minnesotan — was horrified at what she saw. She looked at me skeptically. "You don't think he should be flown to the trauma center? He needs a plastic surgeon!"

I shrugged: "Well, I don't think so…"

On Monday, I took the patient back to the OR. I was able to suture-repair all his wounds. I learned, however, that meanwhile, the CRNA went to the hospital CEO to complain that Schein was doing what he was not supposed to do. It was clear to me who was behind the complaint. The patient's wounds healed beautifully.

A month later, a young boy arrived at the ER. He had fallen while fishing on the river's edge and was impelled by a sharp, long, thick wood stick. The stick was embedded in his chest and abdominal wall — both ends sticking out. The chest X-ray showed no pneumothorax or hemothorax, and his abdomen was soft. I knew that the stick did not involve the chest or abdominal cavities. All I needed was to pull it out, clean the tract, and control bleeding — if any. But to be on the safe side, I told the OR team: "Get ready for a laparotomy — if needed, and have the thoracotomy set to stand by."

I noted the OR nurse's bulging eyes: "Thoracotomy set? We have no thoracotomy sets. We don't do thoracotomies in this hospital. Never, ever."

I tried to reassure the nurses; the same CRNA was present as well. "No, I don't think a thoracotomy will be needed. But shouldn't a hospital like this have a thoracotomy set on stand by. You know, things can happen…"

I needed to enlarge the wounds to remove the impelling stick; all went well, and the boy was home the next day. On the same day, Dr. Garcia, together with the head OR nurse, warned the hospital's CEO with the message: "Schein is crazy. He asked for a thoracotomy set. He thinks he can do chest surgery…"

Not a few weeks later, a young hunter was brought in to the ER, with a shotgun wound to his left chest. They had been hunting for deer somewhere in the woods around town. I immediately recognized that the man was in an agonal state — pulseless, no recordable blood pressure — but there was some electrical activity on the EKG. "I'm going to open his chest," I said. "Intubate him now. Get me the OR team with their instruments. Hand me a scalpel… fast!"

I put on a sterile pair of gloves, splashed some betadine on the hunter's chest, and sliced his left chest in the fifth intercostal space — a gush of blood came rushing out. I found a large rent in the pericardium, I extended it to expose the heart. I could feel and see a giant hole in the left ventricle, the bullet going through and through — shuttering the right ventricle as well.

Nothing to do.

I looked up. The entire ER team was standing around watching. The OR nurses arrived as well, with their instruments. I asked one of the nurses to retract the ribs and showed everybody the destroyed heart.

On my way out of the ER, I saw the head OR nurse packing her instruments. I walked to her and said: "Now you understand why we need a thoracotomy set in the hospital? If this were a smaller wound, we could have saved him." She nodded: "Yes, I understand." This did not mean that I had become her favorite surgeon.

I managed to 'convert' our CRNA Jessica to my side only later — after her favorite surgeon Garcia was no longer with us. I was planning to do a mastectomy for breast cancer. It went like this: the patient is lying on the OR table, ready to be anesthetized; then Jessica says: "Look at her little jaw, she has micrognathia (an undersized jaw). It'll be a difficult endotracheal intubation. I'll be better using an LMA (laryngeal mask airway)."

"Whatever you think is better… you are the CRNA," I say.

I continue standing at the bedside, watching Jessica. In a small hospital where MD anesthesiologists are unavailable, the surgeon is formally responsible, at least nominally, for whatever the CRNA is doing.

Now the patient is asleep, Jessica inserts the LMA device through the mouth into the pharynx. She inflates the balloon, which has to occlude the lower pharynx, to allow the sleeping gas and oxygen to be pumped into the trachea. She compresses the ventilation bag, observing the chest wall movements. Jessica is unhappy: "It's leaking, the seal is not good, the tube is too big. Let me try a smaller one." She removes the tube and continues oxygenating the sleeping patient with an Ambu facemask. "Now let's try again…"

And she tries again. As I watch her struggling with the mask, manipulating it repeatedly, I say quietly: "Jessica, just forget about it. I can do the mastectomy under local anesthesia and sedation. Look at her little breast, how thin she is…"

But the CRNA continues as if in a trance — *she must succeed* — "just one more try." Suddenly, the face of the patient turns bluish. The oxygen saturation on the monitor falls rapidly: 95, 90, 85, 80, 70… it all happens within sixty seconds. The OR nurses freeze in place as if immersed in deep ice — fixated on the monitor. Jessica removes the tube and turns around — mumbling something about laryngospasm — rummaging agitatedly and desperately through her instrument trays.

O_2 — 60.

Bradycardia. *She's dying.*

I approach the sterile instrument tray, grab a scalpel, and slice the center on the neck vertically below the cricoid — all the way down to the trachea. "Give me a tube, a small one, yes an endotracheal tube, help me, I need an artery forceps."

The scrub nurses emerge from the daze and move around in a flurry.

I incise the two upper rings of the trachea, spread the opening with a clamp, and insert the tube handed to me.

"Here, connect it to your tubing, oxygen!" Jessica does what is required. She has regained self-control. I control the bleeding, and fix the tube in place.

"Take her to the ICU. We will postpone the mastectomy. I am sure the patient will choose another hospital for this purpose," I say, walking out of the OR. The woman recovered promptly. As predicted, her breast was then removed at 'St. elsewhere.' A year or so later I encountered her by chance in the hospital corridor; she hugged me saying, "I know you saved my life."

I never discussed this case with Jessica ever again. She never said a word about it to me. I saw it only in her eyes. She moved over to my side.

The moral of the story: when you move to a new hospital, especially a rural one, you are constantly watched by the critical eyes of the OR team. They compare your practice to the other surgeons (previous and current), irrespective of whether the others are or were 'perfect' or 'assholes.' It doesn't matter how experienced you are — whether you were a professor or a hotshot surgeon elsewhere — you still have to gain their trust and appreciation.

* * * * *

Meanwhile, we immersed ourselves in rural life — enjoying what each season offered. We made a few close friends (John, Debbie, Dan, Lynette, Jerry, Ann) who absorbed us into their midst; they introduced us to canoeing/kayaking on the rivers, cross-country skiing, and road biking around the miles and miles of calm, paved, or gravel country lanes.

I consolidated my fishing aptitudes. Before I got a fishing kayak, I would stand with my rod by the edge of the churning water below the Thornapple Dam on the Flambeau River. I would observe the other fishermen and try chatting with them: "What do you fish for? What lures do you use? What line?" I would watch their technique. Wisconsinites are friendly, easy to talk to, and keen to help and advise. In local terms, they love to 'visit' with others. Fishing is a huge passion for rural Wisconsinites; becoming an aficionado also helped me communicate with patients. You ask any (male) patient, old or young, "What do you fish for?" developing a long dialogue that puts both parties at ease. I started netting big fish: catfish, 50-plus-inch musky — even giant sturgeons. Then, I got myself a fishing kayak.

Fishing in a moving kayak in rapid waters demanded advanced training. Imagine netting a flapping northern pike while the kayak drifts rapidly toward a large rock. There are many pitfalls to avoid: entangled lines, lost tackle, broken rods, runoff fish, an overturned kayak, and the worst — a sharp lure (triple hooks are the most dangerous) lodged in your arm or face.

I realized that, in some way, many aspects of fishing parallel the art of surgery. In fishing, like in surgery, there are good and bad days. If there were no bad days and everything would go smoothly — fish biting every day and all day, gallbladders popping out within five minutes, like sebaceous cysts — then fishing and surgery would not be as exciting, fulfilling, and satisfying. Luckily, however (for the patients), the practice of surgery is a little more predictable than fishing. Surgery, like fishing, is a lonely practice. Whatever the number of assistants, nurses, anesthesiologists, and technicians in the operation room, the surgeon is lonely — the ultimate responsibility for the outcome of the operation, for the patient's well-being, is his or hers. It is the same with fishing, where a fish replaces the patient: whether you catch it depends only on you. There are numerous similarities between the two activities: e*ducation* — books vs. apprenticeship; *timing* — crucial in both surgery and fishing; the need for *patience* — attention to detail!; *preparation* — be ready for anything and everything; *equipment* — this is obvious; *changing strategies* — if it does not work — try another method; *avoid gimmicks* — you do not need a stapler to repair a hole in the bowel; you do not need sonar to catch fish in the river; *technique* — the operation's success, whether you land the fish, depends on how perfect your technique is; *readiness for the unexpected* — the right hepatic artery hiding just behind the cystic duct, the 40-pound musky suddenly hooked on your 4-pound test line. Another striking resemblance is that both anglers and surgeons are imaginative *liars*: both tend to exaggerate the number and size of fish they catch and the complexity and danger of the operation performed. There is one crucial difference however: while some smoking and drinking during fishing can be recommended — this is an absolute 'no no' during surgery…

We purchased a modest cabin on the Flambeau River, some seven miles below town. It was on a deep section of the river, upstream of the Thornapple Dam. In the early morning, I would drive to the cabin, park my car, leap on my bike, and ride to the Clinic, listening to the loud concert of frogs croaking in the marshlands on the sides of the road. Rabbits would dart before the bicycle; deer would freeze and then run away. Occasionally, a bear, large or small, would cross the road like a black rocket. At the end of the day, I would ride back to the cabin, swim up and down the cool river, and drive home. I could be 'on call' off my fishing kayak. I would answer the cell phone, replace the fishing rod in the rod holder, paddle back to the cabin, and drive to the hospital. After long years of sedentary city life, the chaotic hospitals, the long hours of the daily commute — I started shedding off the pounds…

* * * * *

Dr. Armando Garcia's special contract was nearing its end. The leadership's decision that one general surgeon would suffice for the local clinic was now final — the other had to go.

The common perception was that Garcia's contract was up; therefore, he had to leave. Meanwhile, I, hired as a permanent replacement for Dr. Bachir, would stay on. However, it appeared that the seventy-something-year-old Garcia decided that he did not have to go. "If I stop operating, I will die" — was his motto, expressed to the OR staff.

Garcia reasoned, "I'm the top local surgeon, with the Clinic for so many years. Schein's is still waiting for his tenure — he should be discarded..." For three months, Garcia tried to convince the Clinic and hospital leadership that he would be a preferable long-term asset to the system. For his 'campaign,' he mobilized the OR nurses and other allies — mainly from the supporting staff. I observed this passively from the sidelines. I had the feeling that the Clinic doctors would support me, that somehow — perhaps for the first time in my professional life — I had not generated any enemies or bad feelings among the local physicians; that they would vote for me.

I realized that I was right when Garcia asked me for a reference letter for the new job he had applied for in northern Minnesota (remember? "If I stop operating — I'll die"). I followed the rule: "Help him go away if you want him out of your life" — composing a glowing reference for him. I remember the day when Garcia packed his things into the trunk of his big Cadillac. He then took out his MA (medical assistant) and a few other nurses for a farewell lunch. None of the doctors were invited.

The next day, I moved into his spacious procedure room. Soon afterward, the medical assistant who worked for me hitherto decided to leave town. Her replacement, Carla, proved herself a most skilled and dedicated assistant. Her charming ways with the patients compensated for my general grumpiness and improved the popularity and success of my practice for the many years to come. I have no doubt that her loyalty and support contributed to my prolonged professional survival in this job!

So now, finally, I had become the only surgeon in town. All referrals went to me. I could do whatever I thought I could; otherwise, I would refer out. The goal was to have a minimal rate of complications and no postoperative deaths — the motto being: if they are going to die... let them die after an operation performed by someone else. As they say: "Everything in surgery is patient selection — the chief determinant of mortality and morbidity." Writing this, almost twenty years after arriving in Ladysmith, I recall only two postoperative deaths. One was an old lady who developed an embolic stroke a few days after a colectomy for cancer. Probably, the decision by her internist to stop her blood thinner before the operation (she had been taking warfarin for atrial fibrillation) contributed to her stroke. The other death followed an operation I performed in a neighboring town on a ninety-two-year-old man with a strangulated abdominal wall hernia. I blame it on myself.

Another consequence of Garcia's departure was the sudden and permanent drastic decline in the number of colon resections for diverticular disease performed in the county; proving what I had already noticed — that most of those operations he did were for mild diverticular disease (so common in the local obese population) and thus unnecessary. But Garcia was a skilled colorectal surgeon who followed the adage: "If all you have is a hammer, everything looks like a nail." Besides, clinics and hospitals celebrate high-volume surgeons; they appreciate the income. How it is earned is not an issue for them unless too many patients die.

With Garcia gone, with supporting colleagues around, with tolerably irritating administrators (non-irritating administrators are hard to find), and with a superb medical assistant, I felt like I was practicing in heaven. These were good years. These were very good years, that is until Princess Charlotte arrived in 2013. She would be the one to retrieve the ghost of Dr. Armando Garcia from oblivion.

* * * * *

With my medical assistant, Carla Egle.

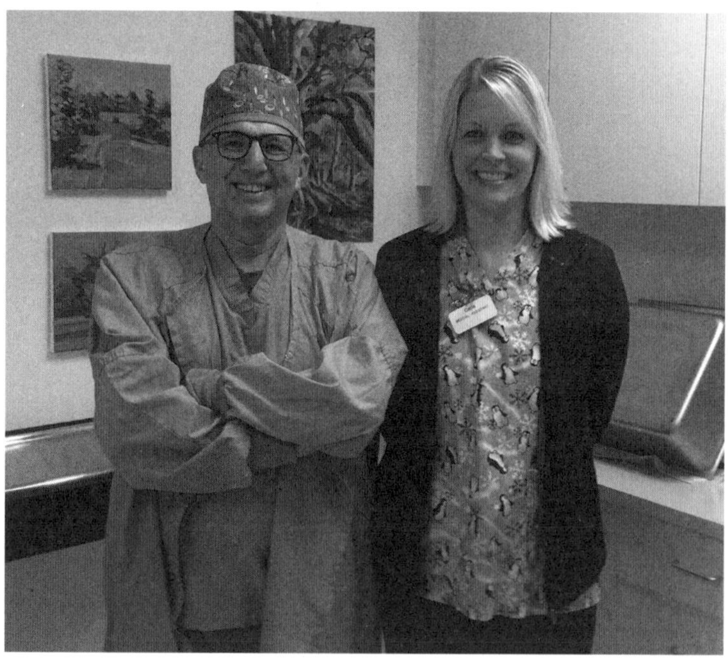

Fishing on the Flambeau River, Rusk County (musky, northern pike, bass).

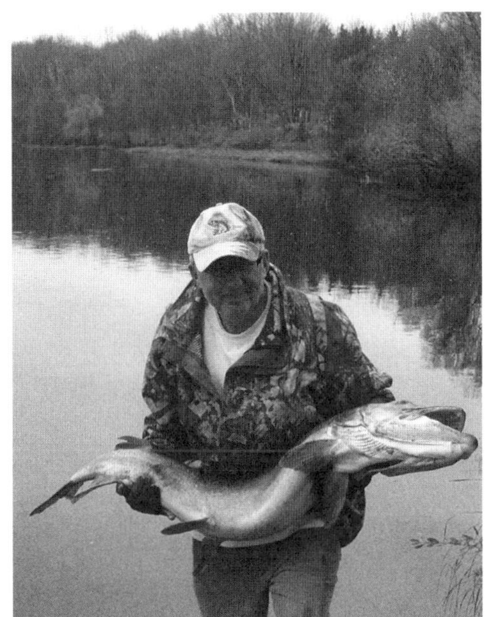

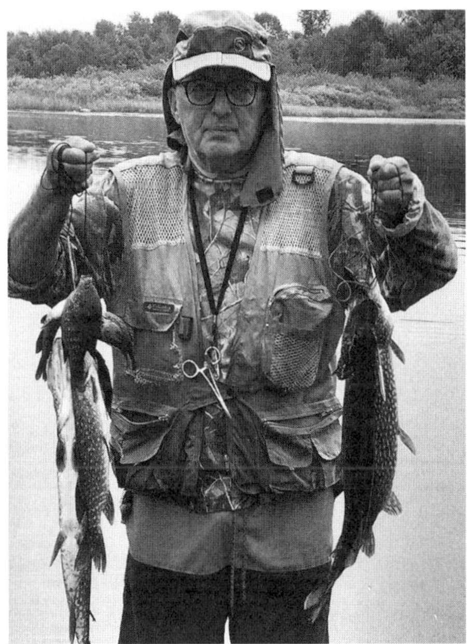

Fifty-eight

The era of Princess Charlotte

We would soon call her "the Princess," but her name was Charlotte Oakwood. She was nominated by the County Board as the new CEO of the County Hospital in 2013. Her qualifications for the job were fuzzy: she was trained in occupational therapy, received some master's degree from an obscure Midwestern entity, served as a director of some rehabilitation center, and, finally, was a vice president of 'something' in a large HMO. However, her primary qualifications soon became apparent: she looked good and could speak! Yes, the woman was some orator! This would explain how and why she managed to impress the bunch of old white country boys (e.g., the retired bank manager, the owner of the feed store, or the wealthy retiree from Chicago — no one knows what he did before) who sat on the County Board and confirmed her appointment.

I first met Charlotte in her office when I dropped in to introduce myself. She walked out from behind her vast desk and shook my hand warmly. I saw a slim woman of an average height, in her mid-fifties but very well preserved.

Her long, light brown hair was elaborately coiffured — like a Southern country belle from the old movies, I thought. She had blue eyes and a charming smile. Most remarkably, she was elegantly dressed: a beige suit, white silk shirt, and expensive looking patent leather high heel shoes. The jewelry was eye-catching as well. She would dress like this for the next five years — tottering and clicking on her Gucci heels from her Mercedes (or maybe it was a Lexus, I cannot remember) to the office. No one dresses like this in the Northwoods of Wisconsin — only self-appointed Princesses…

I do not recall precisely what I said to Charlotte during our first meeting and our frequent encounters over the next six months. Only that our honeymoon period was cordial. *Why not give her a chance,* I thought — why not steer her in the right direction, help her to improve the hospital? Perhaps now is the time, when you are older and wiser, to join the 'establishment' rather than simmer in the 'opposition' — as you have done all your life, I tried to convince myself. Hence, in the beginning, I used to drop into her office occasionally for an informal chat, offering a perspective on the hospital, the community, and what had to be done. She was always polite, nodding her head and pleasantly smiling. Once, I even hugged her...

The five-year reign of our new Princess created a microcosm of dictatorship. A keen observer from the sidelines could watch how a totalitarian regime was rising, how it was sustained, how at the end – if luckily the end arrived – it can rapidly collapse and be forgotten within a few days, without anyone paying the consequence for the crimes committed.

Like any new president entering the White House, the Princess started firing, hiring, and re-shifting personnel; first, the administrative staff, then the doctors. Over a few months, the number of the hospital's supporting staff (i.e., those not directly involved in patient care) was more than tripled. Some days, the ratio of hospital patients to administrative staff was 1:5. New departments mushroomed, like public relations with its three-team staff.

In the current American hospital scene, non-physician CEOs and administrators increasingly control medical affairs (an area previously left to medical staff bodies), and the Princess did the same. But she had a problem: all her hospital doctors were employees of the Clinic. Realizing that "if you don't pay them – you can't control them," she moved fast to get rid of them. To do this, she had to pick a fight with our clinic – the system that essentially dominated medical care in this part of the State.

First, she fired the full-time emergency room doctors – the backbone of any rural hospital, the gatekeepers who provide emergency care to the entire community. To replace them, she had to depend on one of those 'agencies' that supplied locum docs and nurses to any hospital in need. (This is yet another prevailing trend in the American healthcare system: agencies serving as an intermediary between healthcare providers and hospitals – obviously skimming a fair share of the fees paid by the hospital.) Not a few of those medical 'nomads' (some of them already 'discarded' elsewhere) were poorly vetted and not up to the task – as we were soon to realize when the replacement physicians took over the ER.

I started noticing bizarre attitudes and faulty treatment – and consequently poor outcomes – of patients treated in the ER. One case was unforgettable – a middle-aged person presented with features of small bowel obstruction. In the past, he had undergone a Nissen fundoplication procedure (involving a wrap of the stomach around the lower esophagus), which made him unable to vomit and decompress his hugely distended stomach (as visualized on CT) and the blocked intestine below it! As in most such cases, I learned the whole story indirectly, having heard about it through the grapevine – from ER nurses and reviewing the electronic chart. The ER doc tried to insert a nasogastric tube (or most probably told the nurses to do it), but, obviously, the tube did not slide in; *obviously*, because the 'tight' Nissen, which prevented the vomiting, also did not allow placement of the tube. So, the patient was placed in the ambulance and transferred to a tertiary care hospital — where, again, the placement of the nasogastric tube failed. The next afternoon (the surgeon on call was allegedly busy with an elective case in the morning), the patient's abdomen was opened to find the stomach and entire small bowel necrotic — dead! Nothing to do — this was a death sentence! What unsettled me most in this tragedy was that I was only five minutes away from the ER. I was on call; if summoned, I would have taken the patient directly to the OR, decompressed his stomach, and relieved his obstruction. But the system under Princess Charlotte was already failing. Poorly qualified ER docs took over, came and went, and no one bothered to inform them about our local facilities — that we have a surgeon on call.

I was a member of the three-doctor Privileges Committee, scrutinizing the qualifications of any provider applying for privileges to practice in the hospital. However, now the hospital bylaws had become 'Charlotte's laws': a thick file of the nominee was placed on the desk, and we would browse through it and vote to approve. *Next file. Approve. Next...* Initially, I would attempt a mild dissent, e.g., "We need more information... shouldn't we look into this guy's records from California?" Charlotte would brush me off with, "Moshe, we need ER coverage. This appointment is temporary..." Another committee member would look at the wall; the third was always absent. We signed. Our honeymoon was doomed, but I did not feel like terminating it prematurely.

At the same time, Lady Charlotte drove the clinic-employed doctors out of the hospital. In larger hospitals, in-hospital patients are managed by the so-called "hospitalists"— usually qualified internists, MDs. However, unable to recruit and pay suitable doctor-hospitalists, Charlotte had a bright idea, which she borrowed from somewhere: why not use nurse practitioners (NPs) instead... let's call them "nurse-hospitalists." Soon, we saw an ever-changing procession of NPs of different backgrounds and quality in the role of hospitalists. The scene was set for a dysfunctional hospital: patients were maltreated in the ER, often sent home to come back the next day much sicker. Then they would be admitted to the hospital to be looked after by NPs who lacked 'depth' — the experience and knowledge to treat complex cases — only to be shipped south a day later, in worse condition, to a larger center.

Meanwhile, the hospital underwent a facelift: soft carpets replaced the old linoleum in the corridors, rooms were refurbished, and walls were repainted. Original oil paintings by local artists depicting lakes, boats, wooden huts, deer, bears, geese, and dogs were purchased and hung all over. The garden surrounding the building was beautifully landscaped. Bright electronic advertising signs appeared on the roads accessing the hospital. It started to look like a new, small-town Holiday Inn.

In addition, in a side wing of the hospital, an outpatient clinic (aptly named the Riverside Clinic) opened to compete with the adjacent clinic. A few family doctors were hired to work on the new site — they were loudly advertised in the local media and wallboards. However, the local population could not be fooled. News and perceptions circulate rapidly in a small town. Bizarre ER docs, a doctorless hospital, and a few horror stories — exaggerated or not — and the population started voting with their feet and going elsewhere. Those who could drive 45-60 minutes to another center would go there — the less privileged have no choice. The number of patients was falling.

Where was the Board of Trustees? Where was the County that owned the hospital, one would ask? Well, they were all eating crumbs out of Charlotte's hand. Lavish dinners at the golf course, honors, write-ups in the local newspaper with the standard photograph — a group of well-fed dignitaries smiling alongside the Princess. *The hospital looks great, our CEO is great. Aren't we happy!*

With the help of her new director of medical staff (over a few years, the Princess picked up a few of them, including an out-of-town ER doc and a visiting radiologist), Charlotte managed to change the hospital Medical Staff Bylaws, granting NPs an equal status to doctors — including the right to vote. Now, she had no opposition — all decisions were taken by her and approved by the obeying rubber stamp of the staff. A small dictatorship. Yes, some people grumbled in the background, but no clear voice of dissent was heard. The Princess inserted her chosen allies in critical positions, buying their loyalty with flattery and unique benefits. Undoubtedly, the main reason why any CEO dictator succeeds is that people fear losing their jobs, especially in a small town where the choice of employment is limited.

So, what was my status within Charlotte's court? Was I her collaborator, a yes man? Was I a passive bystander? Or did I belong to the opposition — the 'resistance?' The truth is that I belonged to all of the above, in phases — like some characters in the movie *A French Village* under the German occupation. Initially, I tried to collaborate, to be her 'counselor.' It did not last more than a few months as I soon realized she was looking through me and already knew what she wanted and needed. During the next brief phase, I sought to stay out of the fray: *do my job, and let the politicians do whatever they wanted. Why should I care?* This period was also relatively brief. First, it is against my nature to be neutral and passive, and to not take sides. Second, my professional standing came under attack. Unfortunately, I could not join the 'resistance' because no such entity existed in the establishment. The almighty Clinic, my employer, seemed to observe the situation from the sidelines. Ours was only one of their many large and small centers. I think they had decided to let Charlotte run the hospital into the ground, self-destruct… and then take it over — which eventually would occur.

I plodded along, and I wrote to Charlotte: "In view of my utter lack of ability to influence the hospital politics and the inherent differences in style and world view between myself and your leading team, I have decided that excluding myself from any administrative duties would be beneficial to both sides — reducing tensions and preventing conflicts…"

I was hoping to be left alone. But this is not what happened.

* * * * *

Suddenly, one day, Dr. Armando Garcia, my previous 'partner,' reappeared, walking the hospital corridors, smiling, announcing that "I am coming back soon…"

Some background. After leaving our hospital five years prior, the old surgeon found a job in a remote lakeside town in northern Minnesota. (Remember what he had said repeatedly: "If I stop operating, I will die.") Each year during the October meeting of the American College of Surgeons, I would spot him shuffling along the endless carpeted corridors of the convention center. He would try to avoid eye contact, but I stopped him for a brief, terse chat. I had wondered when he would retire, noticing his unsteady gait. And now I asked myself: what is he doing back in Ladysmith, well into his late seventies?

I started my investigations with the Princess. I strolled through the open door of her office, ignoring her secretary's objection, "Charlotte's busy."

"I hear that Dr. Garcia is coming back," I fired off immediately. I watched her face stiffening behind the permanent smile. Her left shoulder jerked. I had observed it previously during meetings — the jerking of the shoulder. She is surprised that I know, I thought; she was planning a bombshell.

"Well, doctor… yes, Dr. Garcia showed interest in returning. We had some preliminary confidential meetings. May I ask how you knew about it?"

"Everybody knows about it. He's walking the corridors advertising his return."

"I understand," she replies, her residual smile evaporating. "We think that it could benefit the hospital. As you know, Dr. Garcia is a leading colorectal surgeon. He'll attract more cases. You and he will be partners…"

"Partners? I decide with whom I want to be a partner." Only thinking about having to deal with Garcia again irritated me. "And anyway," I continued, "do you know how old he is? He must be over seventy-five years old. Yes, he may have been a leading colorectal surgeon. But people deteriorate with age. Did you investigate his recent past? What has he been doing over the last five years? What is his health status? Even five years ago, he wasn't a symbol of healthiness."

The Princess looked directly at my eyes. "Please, doctor, we don't talk about age. No age disqualifies a candidate. Dr. Garcia is in good health, as documented during a recent physical. He comes with excellent references from his colleagues."

"I still don't understand why he suddenly left Minnesota," I persisted. "Did you speak with his employers? People tend to write nice references, but you may hear what's not on paper when you talk to them. And by the way, you know that routine physicals cannot capture the finer points in physical and cognitive deterioration."

The Princess interrupted: "Dr. Garcia would like to relocate back to Wisconsin because it will bring him nearer to his permanent home and extended family. And yes, we have reviewed his references and found them reliable." She turned back to the papers on her desk. "And now, please, excuse me. Please schedule it with my front desk next time you decide to talk to me."

I did not move. "I have a suggestion," I said. "The Sinai Hospital at Baltimore runs a so-called 'Aging Surgeon Program.' They offer a set of tests, assessing old surgeons' performance. You know, whether their head is still well connected with the hands."

The Princess kept staring at me.

"Would you let a seventy-seven-year-old surgeon remove the rectum of your mother?" I persisted. "Would you want to fly with a seventy-seven-year-old untested pilot? If you want to employ him, then send him to Baltimore. It will cost you a few thousand bucks. Not a big deal."

"OK, doctor, we will look into it." Which I knew she wouldn't.

"Could I please see Garcia's application for hospital privileges? Including his list of references," I said.

"Sure. The Executive Secretary will hand you Garcia's file. Have a good day, doctor." Now the other shoulder was jerking as well.

I locked myself in my office, with Garcia's list of references, and called each of Garcia's alleged supporters. I took careful notes.

The first was Dr. Sarah T., a family doctor who recently worked with Garcia in Minnesota. She said: "Dr. Garcia is such a beautiful person... he was permanently on call. No, he did not do any colectomies in our center; he did many appendectomies. I'm not aware of any special problems with him. No, I am not sure why he has retired. I am very fond of him..."

Next, I called Dr. Donald N., another family practice doctor at the same center. He said: "Oh yeah, old Armando is a good friend of mine. He was always available. We already miss him, a rare person, great with patients and their families." As I burrowed deeper into specific areas of the old surgeon's practice, Dr. Donald N. replied: "Yes, he was doing endoscopies initially, but he had to give it up because of problems. I think there were a few missed diagnoses of cancers." When I asked about Garcia's advanced age, the doctor replied: "As a friend, I wish he would agree to retire. Life is catching up with him. But he refuses — he thinks that if he does, he'll die."

Dr. Donald N. denied knowing anything about why Garcia had left his position hastily. He said: "This area belongs to the Chief of Surgery; I am just a family doctor and a good friend."

I had to speak with the Chief of Surgery, whoever he was — his name was not included in Garcia's list of references. I Googled the Chief of Surgery for the system that had employed Garcia. I dialed, and surprisingly, the Chief was immediately available, friendly, chatty, and forthcoming. He said that whatever he would say had to be on a confidential basis… because the termination agreement reached with Dr. Garcia two months ago did not allow him to describe the details. However, he agreed "that such an informal chat between professionals is crucial to help to avoid hiring 'problem candidates.'" On further questioning, the Chief said, "Over the last two years Dr. Garcia's practice was 'restricted'; he was not permitted to perform major surgery (e.g., colectomies); nor was he permitted to do colonoscopies." To my question, "why?" the Chief declined to provide specific reasons but said that there were "serious concerns." When I asked, "why exactly was he terminated?" the Chief replied that "Dr. Garcia's age is catching up with him… his age is showing itself." He added: "We offered him a graceful exit, but he resisted… not showing insight — thus he was terminated." The pleasantly talkative chief concluded: "I hope that you and I when our time comes, will know when to gracefully put down the scalpel before being forced to do so."

"You are right, sir. Thank you very much." I hung up.

Wow. I got what I needed.

Next, I wrote to the Princess with a detailed transcript of each of the conversations I had with Garcia's referees. I concluded: "I respectfully suggest that Dr. AG's application is not presented to the general medical staff meeting next Tuesday."

The following day, I was urgently summoned to see the Princess. Arriving at her office at the scheduled time, I was surprised to find the head administrator of our local clinic sitting opposite the Princess' desk.

"I invited Tim as a representative of the Clinic, your employer, to hear what I have to say," the Princess explained. She placed a document on the desk. "Please read it." I skimmed a cliché-laden narrative admonishing me for unauthorized contact with Garcia's referees, which was unnecessary because even though Dr. Garcia had applied for a job in her hospital, she did not consider him at all. Early on, she realized that the surgeon was not qualified for the position. In fact, she had already called him to tell him so…

I froze for a moment. I dropped the letter on her desk with disgust.

"Charlotte," I said, "you know what you are? You are a liar!" I remember repeating the "liar" a few times to emphasize my disgust.

I watched the CEO's face turn white. Tim, the local clinic's administrator, hissed angrily: "You cannot use such terms. This is unacceptable. You have to apologize now!"

"Why should I," I said, standing up. "She's a liar, she lies all the time." I walked out the door.

Funny, I thought, the Princess has been engaged in endless wars with our clinic. But when it comes to a conflict between administrators and clinicians, the administrators close ranks. From now on, I understood that the Princess would be my sworn enemy. I would have to be careful not to give her any excuse to eliminate me.

I perceived that her mini-dictatorship was unsustainable in the long term and that, eventually, she would abort the ship. I aimed to outlive her. To stay out of trouble. I tried. Nevertheless, I could not stay out of political strife for long. That is when the Princess would go after my jugular.

* * * * *

Let me now introduce Dr. Lorene Green, one of the family doctors recruited by the Princess two years earlier. She was hired, with great fanfare, to practice in Charlotte's Riverside Clinic. Her other roles were the hospital's chief medical officer and the supervisor of the nurse-hospitalist team. From the start, I perceived Lorene as a clever physician and a pleasant person I could work with.

Lorene's story in brief: a Jewish girl from Long Island, a daughter of Holocaust survivors. She attended medical school somewhere in New York. She married an anesthesiologist and moved with him to the West Coast, where she trained to become a family practice doctor. A son was born. It seems that the husband was cruel and abusive, and at some point, they divorced.

She moved to Oregon, where one day, in a bookshop — she described the scenario to me a few times — she met Brad, her current husband. At least twenty years younger, Brad could be described as a 'hunk.' Tall, heavy but muscular, his features were Native American; he sported a pitch-black long ponytail. Lacking formal education, he was an autodidact: eloquent, prone to conspiracy theories, and, it seems, thriving in the bitcoin domain.

The corpulent, middle-aged Jewish girl from Long Island and her giant, longhaired descendant of some Oregon tribe made an unconventional couple. At first glance, she was the bread earner — bringing the dollars in from the hospital; he her caregiver, the glorified butler — cooking, shopping, cleaning, driving her around. But if one bothered to look deeper, one would perceive the bond and loyalty developing between two injured humans — she a battered wife, lonely (after her parents died, she lost contact with her brothers on the East Coast); he an ex-foster child — both seeking warmth, love, and support.

We 'adopted' this likable couple into our social milieu. This resulted in long, boozy dinners at our home, the homes of our friends, and eventually at Lorene's renovated lakeside house. During such dinners, I milked out Lorene's life story bit by bit. Later, after the couple had left, we reflected that not even once during those long dinners, extending over a few years, did Lorene or Brad ask any of us any personal questions. "All she knew about me was that my name is Dan," said one of our friends.

Initially, the couple seemed to settle well in their beautiful house. We observed that Brad desired big toys and that Lorene hastened to fulfill all his wants: a huge brand-new super duty truck, a giant pontoon, a modern home gym in their basement, a super-size German Shepherd, and a series of not-so-huge additional toys.

At the hospital, Lorene took over multiple clinical responsibilities as well as a growing list of administrative roles, constantly heaped on her by the Princess. As time passed, I noted Lorene developing signs of attrition — that, predictably, the Princess, with her incessant demands and criticism, was grating on Lorene's nerves. Lorene was gaining weight and repeatedly staying at home 'sick.' After a glass or two of wine, she would grumble about the Princess and mock her in private. "Charlotte's hospital is like the North Korean regime," she would say. However, she enjoyed a decent income; they had a new home and many toys to pay for — she had to be committed to her contract and the Princess.

* * * * *

My détente with the Princess and the friendship with Lorene and Brad ended in May 2017. Here is the story of what took place…

Saturday, early afternoon. Nicole, one of the 'out of town' nurse-hospitalists, calls me at home. She tells me about an elderly man admitted during the previous night with painful gallstones. "His pain has resolved, and he wants to go home."

"OK, let him see me on Monday in the Clinic to discuss an elective cholecystectomy," I reply.

Sunday. Nicole calls me again just before lunchtime: "Listen, I could not discharge the guy. He is not well, spiking a temp., he has right upper quadrant pain and an elevated WBC count." It sounds to me more like acute cholecystitis, and so, while not formally on call, I drive to the hospital to assess the patient. As expected, I diagnose acute calculous cholecystitis. He is an octogenarian but in relatively good shape despite a history of heart disease. I start him on antibiotics and arrange for a laparoscopic cholecystectomy the following morning. Nicole agrees with the plan and promises to 'clear' the patient for anesthesia. The OR is informed — lap cholecystectomy, Monday 9:45. The patient concurs with the plan and signs the consent form.

Monday. I arrive at the hospital around 8 a.m. I go directly to see the patient to check whether he is ready. I find him tachycardic and more tender in the right upper quadrant than the previous day. I am convinced that his gallbladder is now necrotic and needs to come out ASAP. I look for Nicole but to my surprise, she is gone — another nurse-hospitalist took over last night. She is Celene, a pale-looking forty-something woman I had never met before (in the Princess' Kingdom, new nurse-hospitalists appeared — and rapidly vanished — quite often). She says the patient had a spell of dizziness, tachycardia overnight, and a "bump in his troponin levels" (cardiac enzymes).

"Sure, he is septic," I reply. "His gallbladder is probably necrotic and has to come out soon." I add that I am not worried about the troponin levels — false-positive elevations are common in patients with acute gallbladder disease.

I go over to the OR and speak with the head nurse about the operative plan; they are setting up the room. I still have half an hour for a coffee in my office, scanning *The New York Times* online.

At 9 a.m., I put on my scrub cap, ready to walk to the OR, when the phone rings. It is Celene, the new nurse-hospitalist. "Doctor, your operation has been canceled. The patient has to be shipped immediately to cardiology in Eau Claire..."

"WHAT?!" I interrupt her, my blood already boiling — it's even simmering now, years later, when I'm writing this — for how can anybody decide to cancel an indicated emergency surgical procedure a minute before it should begin without consulting the responsible surgeon?

"Who decided?" I ask, trying to suppress my anger, "On what grounds?"

"Well, Dr. Green did, you know, Lorene. It's her decision. She's worrying about his heart. Like, we think he's developing a heart attack. The troponin..."

"Oh, just forget about the troponin, his gallbladder is necrotic..." I realize there is no use in shooting the messenger, so I hang up on her in midsentence.

I pick up my cell phone and dial Lorene's number. "Good morning," I get directly to the point. Why did she cancel my case without talking to me? I explain that the patient is septic from his necrotic gallbladder — a diabetic patient with acute cholecystitis needs an urgent cholecystectomy — not cardiology.

Lorene is not impressed. "He has to be shipped out," she insists. No discussion.

"Where are you? Can we meet at the bedside and discuss it further?" I ask.

"No, I'm at home…"

"So, you cancel my patient's operation without even examining him? Based on what some nurse tells you over the phone?" I wait for a reply and hear none.

I hang up.

I am furious. It has never happened to me in forty years of surgical practice — a decision to cancel an emergency case behind my back. But I cannot change the verdict. Lorene is the Chief Medical Officer. She decided that the patient was not fit for anesthesia and that he had to see a cardiologist urgently. I cannot force the anesthetist to put him to sleep.

I walk back to the patient's room to inform him — no one else had bothered doing so — that his operation must be canceled, and he is to be transferred to a large hospital in Eau Claire. Where, on the same day, he undergoes a cholecystectomy, during which the gallbladder is found to be purulent and necrotic. He goes home two days later. Of course, there is no problem whatsoever with his heart.

I could not fall asleep the following night, replaying in my mind the day's events, trying to rationalize what happened. After 'sleeping over the case' and listening to my wife's advice, I decide to discuss it with Lorene Green face-to-face. We have been good friends for more than two years, so why shouldn't we be able to settle our dispute without involving any third party? In the morning, I sent her an e-mail asking for a chat. She does not reply. Around noon, I walk up to the Riverside Clinic and find Dr. Green in her office behind a large desk. Her medical assistant stands at her side.

"Can we talk?"

"I am busy," Lorene replies.

"Just five minutes," I persist.

She agrees reluctantly. We move to an empty office on the other side of the corridor and close the door behind us.

Even before we sit down, Lorene says: "You have to apologize. You hung up the phone on me." She is pale. I perceive that she is furious.

I say: "I apologize. I'm sorry for hanging up the phone on you. But you have to understand that you have pissed me off in a big way. No one has ever canceled an emergency operation behind my back… without talking to me. You can't do such things to me…"

"That patient had to fly out of here…," she says, not looking at me. *Is she detached?*

"You could have called me, discussed the matter with me… it would have taken five minutes to explain to you…" I am trying to be calm. Treat her as an equivalent of a shell-shocked soldier.

"I don't have time to talk to you," Lorene replies.

This is the provoking trigger. Now, I am agitated. *What — she does not have time to speak to me!*

I stand and raise my voice: "Lorene, you have not even seen the patient. You didn't examine him, a patient I was working on over the weekend. It is unacceptable..."

Lorene stands up and opens the door. On the way out, she turns her head around. "I don't have time to examine every patient. I just knew that he should be shipped out." I follow Lorene into the corridor, screaming behind her back; I do not remember the exact wording of my angry rants, but bystanders would report later hearing something like "move your fat ass." Her assistant would later report seeing Lorene crying in her office.

Repercussions arrived the next day.

Three years after the Armando Garcia 'affair,' the Princess has finally spotted a chance to hit back at me. To take revenge! For a woman of such character would never forget and forgive being called "a liar" in public.

Complaint letters were immediately drafted by the Princess — signed by Dr. Green and NP Celene — implying that I abused them verbally and they "felt physically threatened." The Princess walked around the hospital collecting 'negative observations' about me from her cronies — that she summarized in another letter. That included the OR head nurse's opinion that "It is not unusual for Dr. Schein to complain when things don't go his way." The head ER nurse (whose husband's large hernia I had fixed just the previous year) said: "He often comes in to complain when patients are transferred out without his knowledge..."

It gave me a déjà vu feeling — back to Indira of Keokuk, the Keokuk Hospital, and its kangaroo court of more than ten years ago. Luckily, my circumstances were much more favorable this time — I was not the Princess's employee; I belonged to the Clinic, and it stood by me. Meetings were conducted; I was reprimanded and 'warned' by the hospital's medical staff — all Charlotte's appointees. To appease the Princess, the Clinic arranged for me to be evaluated by their head psychiatrist (humiliating!), who in turn referred me for a few sessions with a counselor on "interpersonal relationships at the workplace." I was asked to read and discuss *Emotional Intelligence 2.0*, a book I enjoyed.

What happened to my friend Dr. Lorene Green? A week or so after our 'incident,' Lorene went on medical leave. A few months later, she resigned. She and her hunk were not seen ever again.

* * * * *

Before we exit the era of the Princess, there is one more piece to mention — something that had been bothering me. It concerns the Princess's attempts to bring religion, her faith, into the workplace.

A little church stood at one of the wings of the hospital that employed a part-time Catholic chaplain. The first hospital chaplain that I knew was killed in 2007 by a drunken driver while crossing the road opposite the hospital. He was replaced by a tall and robust man, always meticulously dressed, wearing a large cross hanging low on his chest. I would encounter the chaplain sporadically — in the ER comforting a bereaved family, at night sitting with an old man awaiting a laparotomy — but usually, I would meet him in the corridor. We would stop, shake hands, and exchange pleasantries. At some point, I fixed his hernia.

It was well into the Princess' reign when the chaplain decided to retire. A farewell ceremony was organized in the hospital dining room. I decided to show my face because I liked the guy, because he had been my patient, but mainly because it seemed the right thing to do. I entered the crowded room just as the Princess ended her long speech. I heard her saying: "Now, Father, please lead us in a prayer… join your hands, everybody…"

I saw people forming a circle, holding hands. Someone grabbed my right hand, and another nurse tried to capture the left one. What should I do? The door was a few feet away — I still could escape. The chaplain was looking at me, smiling. "Hello, doctor," he said. *How can I leave now?* So, I surrendered my hands on both sides and observed the proceeding. Everyone closed their eyes and looked at the floor while the chaplain recited a prayer. I did not listen to his words. I was thinking how uncomfortable I was — a non-practicing Jew — holding hands with a bunch of praying Christians. Not that I had anything against them or their faith; I respected their faith. However, this should not have happened in a public American hospital supported by federal funds.

A year later, the Princess hired a consulting agency to advise on the hospital's situation and recommend how to rescue it from its financial decline. The two consultants arrived from Boston, a middle-aged smiling man and a younger pretty woman. Both presented themselves as previous senior medical administrators. They spent two days walking around, smiling a lot, and asking questions. Then they left to write their report (predictably stating that the hospital was in poor shape and "drastic changes are needed"), taking a fee of a hundred grand, paid by the County.

A few weeks later, I was invited to a dinner at the local golf club: "The consultants will return to share their findings and recommendations with us." All the city's dignitaries and who's who were invited. I looked at the event's program: "Cocktails, benediction (by our retired chaplain), dinner, introduction by the CEO, consultants' report."

"Benediction." Yet again, the Princess mixes religion with the hospital business. I told myself this time I would not be caught in it. Let them drink, pray, and eat, and I will stroll in towards the end, only to feign interest in what the consultants say.

I walked into the golf club bar at about 7:30 p.m. Through the open doors, I could see the dining room, the cacophony of a large group of dining people reaching my ears. I got myself a bourbon on the rocks and waited at the bar. Once I heard the voice of the Princess on the microphone, I walked in and scanned the dining room. There was an empty seat by one of the front tables nearest the door. I sat down, nodding to the other occupants, still busy with their coffees and desserts.

The Princess was already giving her introductory speech. We made eye contact. "Dear friends, at this time, let me call on chaplain Rogers for the invocation…" *Fuck, he should have done it before dinner.* Before the chaplain opened his mouth, I walked out of the door back into the bar, where I refilled my glass and waited patiently until I heard the end of the prayer. Then I strolled back, looked around the tables, sensing that everyone had noticed my exit and return, and sat down at my place.

The program continued. The consultants went to the podium one by one. Each presented a slide show. I guessed the same PowerPoint show they use repeatedly at each hospital they consult. With the same conclusion: the model of a small independent rural hospital is viable no more – your hospital has to merge into a larger system. As if we did not know it…

We did not know it at that time, but already then, the Princess had been designing her exit. At the end of 2017, she had 'accepted' a CEO position in a larger hospital south of us. She did not last long at her next job. A year later, she moved back to her hometown in Nebraska. A Google search shows that she runs a consulting firm and is a prolific advocate and public speaker in healthcare, servant leadership, spiritual formation, as well as women's issues. She would travel to provide advice on hospital management. Fittingly, she sits on the local chamber of commerce.

Who was Charlotte really? The character I attempted to paint is rather superficial. Could she truly be stereotyped as an immoral dictator – a minor equivalent of our 45th President? I observed only her professional side; I knew almost nothing about her inner life. What I recognized was a charming socialite, a gracious host and probably a loving wife and mother. She was a product of her time and place: a product of a small-town, middle-class upbringing, within a conservative, consumer-capitalistic, parochial, religious-Republican environment. She was ambitious! It must have been tough for a pretty, outspoken girl (probably a local *wunderkind*) to advance in what then was mostly a male dominated world. She had to be ruthless and tough! However, in terms of her performance as a CEO of a rural hospital she provides another example of what is wrong in the American healthcare system.

The Princess left a 'dying' hospital, both financially (with 'doctored' books) and depleted of essential staff, bursting at the seams with paper pushers. But I was relieved. Another 'enemy' had left, and I had survived. I remembered what Tolstoy wrote: "Patience is waiting. Not passively waiting. That is laziness. But to keep going when the going is hard and slow – that is patience. The two most powerful warriors are patience and time."

* * * * *

Fifty-nine

The closing years

The post-Princess years were relatively uneventful. That is, if one considers minor political upheavals and 'routine' clinical dramas as just standard background noise within the prevailing chaos of American medicine. At that stage, I was turning sixty-seven years old. I felt great, but I realized that the end of my surgical life was written on the wall. The only question was when...

Reading memoirs by others, I am always struck by how the quality of writing, the charm, and the eloquence diminish as the narrative reaches the end – not that I can claim that what I wrote hitherto is overly charming or eloquent. Gradually, as events become more recent, the storyline becomes impassive, technical, stale, and dull. Hence, I will fast-forward through the closing years leading to the final steps of my surgical life.

In parallel with the departure of Princess Charlotte, the hospital that she had managed to devastate was purchased by our clinic. Now, finally, the almighty Clinic was in control of both entities. Typically, such mergers are followed by significant changes. The most enormous consequence to me personally was the closure of the hospital's operating room in the evenings, nights, and weekends. Consequently, all emergencies arriving at the emergency room were to be shipped out to one of the larger hospitals owned by the Clinic. I had to start sharing calls with the general surgery group at the Rice Lake Hospital, situated some forty miles west of us.

It was a significant change: after more than ten years of solo practice, I had to get used to working with partners yet again. It turned out well. The Rice Lake Hospital proved to be a state-of-the-art, well-run facility. My new partners, a changing assortment of surgeons, were mostly decent chaps and sound surgeons. Phil M., some twenty years younger than me, was my favorite – a model of a solid small-town surgeon. The even younger Bill K. and Phil K. proved superb – it is reassuring that our modern training systems can still produce some solid, clinically orientated, and ethical surgeons.

My quality of life improved: whereas previously I had always made myself available for emergencies, now, on call 1:4, I could 'switch off' and relax. The tradeoff consisted of longer drives to the hospital at night, especially in bad weather, and long weekends on call in one of Rice Lake's motels: little kids running through the corridors, screaming, dripping water — from the pool to the room, back to the pool, their parents sipping light beer and watching Fox News. It was a relief to be called in for an acute appendix or a rotten gallbladder.

* * * * *

And so, the years continued passing by while I was brooding about retirement the 'next year.' Old colleagues were gradually retiring, and I found myself working with people 30-40 years younger than me; in fact, I became the oldest 'provider' around. But because I relished the role of the 'old' surgeon (and managed to adapt to the pace and magnitude of my practice), the 'next year' never arrived. That is, until I was diagnosed with the 'old man's cancer' — prostate cancer. My cancer appears localized and is potentially curable; statistically, at least, it shouldn't shorten my longevity on this earth. However, it was a wake-up call that the end is not elusive — it will arrive sooner than later. So perhaps one should allow more time with the grandkids…

I could dedicate a whole book about my experience with prostate cancer. Many others, patients and doctors, have done it already (like Henry Marsh, the bestselling British brain surgeon in *And Finally: Matters of Life and Death*, 2022). I will only mention this: navigating the options and decision-making is complex — even for such a relatively common condition. It has become more complex in the era of the Internet, where misinformation dilutes reliable information. It is even more difficult for someone familiar with medical literature to perceive the risks and benefits of any management modality chosen. I was already scheduled for a robotic prostatectomy ("let's remove the tumor… you will be home the next day"), but I chickened out! I canceled the operation and decided to undergo six weeks of radiation therapy instead. It is well known that surgeons are less inclined to choose an operative approach (for any disease where there are other options) for themselves and their families — they know better. I was advised by an excellent oncologist to receive a prolonged course of medication to suppress/abolish my testosterone levels "because studies show it to improve long-term results," but I decided to stop the injections of Lupron after two months. Unpleasant side effects developed within a few weeks; I knew more would follow.

Why suffer now, I thought, when I am healthy and fit, for the (statistical) probability that the drug would prolong my life by a few percent? Statistically, my prognosis should be excellent. But who knows…

* * * * *

I promised a book about a surgical life. But now, as we arrive at the end, I notice that I skipped not a few topics that occupied my professional life. My take on any of those topics could be, or was, a subject for a book by itself. Here, I will dedicate a few pages to it.

I spent a lot of my 'free' time researching, writing, publishing, editing, and reviewing work by others. It was a satisfying hobby. I believe that the advice in our book (with Abe Fingerhut and the late John Farndon), *A Surgeon's Guide to Writing and Publishing* (2001), is still pertinent today. Our book *Schein's Common Sense Emergency Abdominal Surgery* (with Paul Rogers, Danny Rosin, Mark Cheetham, Ari Leppäniemi, and Ahmad Assalia) has now reached its 5th edition. It has been translated into numerous languages; from the feedback we receive constantly from readers, it seems that the book has achieved 'cult status' among young surgeons in some places. My book *Aphorisms and Quotations for the Surgeon* (2002) has been selling well for years — probably one of those immortal books.

I published hundreds of articles in professional journals until I left New York and 'academia.' Over the years, however, my enthusiasm dwindled. I became cynical, skeptical, and suspicious — my trust in published medical literature deeply eroded. The Internet and electronic revolution have been killing medical publications' prestige, quality, and reliability, flooding us with untrustworthy and often unreadable information. During my last years as an Associate Editor of the *World Journal of Surgery*, searching for a publishable submission was like finding a needle in a haystack. Many of the submissions, mostly cliché-ridden, read like politically correct fiction. I resigned.

About the politics, intrigues, and social aspects of academic life, which I tasted in limited portions, others, more experienced, can write better about this (for a comical version of it, try David Lodge). I traveled extensively during the New York years, giving talks, sitting on panels, etc. Moscow, Bangkok, Ghent, Mumbai, Santiago, Gdansk, Halle, Hong Kong, Lucerne, Cartagena… come to mind. Some of the gathered adventures would deserve a travelogue. The endless nights of Moscow, Gdansk, Mumbai, or Cartagena would belong to a different genre. Around the world, I made not a few friends: most transient, a few for life (e.g., Paul

Rogers of Glasgow, Ari Leppäniemi of Helsinki, Wojciech Górecki of Krakow, Denis Arkhipov of Moscow).

Another special friend was Boris Savchuk, a Russian surgeon of Ukrainian origin. His career shined under the Soviet system, but deep inside, he definitely was not a *Homo Sovieticus*. He had led the Russian medical aid efforts in war-torn Ethiopia, later to become the Surgeon-in-Chief in the famed Kremlin Hospital that served the Soviet elite — the *nomenklatura*. His excellent English, frequent foreign travels, large fancy apartment, and new Volvo suggested he was well connected higher up. In Moscow, he treated me like a father. In the mornings, he would pick me up at the giant (2272 rooms), now demolished, Rossiya Hotel, immediately stopping at a kiosk to buy me a cold beer ("it will help you to recover"). In the evening, after a day of activities, he would drop me off back at the hotel but never join me into the stormy nights ("I'm too old for it"). Initially, Boris had promised to travel with me to Western Ukraine by train — to visit his parents' graves, "perhaps the last time," he said. But on the day of departure, he arrived at the hotel and formally announced that he could not go because "his heart is not too well." Before my departure to the railway station, he made us sit around a table at the lobby and observe a minute of silence: "This is how we do it in Russia," he said, "before parting, we sit together silently and contemplate, for one never knows whether this is our last meeting." He drove me to the railway station, shoved a large bottle of the "best Russian vodka" in my hands, and we said our last goodbye — a kiss on each cheek and a bear hug — the Russian way. A few months later, in March 2004, Boris e-mailed me from Moscow: "Couple of words about myself: during the last year I acquired some cardiac problems. Next week, I should be admitted to the National Center of Cardiology for a surgical intervention. I hope I can inform you in detail after the intervention. Curse me (Russian token), or pray for me, please! Your devoted friend Boris." Boris never woke up after the operation. He was seventy-one years old. He was a real Russian gentleman — polite and correct, knowledgeable in medicine, surgery, literature, art, music, and life — and with a large, warm, and sensitive heart — he belonged to a vanishing generation of great surgeons. Although 100% Russian down to his bones, unlike most of his peers, he dared to look beyond the boundaries of his vast fatherland; thus, his departure was a loss to international surgery. One can read more about Boris's fascinating life in the *World Journal of Surgery* (A Great Russian Surgeon: Boris Dmitrievich Savchuk (1933-2004). *World J Surg* 2005; 29: 676-8).

What do I think about our current medical system?

I decided not to bore you with the maladies of the US medical-industrial complex. So much has been written about the chaos, the corruption, the greed, the overbilling, the inequality, the deficient access, about what the EMR does to our practice and brains — so many articles and books are dedicated to these problems, but politicians driven by interest groups obstruct remedies. I summoned my thoughts in an article published in the *Scandinavian Journal of Surgery* (As We Continue to Drift Into a Totalitarian Medical System: A View of a Country Boy. *Scand J Surg* 2018; 107: 3-5). My good friend Ari L. of Helsinki, who served as the journal's Editor, agreed to publish it anonymously. The full version is available online: https://journals.sagepub.com/doi/full/10.1177/1457496918757579.

I cannot, however, avoid mentioning the horrible fee-for-service system that dominates American medicine (and other regions of the world) in some form or another. Wherever you work, the system wants you to be productive or, in other words, to do more. You are not compensated for your value to the community in preventing and alleviating morbidity and suffering. Instead, your compensation is based, directly or indirectly, on the volume of your production. Undoubtedly, this constant pressure to 'produce' is responsible for the common phenomenon of unnecessary surgery — in fact, surgery and any procedure — and the escalating costs. Consequently, some surgeons would repair any asymptomatic inguinal hernia (which could be safely left alone), and a cardiologist would insert a stent in any narrow coronary artery, whether it is indicated or not. By deciding to 'do' something rather than leave it alone, the physician earns manifold more; actually, one is 'punished' for practicing ethical surgery. This phenomenon, I believe, poisons US medicine.

In a few years, my generation will enter the ranks of the elderly patient population. It is a scary proposition — becoming a sick patient and having to navigate the future (or current) healthcare environment can be frightening. In my mind, there is no partial remedy for the system. No method of palliation would eradicate the cancer. Only radical resection: replacing the system with a single-payer system would have a chance to work. But it is wishful thinking. It will never be allowed to happen in this country. The totalitarian medical system and its friends are too strong.

Serving as an expert witness on medical malpractice cases became a side hobby of mine. In the vast majority of cases, I served supporting the plaintiffs' cases — the claims of the harmed patients against the medical system that maltreated them. Most doctors consider experts who testify against them as traitors. Some call them "legal whores" — as if the experts defending the doctors are not equally well-paid "whores." I saw it differently: if the patient is harmed, if the consequences of the harm are permanent, and if the damage was caused by a breach in the so-called "standard of care," then the patient deserves to be compensated. And to be compensated, he must have a solid expert witness on his side.

I was recruited to this field by Avi Rubinstein. Avi has been a close friend from our medical school years in Jerusalem. Later, he trained to become a neurosurgeon and studied law simultaneously, becoming a leading malpractice lawyer in Tel Aviv. I supported numerous surgical malpractice claims with Avi and later other lawyers in Israel. We won in all of them. None was ruled in favor of the defendants. The secret, I learned, is to be objective, impartial, and selective — to support only cases of individuals genuinely harmed by an apparent, demonstrable deviation from what one believes (based on experience and the literature) is the standard of care (SOC). The latter is defined as "the watchfulness, attention, caution, and prudence that a reasonable surgeon under similar circumstances would exercise." Failure to meet the SOC means negligence.

This legal work, dissecting the medical records and finding how to prove the allegations, gave me more than intellectual satisfaction. It was a constant reminder of how to avoid, in my practice, all those pitfalls and errors committed by those surgeons whom we litigated. It provided examples for our book, *Schein's Common Sense Prevention and Management of Surgical Complications* (2013). Besides, I always find it a pleasure to go against the 'establishment' — the system armed with big pockets, big lawyers, and big-name professors serving as experts for the defense. Add to it some *schadenfreude*. The director of the hospital in Haifa had said that I was not good enough for them. Remember? Now it was time for karma!

I engaged in similar legal activities in the USA but to a lesser extent — perhaps a case or two a year. Also, in the USA, we have won all our cases except one — I wrote a short book about it: *Justice in Biloxi. Anatomy of a Malpractice Case.* You can find it on amazon.

SURGINET has enriched my professional life for many years. SURGINET is an international online discussion group for general surgeons. It was founded in 1995 by Dr. Tom Gilas from the University of Toronto. From its early days, I became one of SURGINET's prolific contributors, contributing, I believe, more than a million words. However, SURGINET gave me much more than I gave it. It provided me with real-time, almost instant advice for any clinical dilemma — I found the input from a bunch of surgeons worldwide more valuable than listening to the 'dogma' preached by local colleagues. Furthermore, I constantly used it as a 'testing ground' for ideas for publications; I valued the CME I got from it much above that imparted from the literature or meetings. Unfortunately, SURGINET is aging along with its members. The emerging new *Homo Chirurgicus* seems less altruistic, and less inclined to invest effort in sharing ideas and wisdom and educate others. He or she is less inquisitive, more prone to dogma — as much an admirer of guidelines as a product of them. All the wisdom they need is available on Google, YouTube or one of the UPDATE apps. However, I cannot blame the new generation, for they are overwhelmed, drowning under a constant flood of office e-mails, administrative mandates, and mandatory education (e.g., the same videos about sexual harassment, computer safety, and numerous other topics each year); they have to retrain in ever-changing versions of the EMR, they are pressurized to be productive and generate RVUs (Relative Value Units) — who has any time left for anything else?

There could be so many other items to discuss. For example, the horrendous obesity affecting the population in this part of the world constantly occupied my 'surgical' mind. As professionals, surgeons tend to be politically correct, but I will be blunt: the average American eats and drinks crap uncontrollably. Thus, he or she is fat! You can see morbidly obese Americans everywhere, young, and old, and even little children weighing as much as an overweight adult. In contrast, stroll about Italy or Spain or France: if you see a really huge man, be assured that he is an American tourist. Yes, often it's 'not their fault' — blame the 'environment,' the food industry, the prevailing 'food culture' or their 'DNA' (even though their 'genetic cousins' in Scandinavia, Germany or Poland are spared). But the bottom line is that Americans eat themselves to death. Walk into any clinic, and you will note the high proportion of obese individuals in the waiting room. For they, and their numerous obesity-related maladies, devour a significant chunk of our medical resources.

Surgeons hate operating on 'fatties' — except, obviously, those surgeons who make their living in the bariatric industry. Taking out an appendix or a colon in an obese patient involves double the effort and stress than doing it in a petite Japanese person. And of course operations on the very obese are associated with an increased risk of postoperative complications. Thus, the first item I look at on the EMR before seeing a potential surgical candidate is their BMI. While the enormous implications of the obesity epidemic are well documented in the literature, they tend to be disregarded by the public and lay media. We have the right to be fat, leave us alone — this is their motto. But the truth is that the obesity epidemic kills more people each year than the COVID-19 pandemic did. Alas, there is no vaccine for obesity. But the denial of the deniers is the same. One thing that I will not miss after retiring is diving into the depths of an immense abdomen, trying to remove a perforated colon covered by tons of fat. Enough said.

In addition, I will not miss the constant worrying. Like any professionals holding responsible jobs, surgeons worry a lot. Often I would wake up in the middle of the night and worry. Worry about the operative case awaiting me the next morning (*Is he ready? Is the operative plan correct?*); worry about the case I did yesterday — replaying in my mind each step of the procedure (*was I too 'aggressive,' should I have done anything differently?*); worry about the patient who developed complications (*should I take him back to the OR, or transfer him out?*). Worry, worry, like more 'normal' surgeons do. But there is something that I have never read in any of the numerous surgical memoirs — the 'surgical nightmares.' The pattern of such nightmares that I experience on and off is constant: I am doing something deep in the recesses of the abdomen but the procedure does not move forward. Torrential bleeding develops up and behind the liver and I cannot control it; I try to suture the intestine but everything falls apart; I ask for instruments but the scrub nurses leave the room; I scream for help but there isn't anyone to respond. All of this happens in slow motion over and over again, and I am helpless… The same dream occurs with many variations. Most likely the 'worrying' will resolve after one retires, but will the nightmares continue?

How about more lessons learned — advice on succeeding in surgical practice, academia, medical politics, and the rural environment? Or how to avoid burnout in our chaotic system? But then this book will become one of those self-help books I have always abhorred.

* * * * *

What is a Jew doing in rural northern Wisconsin? I was asked that question, with a few variations, repeatedly over the years. I had to arrange some formalities at the Israeli Consulate in Chicago a few years ago. The Consul examined my driver's license. "Ladysmith," he asked, "where is this?"

"Northern Wisconsin," I replied.

"Wisconsin, Milwaukee?"

"No, it's five hours north-west of Milwaukee."

"What's the nearest large town?" The Consul asked.

"Eau Claire is an hour south of us."

The Consul looked blankly at me, "Is it near Minneapolis? Any synagogue nearby?"

"We are two and a half hours north-east of Minneapolis."

The Consul seemed astounded — he had never met any Israeli or Jew who did not live in New York, Chicago, or a similar metropolis. He looked at me suspiciously. Yes, Jews live in Florida and California, but a guy living in the remote nowhere of the flyover country — the lone Jew among the Gentiles — must be weird. And indeed, the only other local Jew I met during the years in northern Wisconsin was a urologist who practiced in

Eau Claire. However, occasionally, I would come across a 'hidden Jew' like the old farmer, with a Scandinavian name but Semitic features, who confessed that his mother was Jewish. No, he didn't know anything about her family. She died on the farm when he was a young boy. His father remarried, and all his siblings looked different. Later, his father would explain to him why… Occasionally, I would also spot a 'potential' Jew, like that old farmer: the nose, the swarthy skin, even the body language, unlike the homogenous northern Wisconsin background made up of the German, Scandinavian, and Polish gene pool. "So, Mr. Schniederman, where are your parents from?" I asked.

"My mom was born in Milwaukee; her parents, I think, came from Poland. My father's family came from Germany through Ellis Island before the First World War; they eventually settled here on a farm. I never met my grandparents."

The farmer smiled at my suggestion that he could be at least partially Jewish, saying, "Our Polish priest told me the same; you may be right."

During all my years in the USA, I never had to confront *overt* anti-Semitism. In New York, the Jewish capital of America, I experienced animosities between the various ethnic medical groups: the Italian versus the Pakistani, the Indian versus the Jews, and the Jews versus everybody; the disaccord was not based on racial issues but on control and money. Was there *covert* anti-Semitism — behind my back? Jack and his supporters in Keokuk? Probably yes. Princess Charlotte in Ladysmith? Maybe. However, I never heard an anti-Semitic utterance from patients and their families.

What about xenophobia? To some extent, this is a universal phenomenon. People tend to prefer their kind to the 'otherness.' Such feelings should be more pronounced in homogenous populations like the ones in northern Wisconsin. However, again, I did not experience anything like this personally. Occasionally, someone, a patient, or a family member, would ask, "Doctor, where are you from?" or "Where is your accent from?" But this, I think, manifested only from genuine interest. I noticed that sometimes older patients felt more comfortable seeing white American doctors rather than foreign ones. I remember hearing an old grumpy farmer complaining about having to see "that black woman doctor, whose name I cannot even pronounce." (Being a black doctor in a predominantly white environment makes things more difficult.)

I believe that, on average, foreign-born doctors (including myself) score a little less on patient satisfaction questionnaires than their American counterparts. I realized that a single old, grumpy, hard-of-hearing patient — having difficulty understanding your words — can significantly reduce your patient satisfaction score with negative input.

But these are tiny stains on the big picture that I saw: the northern Wisconsinites are a welcoming people, as long as you adapt to their way of life and culture. Then they will accept you almost as one of them. Henry Kissinger wrote in his memoir: "Nowhere else is there to be found the same generosity of spirit and absence of malice as in small-town America." I found it true in Wisconsin. However, I don't know how accurate such an attitude would be, or is, in a small town in West Virginia or Mississippi.

I have never lived and worked in one place as long as I did here in northern Wisconsin. These have been the best years of my life.

* * * * *

Boris Dmitrievich Savchuk (1933-2004).

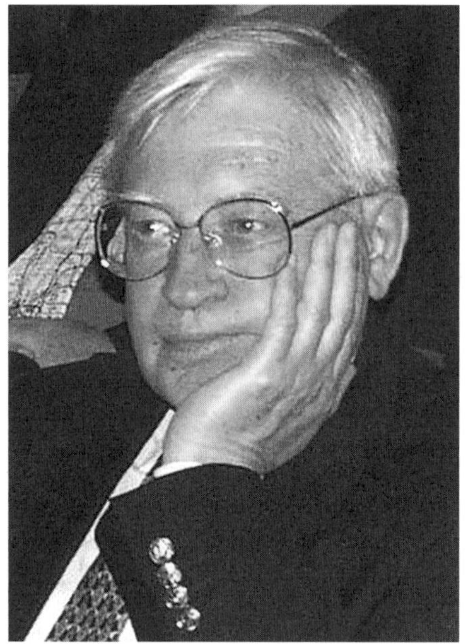

Epilogue

Taking off the gloves

The most difficult decision I have made in my life was when to retire. I am sure that my experience is not unique, as for most of us, being a surgeon is not a mere profession — it is a way of life, an addiction — it is what we are. In other countries or systems (e.g., university departments), the decision to retire is simple: at a certain age, it is mandatory. But around here, the decision belongs to us. You continue as long as you can perform reasonably, and if you cannot, you may eventually hear it from others.

The late Professor David Dent of Cape Town, a very wise man, wrote: "Each surgeon has an expiration date on the wall — everybody sees it but the surgeon himself." It is, however, only partially true, for thoughts of "when should I retire?" and "should I exit abruptly or gradually?" occupy the mind of many older surgeons at some stage. At any rate, it started to occupy my mind early on.

Another aphorism states: "For surgeons, an old man is somebody ten years older than you." Over the years, observing older surgeons, I promised to never stay around as long as they did — and not end up like Dr. Mantzur of Brooklyn or Dr. Garcia of Wisconsin (both discussed in previous chapters). When I arrived in Wisconsin at the age of fifty-six, I was sure I would not be practicing for more than 9-10 years. But ten years passed, and I became the oldest surgeon and one of the oldest physicians around.

The Welsh historian and travel writer Jan Morris wrote: "One of the prizes of old age is its release from competition…" However, I continued to enjoy competition; not competition in the true sense — competition for operative cases, power, money — but competition with myself: can I maintain my surgical aptitude as the years pass by? Dr. Hertzler, a pioneering American surgeon of the 19th century wrote: "Surgeons of old experience… consciously or subconsciously long for the day when they shall do their last operation." But I did not long for such a day — I continued enjoying being a surgeon. I decided to take it year by year, carefully examining my own performance.

I knew what a surgeon has to do to age gracefully, and I wrote a short piece, "50 Tips for Coping With Burnout, Aging in Surgical Practice" (you can find it online: https://www.generalsurgerynews.com/Opinion/Article/02-12/50-Tips-for-Coping-With-Burnout-Aging-in-Surgical-Practice/20116 — *General Surgery News*, 2012). My clinical judgment and acuity remained intact, and so did the steadiness of my hands. But one cannot cheat the creeping age: the growing susceptibility to sleep deprivation, and the increased tiredness after a prolonged operation, which in turn leads to some impatience — the tendency to cut corners. I was aware of the studies showing a steady decline in cognitive abilities (spatial visualization, speed, reasoning, memory but not vocabulary) starting in the twenties and diving well below the average when one crosses the seventies. (Obviously, the magnitude and pace of such decline varies in individual subjects and depends on multiple factors.)

The following is my attempt to outline the average progress of a 'surgical life':

YOUNG (age 30-35): not so 'young,' but this is how long it takes to become a surgeon; lacking confidence or overconfident; tends to 'experiment' and takes risks; 'hungry' for cases; prone to gaffes; needs support and advice, both theoretical and technical.

MATURING (age 35-40): improving but 'not there.'

MATURE (age 40-50): mostly fully independent and confident; still thriving to reach the top and susceptible to adopting various gimmicks.

AT THEIR BEST (age 50-60): having achieved optimal judgment and technical skills — 'mastery' — each at his or her own level; entering leadership roles.

AT THE TOP, BUT DECLINING (age 60-65): at the top of the profession; often considered the 'go-to guru' in his or her environment; while knowledge, experience, and wisdom are unsurpassable, stamina and technical skills gradually decline; some retire or seek a different avenue (e.g., administration).

OLDER, AT THEIR TWILIGHT (age 65-70): getting tired easily; further technical decline; the question "When should I retire?" constantly plays in his or her mind — usually he or she retires.

OLD FART. OLDER THAN 70: further cognitive and technical decline; colleagues and staff asking (behind their back): "When is he going to retire?"

This is, of course, a general view. Not all individual surgeons follow the trend; some surgeons are forever 'locked' in the maturing phase; others reach the best years much earlier; and some older surgeons or even old farts stay at the top of the profession. It also depends on the specific surgical environment: for example, 'top' aging surgeons working in ivory towers are often supported by an army of residents and younger partners who serve as a crutch, thus prolonging the old man's surgical life (e.g., Michael DeBakey, mentioned in Chapter 31, operated until the age of ninety). On the other hand, a community or rural surgeon depends only on themself.

Either he or she can do it or not! Psychopaths, a few of them mentioned in previous chapters, represent a completely different story.

Myself, I reached the bottom of the list — I was becoming an old fart. Returning patients would ask me, "Are you still here? We thought you had retired." So, I was gradually adapting my practice to suit my decline. Just before my seventy-fifth birthday I stopped taking emergency calls, limiting myself to elective operations — of which the complex, high-risk cases I referred to my partners or shipped out to the ivory towers. Meanwhile, I took on 'wound care,' hoping that such a 'hobby,' in addition to the usual office, lumps and bumps and skin cases, would keep me busy for a few more years.

A careful reader might ask: at the start of the Prologue the author was describing "his last day at work," so how come he's still working? Well, some two years ago, when I began working on the final version of the manuscript, I was convinced that this book would be published only after my full retirement. But over time situations and decisions tend to change. That is why the Prologue states: "this is how he *imagined* his last day at work to be..."

* * * * *

So much has changed over the fifty years since I entered medical school: the world of medicine and surgery has undergone a total metamorphosis. Can you, or any of our young colleagues, imagine diagnosing and treating patients without modern imaging technology such as ultrasound or CT? When I was a resident, all we had was basic radiographs, contrast studies, and primitive non-video endoscopy. Endoscopic retrograde cholangio-pancreatography (ERCP) was considered an 'emerging magic.' The abdominal cavity was like a 'black obscured box' — we examined patients and took a history — this is all that we had to deal with the 'acute abdomen.' We bypassed clogged arteries and resected arterial aneurysms through long incisions, sometimes in heroic blood baths — stents and endovascular procedures were not even dreamed of. The current brave new world was achieved solely due to advances in technology. The industrial-medical complex took over medicine. The revolution is only starting. I look at my young colleagues, sitting at the edge of the operating room, repairing the humble inguinal hernia with a robot (through the abdomen), and I know that soon, most abdominal operations will be performed robotically, with the surgeon in his office or at home, or even with the robot controlled by AI. Will any surgeon be available (and capable) to open the abdomen and save the patient when the robot misfires? Unlikely, as the 'open surgeon' is a dying species. The world of medical academia has metamorphosed as well: who remembers the days when we sat in the basement of the library digging into thick volumes of *Index Medicus,* searching for a relevant article? At that time 'high-impact' journals and leading books were considered *authoritative* — all this has now almost been replaced by surgical YouTube stars...

The only thing that hasn't changed is human nature. Humans continue to love, hate, struggle, fight, succeed, or fail; some are altruistic, others greedy. And this applies to us surgeons, making life and surgery unpredictable and chaotic like it always was. Today, we can visualize everything and see everything. Information and communication are instantly available at the tip of our fingers. But, being humans, we still commit the same mistakes as we always did. The fact that Electronic Medical Records and Google can provide us with so many details does not always help because the volume and character of our brains have not increased or improved. Often, the reverse is true. Would AI help, as suggested by experts? I don't know, but time will tell.

* * * * *

At what point in time should a memoir stop? In most memoirs or autobiographies, the beginning tends to be idyllic, charming, nostalgic — adverse experiences portrayed as adventures rather than disasters. Most insignificant details disappear from memory, and some are inflated to become significant. But as the memoir progresses, it gradually becomes, or sounds like, an unedited logbook. The element needed to transform a diary into a memoir is time — some distance from the events described. Only time and distance provide perspective — maturing and modifying acute emotions — and allow for a more balanced version of events; forget about objectivity, which is never attainable. It is true for most memoirs and autobiographies I have read — even those written by great writers and intellectuals. The first half is enchanting; it reads like one of their best novels, but then, as the narrative nears the actual time of writing, the charm evaporates, replaced, for example, by long lists of all the honors, prizes, and invited trips now enjoyed, and cherished, by the successful author. But great authors (e.g., Tolstoy, Nabokov) knew when to stop their memoirs, waiting for others to dwell on their completed lives. I am sufficiently sane not to expect anyone ever to find my life story interesting enough to warrant a biography. Thus, I have written my own and will stop here. Perhaps someday, it will continue. We each have more than one memoir in ourselves — so the future could expose more layers of the story and, perhaps, even change versions.

According to James R. Hagerty, the key to writing obituaries (or memoirs) can be summarized in three questions: *What were you trying to do with your life?* — here we speak about the professional life. *Why? And how did it work out?* My answers to these questions would be: I tried to be a good surgeon, saving lives, alleviating suffering, and inflicting as little damage as possible. *Why?* I don't know. *Did it work out?* I don't know whether my life and professional journey can be considered a story of success or failure; I have to leave it to you, the reader, to decide. Typically, however, most lives represent a mixed picture of achievements and disappointments. Whatever the moral of my story might be, I hope it provided some insight and perhaps entertainment to some readers.

Let me conclude then with my favorite quote by Winston Churchill: "Success is the ability to go from failure to failure without losing your enthusiasm."

And another one by Béla Schick: "Every Chief of Service should have a pet dog, like Ulysses had. When he retires he should leave his dog on the floor of the department he served, because when he returns the only one who will recognize him will be his dog." Luckily, I have two loving dogs at home!

* * * * *

Mishka (left) and Patsy (right).

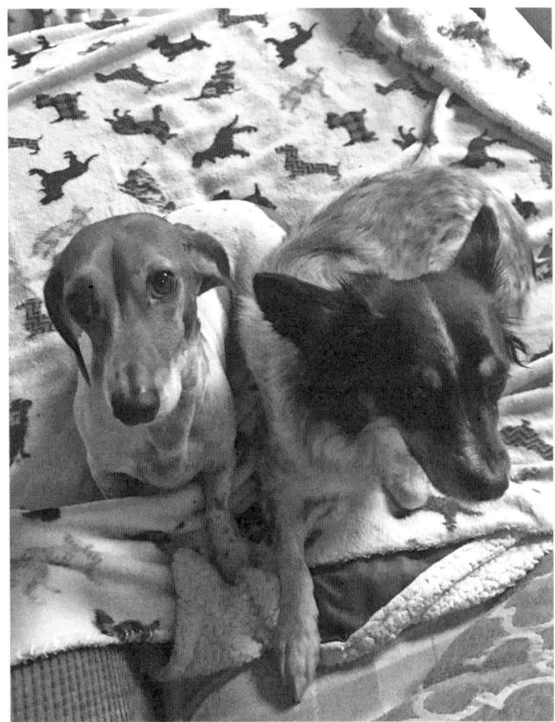

Acknowledgements

It was Dr. Abraham Verghese (California) who for years encouraged me to publish this memoir. Thank you Abe!

I am indebted to Nikki Bramhill (tfm publishing, UK) for taking the risk to publish a book of such low commercial potential. In addition to her unsurpassable editing skills Nikki managed to persuade me to 'tone down' the narrative, rendering it less politically incorrect. I am thankful to Daria Diehtiarova (Kyiv, Ukraine) for being such a careful reader, and to my son Omri Schein (San Diego) who proofed large chunks of the manuscript.

During a journey of many years, one meets and interacts with countless individuals who have a direct or indirect impact on one's life and career. Many faces are entrenched in the memory — the names of some less 'significant' individuals have faded away. Not a few such individuals had a 'negative' impact on my career (some mentioned in the various chapters) — I won't be mentioning them here. So the following is the list of people (the deceased are marked with a "D") whom I wish to thank for their help, company and friendship. It's in alphabetical order, according to the country (their current location); spouses are included selectively.

Israel:

Yaakov Aginski, Ahmad and Anat Assalia, Jack and Tova Baniel, Shabtai Beni, Yossi and Ayelet Berger, Jacob "Bubi" and Memi Daube, Shmuel "Shmil" Eldar (D), Moshe Fliegelman, Michael Friedman, Gideon and Sarah Fuks, Yuval and Joan Gelfand, Yossi Grosberg, Moshe Hashmonai, Dudu and Shuli Hendel, Shlomo Isserlish (D), Dean Lutrin, Eli and Daniela Mavor, Eran and Orli Perlman, Yitzchak Pfeferman, Amikam and Rachel Reshef, Danny and Gilly Rosin, Aviel Roy-Shapira, Avi and Sari Rubinstein, Yossi and Nilli Schein, Yochanan and Michal Schiffman, Zvi Schiller, Uri Teitelman (D), Shmulik and Chaya Yonai, Eitan Zion.

South Africa:

Angelo D'Edigio, Carlos De Nobrega, George (D) and Margaret Decker, David Dent (D), Moshe and Miriam Fayman, Wolf Frankel, Emerik and Eva Frohlich, Herman Gerding, Ruth and Zach Gershoni, David and Estelle Hatchuel, Jim Howell (D), John Jamieson (D), Jan Christoph and Angela Meister.

USA:

Rebecca Allen, Charles Aprahamian (D), Lynette and Dan Bale, Joseph and Myrna Bashir, Harold Bernanke (D), Judith and David Bernanke, Stephanie Bixler, Cedrick Bremner, Ron (D) and Marge Charipar, Doug Condit, Robert Condon (D), Bob Crochelt, Karen Draper, Carla Egle, Bashar Fahoum, Erik Frykberg (D), Syed Gardezi (D), Gary and Jacki Gecelter, Lloyd and Danna Gold, Bob Goldman, Piotr Górecki, Joyce Griffith, Milton A. Gumbs, Asher Hirshberg, Joseph Holt, John and Laura Hunter, Samir Johna, John Kennedy, Satish Khaneja, Samantha Klebe, Adam Klipfel, Philip Kramer, William Krause, Narong Kulvatunyou, Pasquale Lapalorcia (D), Jon Lloyd, Shannon Martin, Philip Mofle, Navid Monajjem, Robert and Deb Nogler, Jody Nordine, Ramesh Paladugu, Brandon Parkhurst, Tom and Jan Paulson, Stan Pepple, Graeme and Tracy Pitcher, Kellsey Provos, Heather Repka, Kenneth Retzlaff, James and Nancy Rucinski, Thomas Salach (D), Jerry Steiner, Howie and Amy Sutlive, Barbara Syrakos, Abraham Verghese, Kristin Verville, David Waddel, Vicki and Steve Weiss, Jerry Wilkes and Ann Mershon, Katie Winiarczyk, Leslie (D) and Amal Wise, Dietmar and Heide Wittmann, Al Zastrow, John and Debbie Ziemer.

Australia:

Barry (Baz) Alexander, Ramana Balasubramanian, Stephen Clifforth, Afif Hadj, Matt Oliver, Anil Thakur (D).

Canada:

Tom Gilas, Mohammad Keshoofy, Robert Lane, George (D) and Kathy Louridas, Angus and Janis McIver, John Marshall, Roger and Vivian Saadia.

Chile:

Hernan Diaz, Alfredo and Ximena (D) Sepúlveda.

Cuba:

Rolando Ramos, Edelberto Fuentes Valdés.

Czech Republic

Leo Klein.

Denmark:

Annette Jensen, Liselotte Kring, Susanne Sas Hvas.

Finland:

Ari and Eija Leppäniemi.

France:
Bernard Cristalli, Hafez Serhal.

Germany:
Artur Bauhofer, Stephanie Benko, Uli and Ulrike Elben, Ralph and Gabi Heemken, Agnes Heinz, Frank Hoermann, Mathias and Katrin Kalkum, Yanina Lippal, Marian Littke, Wilfried Lorenz (D), Ulrich Schoeffel, Alexander and Dace Schoucair.

Italy:
Francesco Gammarota, Luigi Lapalorcia, Bruna Pasticci, Fausto Pistoni, Zigi and Lena Riegler (D).

India:
Sayandev DasGupta (D), Vinay Mehendale, Kuldip Pandey, John Thanakumar.

Iraq:
Mazin Abdulsattar Abdulla.

Ireland:
Ray McLaughlin.

Pakistan:
Amjad Siraj Memon.

Poland:
Wojciech and Eva Górecki, Dominik Walczak.

Portugal:
Vitor Ribeiro.

Russia:
Denis Arkhipov, Evgeniy (Perya) Perelygin, Yuri Plotnikov, Boris Savchuk (D).

Surinam:
Rob Does.

Sweden:
Roland Andersson, PO Nyström.

Switzerland:
Carl Faas and Franziska Brenn, Brigitte and Armin Hafner, Viatcheslav "Slava" Ryndine, Erik Schadde.

Turkey:
Metin Çakmakçı.

Ukraine:
Alex Berzoy, Daria Diehtiarova.

United Kingdom:
Maryam Alfa-Wali, Nikki Bramhill and Paul Lawrence, Mark Cheetam, John Farndon (D), Yasser Mohsen, Paul and Jackie Rogers, Mark Rogers, Simon Shaw, Mark Taylor.

Uruguay:
Luis Carriquiry.

Unfortunately missing from the above lists are the numerous colleagues, residents, nurses, scrub techs, secretaries, orderlies, and maintenance guys, who made my long trip possible through the many hospitals.